Abdominal Sonography

Abdominal Sonography

Eric E. Sauerbrei, B.Sc., M.Sc., M.D., F.R.C.P.C.
Professor of Radiology

Khanh T. Nguyen, M.Sc., M.D., F.R.C.P.C.
Associate Professor of Radiology

Robert L. Nolan, B.Sc., M.D., F.R.C.P.C.
Associate Professor of Radiology

Queen's University
Kingston General Hospital and Hotel Dieu Hospital
Kingston, Ontario, Canada

RAVEN PRESS 🐦 NEW YORK

Raven Press, Ltd., 1185 Avenue of the Americas, New York, New York 10036

Made in the United States of America

Library of Congress Cataloging-in-Publication Data

Sauerbrei, Eric E.
    Abdominal sonography/Eric E. Sauerbrei, Khanh T. Nguyen, Robert
  L. Nolan.
        p.   cm.
    Includes bibliographical references and index.
    ISBN 0-88167-917-8
    1. Abdomen—Ultrasonic imaging.   I. Nguyen, Khanh T.   II. Nolan,
  Robert L. (Robert Louis)   III. Title.
    [DNLM: 1. Abdomen—Ultrasonography.   WI 900 S255a]
  RC944.S29   1992
  617.5'507543—dc20
  DNLM/DLC
  for Library of Congress   92-3495
                                                                CIP

9   8   7   6   5   4   3   2   1

To Karen, Tyler, and Peter and my parents, Jack and Verna Sauerbrei
EES

To Hau, Daphne, Jade, and Peter
KTN

To Rose, Erin, Kathryn, and Lisa
RLN

Contents

Color plate section A appears following page 50.
Color plate section B appears following page 242.

Preface

This book provides a concise, organized, and well-illustrated text that covers most of the normal and abnormal structures encountered in the hospital, clinic, and office practice of abdominal sonography. The book is useful in schools of medical sonography for student sonographers, in radiology training programs for radiology residents, and also in medical schools for students. It is also a helpful guide, reference, and refresher for physicians and sonographers already practicing abdominal sonography.

We have emphasized high-quality images to give the reader a visual portrayal of most normal and abnormal structures encountered in practice. Where possible, different manifestations of the same pathology are included. Color Doppler images of several normal structures and some pathology are also included.

A consistent chapter organization and style allows easier reading and comprehension; each chapter has the following sections: Introduction, Scanning Techniques, Normal Anatomy and Variants, Pathology, and Pitfalls, Artifacts, and Practical Tips.

Eric E. Sauerbrei
Khanh T. Nguyen
Robert L. Nolan

Acknowledgments

The authors would first like to thank the sonographers at the Kingston General Hospital and Hotel Dieu Hospital for their support in providing the quality scans that form the majority of illustrations in this book. These sonographers include Cathy Marshall, A.R.D.M.S. (Chief Sonographer), Leslie Campbell, A.R.D.M.S., Anne Joslin, A.R.D.M.S., Marie Scott, A.R.D.M.S., Dawn Fletcher, A.R.D.M.S., Angie Henson, A.R.D.M.S., and Jan Veenstra, A.R.D.M.S.

The processing of scans to prints was performed capably by the Department of Medical Photography of Kingston General Hospital (Christopher Peck, Leo MacDonald, and Ron Irvine), and the artwork was produced by Andrew Pedersen.

We wish to thank Claire Chow and Nancy Cutway for their fine work in producing draft after draft for the text.

Several scans were obtained from other ultrasound departments in Canada and these are acknowledged individually in the illustration legends. These include scans from Drs. Peter Cooperberg, Vancouver, Ian Hammond, Ottawa, David Martin, Ottawa, Sigrid Jecquier, Montreal, Howard Greenberg, Winnipeg, John H. K. Wallace, Saskatoon, and Linda Hutton, London. Some scans of normal anatomy were obtained from the radiology residents at Queen's University, Kingston and they are also acknowledged in the figure legends. These include scans from Drs. Patrick Llwellyn, Stephen Valentine, Kenneth Sutherland, and Wayne Tonogai. Other normal scans were graciously provided by two young patients: Tyler and Peter Sauerbrei. Advanced Technology Laboratories (ATL) provided three color pictures, and the source physicians are acknowledged in the legends. We thank ATL for financial support in publishing expenses of these three color illustrations.

A special thanks goes to Siemens Quantum Corporation for their generous support in publishing 37 color Doppler scans obtained on the Quantum 2000 Color Doppler Ultrasound Machine.

Abdominal Sonography

CHAPTER 1

Guidelines for the Performance of Abdominal Sonography

The American Institute of Ultrasound in Medicine (AIUM) currently publishes seven guidelines for the performance of diagnostic ultrasound examinations for the following areas:

1. abdominal and retroperitoneal ultrasound examination
2. renal and retroperitoneal ultrasound examination
3. antepartum obstetrical ultrasound examination
4. ultrasound examination of the female pelvis
5. scrotal ultrasound examination
6. ultrasound examination of the prostate (and surrounding structures)
7. pediatric neurosonology ultrasound examination

The Guidelines for Performance of the Abdominal and Retroperitoneal Ultrasound Examination provide guiding principles for the performance of a basic complete abdominal sonogram. These guidelines comment on equipment, documentation of the study, and the actual performance of the scan. The following guidelines are quoted from the AIUM *Guidelines for Performance of the Abdominal and Retroperitoneal Ultrasound Examination.*

PART I: GUIDELINES FOR EQUIPMENT AND DOCUMENTATION

Equipment

Abdominal and retroperitoneal studies should be conducted with a real-time scanner, preferably using sector or curved linear transducers. Static B-scan images may be obtained as a supplement to the real-time images when indicated. The transducer or scanner should be adjusted to operate at the highest clinically appropriate frequency, realizing that there is a trade-off between reso-

lution and beam penetration. With modern equipment, these frequencies are usually between 2.25 and 5.0 MHz.

Documentation

Adequate documentation is essential for high quality patient care. This should be a permanent record of the ultrasound examination and its interpretation. Images of all appropriate areas, both normal and abnormal, should be recorded [on] appropriate imaging or storage format. Variations from normal size should be accompanied by measurements. Images are to be appropriately labeled with the examination date, patient identification and image orientation. A report of the ultrasound findings should be included in the patient's medical record regardless of where the study is performed. Retention of the ultrasound examination should be consistent both with clinical need and with relevant legal and local health care facility requirements.

PART II: GUIDELINES FOR THE ABDOMEN AND RETROPERITONEUM ULTRASOUND EXAMINATION

The following guidelines describe the examination to be performed for each organ and anatomic region in the abdomen and retroperitoneum. A complete examination would include all of the following. A limited examination would include only one or more of these areas, but not all of them.

Liver

The liver survey should include both long axis (coronal and sagittal) and transverse views. If possible, views comparing the echogenicity of the liver to the right kidney should be performed. The major vessels (aorta/inferior vena cava) in the region of the liver should be imaged, including the position of the inferior vena cava where it passes through the liver.

The regions of the ligamentum teres on the left and of the dome of the right lobe with the right hemidiaphragm and right pleural space should be imaged. The main lobar fissure should be demonstrated.

Survey of right and left lobes should include visualization of the hepatic veins. The right and left branches of the portal vein should be identified. The intrahepatic bile ducts should be evaluated for possible dilatation.

Gallbladder and Biliary Tract

The gallbladder evaluation should include long axis (coronal or sagittal) and transverse views obtained in supine position. Left lateral decubitus (left side down), erect or prone positions may also be necessary to allow a complete evaluation of the gallbladder and its surrounding area.

The intrahepatic ducts can be evaluated, as described under the liver, by obtaining views of the liver demonstrating the right and left hepatic branches of the portal vein. The extrahepatic ducts can be evaluated in supine, left lateral decubitus and/or semi-erect positions. The size of the intrahepatic and extrahepatic ducts should be assessed. With these views the relationship between the bile ducts, hepatic artery and portal vein can be shown. When possible, the common bile duct in the pancreatic head should be visualized.

Pancreas

The pancreatic head, uncinate process, and body should be identified in transverse, and, when possible, long axis (coronal or sagittal) projections. If possible, the pancreatic tail should also be imaged, and the pancreatic duct demonstrated. The peripancreatic region should be assessed for adenopathy.

Spleen

Representative views of the spleen in long axis, either sagittal or coronal, and in transverse projection should be performed. An attempt should be made to demonstrate the left pleural space. When possible, the echogenicity of the upper pole of the left kidney should be compared to that of the spleen.

Kidneys

Representative long axis (coronal or sagittal) views of each kidney should be obtained, visualizing the cortex and the renal pelvis. Transverse views of both the left and right kidney should include the upper pole, middle section at the renal pelvis, and the lower pole. When possible, comparison of renal echogenicity with the adjacent liver and spleen should be performed. The perirenal regions should be assessed for possible abnormality.

Aorta and Inferior Vena Cava

The aorta and inferior vena cava should be imaged in long axis (either sagittal or coronal) and transverse planes. Scans of both vessels should be attempted from the diaphragm to the bifurcation (usually at the level of the umbilicus). If possible, images should also include the adjacent common iliac vessels.

Abnormalities should be assessed. The surrounding soft tissues should be evaluated for adenopathy.

CHAPTER 2

Abdominal Wall and Peritoneal Cavity

INTRODUCTION

The abdominal organs are contained in the abdominal cavity, which is surrounded by the abdominal wall. The abdominal cavity is separated superiorly from the thoracic cavity by the diaphragm and is continuous inferiorly with the pelvic cavity.

Many abdominal organs such as the liver, spleen, stomach, and a large portion of the bowel are covered by a thin serous membrane, the peritoneum, which has a parietal and visceral layer. The parietal membrane lines the inside of the abdominal cavity; the visceral membrane is reflected over the organ with which it forms an integral unit. The potential space between the parietal and visceral membranes constitutes the peritoneal cavity.

Real-time sonography provides an excellent screening technique in the evaluation of the abdominal wall, diaphragm, and peritoneal cavity. It performs better than CT in evaluating diaphragmatic motion, in detecting small amounts of ascites, and in distinguishing fluid-filled bowel from cystic masses. It also provides a quick, safe guide to percutaneous aspiration or drainage of fluid collections. For the critically ill, the examination can be performed at the patient's bedside with portable equipment.

Abbreviations: **CDH,** congenital diaphragmatic hernia; **CT,** computed tomography; **GI,** gastrointestinal; **MHz,** megahertz; **MR,** magnetic resonance.

2.1 SCANNING TECHNIQUES

Scanning the abdominal wall, diaphragm, and peritoneal cavity requires no special patient preparation. The patient is routinely scanned lying supine. Scans may also be performed in the decubitus or erect positions, or both. Certain surface landmarks serve as useful guides to target specific organs: Murphy's point in the right upper quadrant refers to the gallbladder; McBurney's point in the right lower quadrant refers to the appendix.

The skin and the anterior abdominal wall are best scanned using a 5-, 7.5-, or 10-MHz linear array transducer. To avoid the "bang effect" of direct transducer placement on the skin and to obtain the best resolution, various standoff techniques have been developed to scan the superficial cutaneous layers. Flotation pads, which are liquid-filled microcell sponges, synthetic polymer blocks, and silicone elastomer blocks are excellent standoff pads (1–3). These substances are dense enough to stand alone; they have a uniform consistency to minimize artifacts. Scanning over a surgical wound can be performed by applying an adhesive plastic membrane (Op-site) over the wound after removing the dressing (4). Scanning the diaphragm is best achieved with a 3.5- or 5-MHz real-time sector probe. Coronal and sagittal views are obtained in quiet respiration. Sniffing or coughing tests may be used to elicit paradoxic motion.

Scanning the peritoneal cavity constitutes an integral part of the routine survey of the upper abdominal organs and follows similar steps. Once pathology is identified,

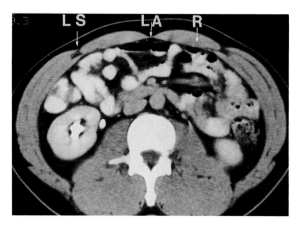

FIG. 2.1. CT scan of abdomen: normal anatomy of abdominal wall. *LA,* linea alba; *LS,* linea semilunaris; *R,* rectus abdominis muscle.

attempts should be made to determine its extent and its location in relation to the specific peritoneal compartments. The information provides a useful guide to therapeutic planning.

2.2 NORMAL ANATOMY

Abdominal Wall

The abdominal wall is composed of the skin covering a subcutaneous fat layer and a deeper musculofascial layer (Figs. 2.1 and 2.2). The normal epidermis is a highly reflective layer measuring 1 to 4 mm in thickness (5).

The subcutaneous fat layer is of variable thickness. It is usually hypoechoic and lobulated in contour. The musculofascial layer is composed of the paired rectus muscles in the anterior wall, one on each side of the midline; the oblique and transversalis muscles in the lateral wall; and the quadratus lumborum and erector spinae muscles in the posterior wall. The musculofascial layer is

usually more echogenic than the subcutaneous fat layer (6). However, in thin and athletic people, the reverse may be seen, with the muscles appearing as hypoechoic masses (Fig. 2.3a,b). Points of weakness in the abdominal wall are the linea alba in the midline; the linea semilunaris at the junction of the anterior and lateral abdominal walls (Spieghelian line); and the inferior lumbar space in the posterior axillary line of the mid flank.

In many people, there is a collection of extra-peritoneal fat, which appears lens-shaped in cross section posterior to the linea alba and to the linea semilunaris. It may be very prominent, especially in obese people (Fig. 2.3). Care must be taken not to mistake this for an abnormal mass. It is also the source of the split image artifact, which will be discussed later.

Diaphragm

The diaphragm serves as a partition between the thoracic and abdominal cavities and as the major active muscle of respiration. It is composed of a central crescent- or boomerang-shaped tendinous plate connected to peripheral muscular fibers that attach anteriorly to the lower sternum and lower six ribs and posteriorly to the lumbar spine by the two crura. The posterior muscular fibers are the longest (Fig. 2.4).

The diaphragmatic crura join anteriorly to form the median arcuate ligament; posterior to this and in front of the spine at the level of the tenth dorsal vertebra is the aortic opening or hiatus. The esophagus passes through the medial fibers of the right crux, at the level of the tenth dorsal vertebra and slightly to the left of the midline. The hiatus for the inferior vena cava is on the right side of the central tendon, usually at the level of the eighth or ninth dorsal vertebra.

The normal diaphragm is dome-shaped, with the central tendon forming the dome and with convexity toward the thoracic cavity.

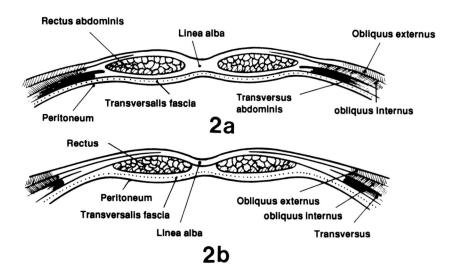

FIG. 2.2. Anterior abdominal wall. **a:** above arcuate line; **b:** below arcuate line. (From Warwick R, Williams PL. Myology. In: Warwick R, Williams PL, eds. *Gray's anatomy.* Edinburgh, UK: Longman; 1973:526, with permission.)

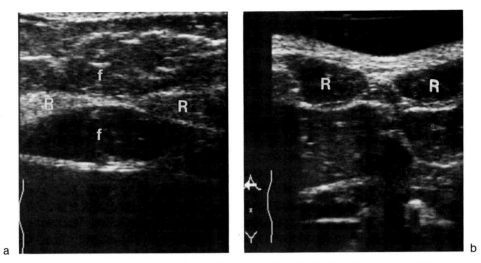

FIG. 2.3. Transverse sonogram of anterior abdominal wall. **a:** Note that the muscles (*R*) appear echogenic. The collection of extraperitoneal fat (*f*) is prominent in this obese person. **b:** The muscles (*R*) appear hypoechoic in this thin person. There is not much subcutaneous or extraperitoneal fat.

On sonography, the diaphragm itself appears as a thin curved echo-poor band. The diaphragm–lung interface appears as a thick echogenic line; reverberation artifacts from air in the lung may occasionally be seen originating from this line. A thin curved line on the abdominal side represents the diaphragm–liver interface (Fig. 2.5). At times, another thin echogenic line may be seen on the thoracic side (Fig. 2.6). It is actually an artifact, a mirror image of the diaphragm–liver interface (7). When there is adjacent fluid from a pleural effusion or ascites, the central tendon is outlined as a thin line covering the dome of the liver. Posteriorly in the sagittal scan and posterolaterally in the transverse scan, the peripheral muscular insertions appear as thick triangular hypoechoic bands (Fig. 2.7). The left hemidiaphragm is more difficult to scan than the right, because of presence of gas in the stomach.

Not infrequently, the muscular bundles or diaphragmatic slips are much more prominent than usual. They may give a lobulated contour to the diaphragmatic surface and produce deep grooves on the liver surface (hepar lobulation) (8). In some patients, however, the diaphragmatic slips appear as focal echogenic masses, which may be round, triangular, oval, or irregularly shaped when seen in cross section (Fig. 2.8a). In this situation, they may be mistaken for focal liver lesions or peritoneal masses. To clarify this, they should be scanned along their long axis by rotating the transducer. In this plane, they become elongated in configuration (Fig. 2.8b). These findings are diagnostic of diaphragmatic slips (8,9).

The diaphragmatic crura lie anterior to the upper abdominal aorta and appear as thin hypoechoic bands that thicken during deep inspiration (8,9) (Fig. 2.9).

Peritoneum and Peritoneal Compartments

There are several peritoneal compartments, which are separated by various peritoneal ligaments and folds.

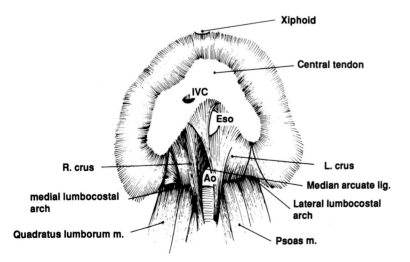

FIG. 2.4. Abdominal view of diaphragm. *IVC*, inferior vena cava; *Eso*, esophagus; *Ao*, aorta.

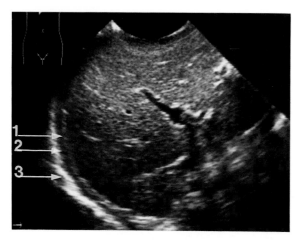

FIG. 2.5. Right hemidiaphragm: parasagittal scan. (1) diaphragm–liver interface; (2) diaphragmatic muscle; (3) diaphragm–lung interface.

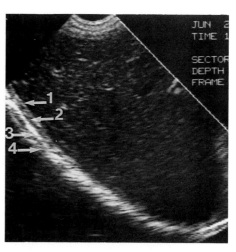

FIG. 2.6. Right hemidiaphragm: parasagittal scan. (1) diaphragm–liver interface; (2) diaphragmatic muscle; (3) diaphragm–lung interface; (4) mirror image artifact.

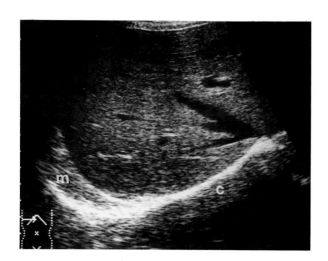

FIG. 2.7. Right hemidiaphragm: transverse scan. c, central tendon; m, peripheral muscle.

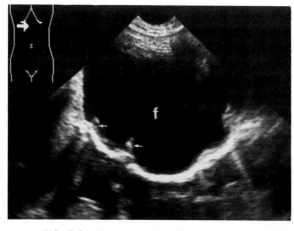
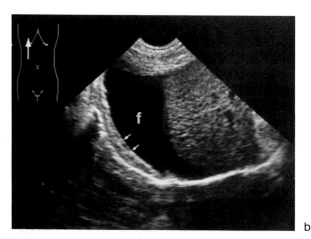

FIG. 2.8. Diaphragmatic slips. a: in cross section; b: in long axis. Diaphragmatic slips appear as small echogenic masses (arrows) in short axis view. When scanned in their long axis, they become elongated. They are particularly well seen in this patient with ascites (f).

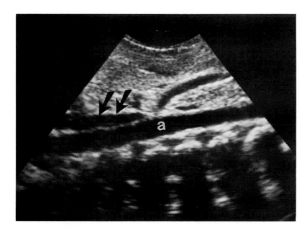

FIG. 2.9. Diaphragmatic crus. In this parasagittal scan, crus of the diaphragm (*arrows*) appears as a thin echo-poor band anterior to abdominal aorta (*a*).

TABLE 2.1. *Peritoneal compartments*

Supra-mesocolic compartment
  Right
    Right subphrenic
    Right subhepatic
    • anterior
    • posterior (Morison's pouch)
  Left
    Left subhepatic space
    • anterior
    • posterior
    Left subphrenic space
    • anterior (perigastric)
    • posterior (perisplenic)
  Lesser sac
    Superomedial recess
    Lateroinferior recess
Infra-mesocolic compartment
  Right space
  Left space
Right and left paracolic gutters
Pelvic cavity
  Pouch of Douglas (rectovaginal or rectovesical)
  Lateral paravesical recesses

They are listed in Table 2.1 and illustrated in Fig. 2.10 (10,11).

The major ligaments and folds are the falciform ligament, the lesser omentum, the greater omentum, the small bowel mesentery, the transverse mesocolon, and the sigmoid mesocolon. The falciform ligament runs in or to the right of the midline, suspending the liver from the diaphragm and abdominal wall. The lesser omentum is a peritoneal fold connecting the liver to the stomach (hepatogastric ligament) and to the duodenum (hepatoduodenal ligament). Its free margin contains the portal vein, the hepatic artery, and the common bile duct. Posterior to the free margin is the foramen of Winslow (epiploic foramen), which provides communication between the lesser and greater peritoneal sac. The greater omentum, the largest fold, extends from the greater curvature of the stomach to hang in front of the transverse colon and small bowel like a curtain. It acts as a storehouse of fat and as a protective barrier against the spread of disease. The transverse mesocolon is a broad fold sus-

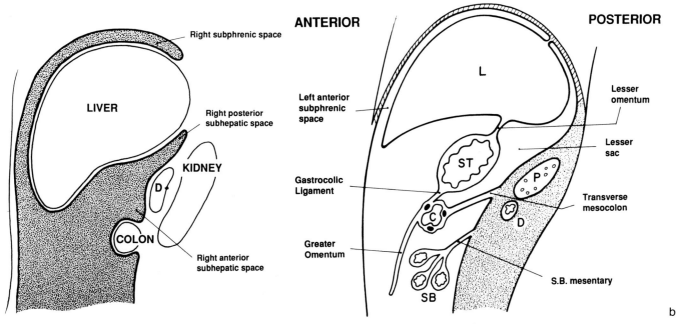

FIG. 2.10. a: Peritoneal compartments: parasagittal view (*right side*). (From Meyers, ref. 10, with permission.) **b:** Peritoneal compartments: parasagittal view (*left side*). (From Siegel MJ. Spleen and peritoneal cavity. In: Siegel MJ, ed. *Pediatric sonography.* New York: Raven Press; 1991:161–178, with permission.) *L,* liver; *D,* duodenum; *St,* stomach; *P,* pancreas; *SB,* small bowel; *C,* colon.

pending the transverse colon from the posterior abdominal wall, in front of the pancreas and behind the greater omentum. The sigmoid mesocolon is a fold attaching the sigmoid colon to the pelvic wall.

The *supra-* and *infra-mesocolic* compartments are separated by the transverse mesocolon.

The *supra-mesocolic* compartment is in turn divided by the falciform ligament into the right and left supra-mesocolic spaces. It also contains the *lesser sac.* The right supra-mesocolic spaces consist of the right *subphrenic* and *subhepatic* spaces. The right subphrenic space lies between the diaphragm and the dome of the liver. It is bounded posteromedially by the right superior coronary ligament, which suspends the liver from the diaphragm. The *bare area* of the liver, not covered by peritoneum, lies medial to this ligament, in contact with the retroperitoneum. The right subhepatic space is inferior to the liver and is composed of an anterior and posterior portion. The anterior portion is adjacent to the gallbladder fossa. The most dependent space in the recumbent position is the posterior portion, also called the hepato-renal recess or Morison's pouch.

The *left* supra-mesocolic space has four compartments: the anterior and posterior subhepatic spaces inferior to the liver, and the anterior (perigastric) and posterior (perisplenic) subphrenic spaces. The left anterior subphrenic space lies high under the diaphragm, anterior to the stomach and extending on both sides of the midline.

The *lesser sac* is a separate compartment lying at a more caudal and posterior plane than the left anterior subphrenic space. It also extends on both sides of the midline. Its superior medial recess is to the right of the lumbar spine, surrounding the caudate lobe of the liver. Its inferolateral recess is larger, extending to the left, separating the stomach anteriorly from the pancreas posteriorly.

The *infra-mesocolic* compartment is divided by the oblique root of the small bowel mesentery into the smaller *right* space and larger *left* space (Fig. 2.10). The right space is bounded laterally by the ascending colon and inferiorly by the ileocecal junction; the left space is bounded laterally by the descending colon and sigmoid mesocolon. The two spaces open inferiorly to the pelvic, cavity, which is the most dependent part of the peritoneal cavity both in the erect and recumbent positions. The pelvic recesses communicate freely on the right side with the supra-mesocolic space via the right paracolic gutter lateral to the ascending colon; on the left, communication is prevented by the phrenocolic ligament at the cephalad end of the left paracolic gutter (10,11). The abdominal and pelvic cavities form an anatomical continuum. Diseases in the abdomen may spread down into the pelvis and vice versa.

The peritoneum contains fat, blood vessels, lymphatics, and nerves. It is composed of a single mesothe-

lial layer that regulates the dynamics of abdominal fluid and solutes. In normal people, the thin peritoneum is not visualized by ultrasound. The potential spaces are seen only when they are filled with air, fluid, or tumor.

2.3 PATHOLOGY

Cutaneous Lesions

Occult recurrent or metastatic melanoma may be detected by sonography using the standoff techniques previously described. Fine needle aspiration biopsies of these lesions may be performed under ultrasound guidance (12). Pigmented nevi and malignant melanoma are clearly demarcated from normal skin. Melanomas typically appear hypoechoic and may demonstrate enhanced through transmission (Fig. 2.11). They rarely occur in the anterior abdominal wall, which is, however, a common site for metastatic cutaneous and subcutaneous nodules (12).

Abdominal Wall Pathology

Ventral Hernia

Congenital ventral hernias include omphalocele and gastroschisis, which can be detected sonographically in the fetus *in utero* as early as 18 weeks menstrual age (13).

Omphalocele occurs in about one in 5,800 births. It is due to a defect in the abdominal wall at the site of the umbilical cord insertion (Fig. 2.12a,b). A mass representing herniated liver or bowel, or both, is seen protruding from the fetal abdomen. This condition is often associated with abnormalities of other organ systems (13). Gastroschisis is one third as common as omphalocele. It is usually not associated with other malformations. The abdominal defect occurs to the right of the umbilical cord insertion, with herniation of small bowel not covered by a membrane (Fig. 2.13a,b). There is normal insertion of the umbilical cord (13).

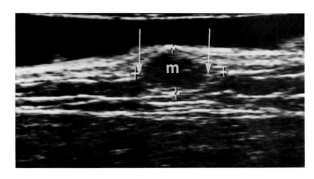

FIG. 2.11. Subcutaneous metastatic melanoma. Lesion (*m*) appears hypoechoic. Note disruption of cutaneous layer (*arrows*).

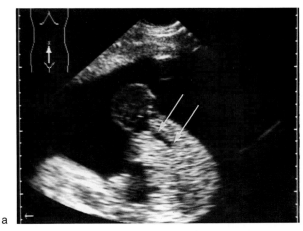 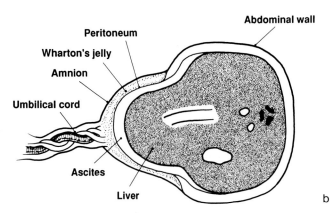

a   b

FIG. 2.12. Omphalocele seen *in utero* (18 weeks menstrual age). **a:** axial view of fetal abdomen; **b:** diagram. Note umbilical vein (*arrows*) running into herniated liver, which is covered by a membrane. There is also polyhydraminos. (From Nyberg DA, Mack LA. Abdominal wall defects. In: Callen PW, ed. *Ultrasonography in obstetrics and gynecology.* Philadelphia: WB Saunders; 1988:240–253, with permission.)

Acquired hernias more frequently affect the obese, the elderly, and patients with previous abdominal surgery or trauma (14). They typically occur at points of weakness where there is absence of muscles, along the linea alba in the midline, along the linea semilunaris on each side (Spieghelian hernia), and in the inferior lumbar space (defect in the transversalis fascia) (15,16). Careful scanning in the transverse plane usually identifies the fascial defect and the herniated contents, which are either omental fat or bowel.

The herniated bowel loops appear sonographically as lobulated masses with strong reflective central echoes representing air in the lumen (Fig. 2.14a,b). When incarcerated, they appear as tubular fluid-filled structures characteristic of bowel loops. Anatomical detail of larger ventral hernias is better obtained with CT scanning. Oc-

casionally, free air (pneumoperitoneum) may be detected simulating a ventral hernia (Fig. 2.15).

Muscle Injuries

The muscles of the abdominal wall may be injured by a penetrating wound, by a blow to the abdomen, or by hyperextension strain. Blunt trauma may cause subcutaneous edema or muscle contusion (Fig. 2.16). The contused muscle appears thickened because of swelling. It is more sonolucent than usual, probably because of edema. Disorganized coarse echoes are seen representing extravasated blood and inflammatory reaction. A similar appearance may be seen in rhabdomyolysis, which is a breakdown of muscle caused by injury (17).

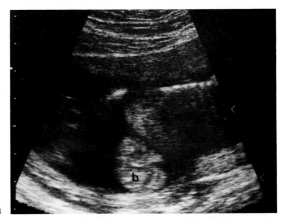 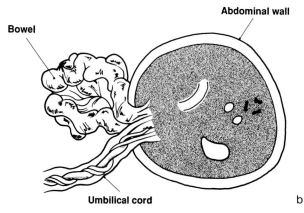

a   b

FIG. 2.13. Gastroschisis seen *in utero* (17 weeks menstrual age). **a:** parasagittal view of fetal abdomen; **b:** diagram (axial view). Mass of herniated bowel (*b*) is not covered by a membrane. Defect is usually to right of umbilical cord insertion. (From Nyberg DA, Mack LA. Abdominal wall defects. In: Callen PW, ed. *Ultrasonography in obstetrics and gynecology.* Philadelphia: WB Saunders; 1988:240–253, with permission.)

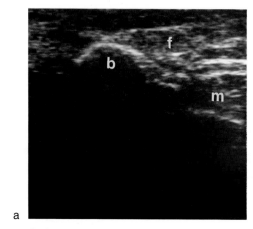
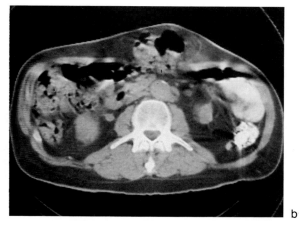

a   b

FIG. 2.14. Ventral hernia. **a:** transverse sonogram; **b:** corresponding CT scan. Gas in herniated bowel (*b*) casts posterior shadowing. *f*, subcutaneous fat; *m,* muscular layer.

When hyperextension strain is violent enough, the rectus muscle may rupture, with tearing of the inferior epigastric artery. There is a tender mass that may be detected by ultrasound as a superficial hematoma.

Abdominal Wall Fluid Collections

Abdominal wall fluid collections are usually seroma(s) (Fig. 2.17a,b), liquefying hematoma(s), or abscess(es), related to previous surgery or trauma. An abdominal wall abscess may arise from infection of a surgical incision or may be an extension of a superficial intraperitoneal abscess. A tuberculous paraspinal abscess may also track along the musculofascial plane into the lateral and posterior abdominal walls. Rarely, an infected urachal cyst or tumor may be seen extending from the umbilicus to the dome of the bladder (18,19) (Fig. 2.18).

Fluid collections complicated by hemorrhage or infec-tion present a more complex appearance, with septations and layering low-level echoes representing blood cells or debris. They may be aspirated under ultrasound guidance, with specimen sent for Gram stain and culture and sensitivity.

In certain cases, it is difficult to differentiate an incarcerated bowel loop of a ventral hernia from a focal fluid collection. In thin patients, it may also be difficult to distinguish between a fluid collection in the abdominal wall and a superficial intraperitoneal collection. In these situations, a CT scan is helpful to clarify the issue.

Rectus Sheath Hematoma

The rectus muscles are enclosed in the rectus sheath, which is formed by the aponeuroses of the two oblique

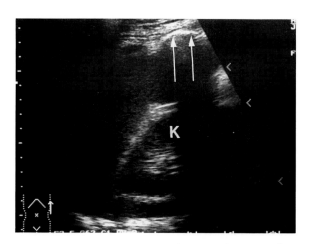

FIG. 2.15. Free air (pneumoperitoneum). This parasagittal sonogram shows collection of air posterior to abdominal wall (*arrows*). It is not associated with bowel or abdominal wall defect. This suggests diagnosis of pneumoperitoneum. At surgery, patient had a perforated gastric ulcer. *K*, kidney.

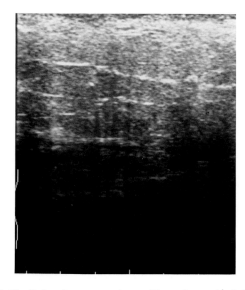

FIG. 2.16. Subcutaneous edema. There is marked thickening with increased echogenicity of subcutaneous fat layer in this patient who had a blow to the abdomen.

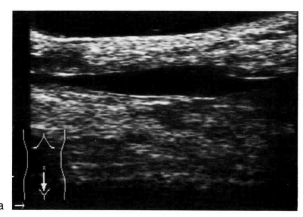
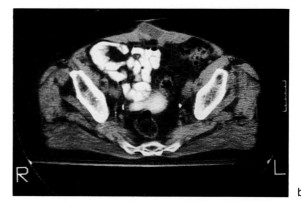

a →   b

FIG. 2.17. Incisional seroma. **a:** parasagittal sonogram; **b:** corresponding CT scan. There is a fluid collection in abdominal wall along incision in this patient who had a recent laparotomy. Serous fluid was obtained from aspiration.

and transversalis muscles. At the lateral margin of the rectus muscle, the aponeurosis of the internal oblique splits into an anterior and posterior lamina. The anterior lamina blends in front of the rectus with the aponeurosis of the external oblique; the posterior lamina blends behind the rectus with the aponeurosis of the transversalis muscle. The aponeuroses join in the midline to form the linea alba. This arrangement extends from the costal margin to the arcuate line, which is located midway between the umbilicus and the symphysis pubis, where the posterior wall of the sheath ends in a curved margin. Caudal to the arcuate line, the posterior layer of the sheath is formed by the transversalis fascia only, whereas the anterior layer is formed by the aponeuroses of all three muscles (Fig. 2.2a,b). The inferior and superior epigastric arteries and veins run posterior to the muscles.

A rectus sheath hematoma may develop after surgery,

a blow to the abdomen, or hyperextension strain, during labor or episode of violent coughing, or in patients with blood dyscrasias or on anticoagulant therapy.

The hematoma is often posterior to the muscles, but it may be surrounding the muscles, enclosed within the sheath. It may be uni- or bilateral. It may be small or quite large, extending along the entire muscles or sheath. Because of gravity and the configuration of the rectus sheath, a hematoma usually becomes larger as it extends caudally across the midline over the lower abdomen and pelvis where it causes external compression on the urinary bladder (20,21) (Fig. 2.19).

In the acute phase, a fluid–fluid level may be seen in the hematoma, with the clotted blood layering in the dependent part and the unclotted blood or plasma floating on top (Fig. 2.20). Rarely, turbulence may be detected in the layer of unclotted blood, indicating active

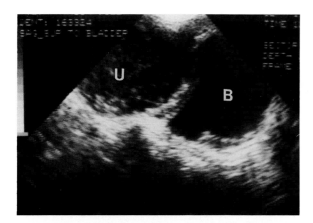

FIG. 2.18. Infected urachal cyst: parasagittal sonogram. This young child has a cystic mass extending from umbilicus to dome of urinary bladder. Urachal cyst originates from a remnant of urachal duct, which communicates externally in region of umbilicus. It may be the site of local infection, carcinoma, or sarcoma. *u,* urachal cyst; *B,* bladder. (Courtesy Dr. Chen Fong, Calgary Children's Hospital, Alberta.)

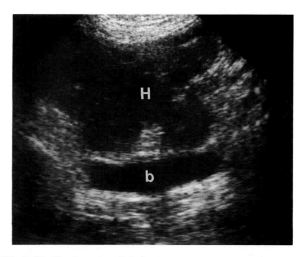

FIG. 2.19. Rectus sheath hematoma: transverse sonogram. Distal to arcuate line, hypoechoic hematoma (*H*) extends across the midline and compresses the urinary bladder (*b*).

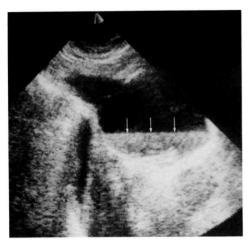

FIG. 2.20. Rectus sheath hematoma: sagittal scan. Note fluid/fluid–level (*arrows*).

bleeding (22). Liquefying hematoma manifests as sono-lucent collection (Fig. 2.21).

Most hematomas, even large, can be managed conservatively, using sonography to monitor their size and resolution. During the resorption phase, the hematoma appears usually hypoechoic. If it liquifies, it becomes sonolucent, with or without septations.

When active arterial bleeding is identified or when the hematoma is complicated by infection, surgery is usually performed to ligate the bleeding artery and to evacuate the hematoma.

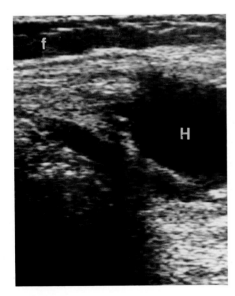

FIG. 2.21. Rectus sheath hematoma: sagittal scan. Liquefying hematoma (*H*) such as this one appears cystic. The hematoma becomes larger as it extends caudally. *f,* subcutaneous fat.

Abdominal Wall Neoplasms

Primary abdominal wall neoplasms are rare. They include lipoma, neuroma, neurofibroma, desmoid tumors, and sarcomas of various types (23). *Lipomas* typically appear as strongly echogenic lesions (Fig. 2.22). This is due to multiple fat–water interfaces. The other neoplasms have no specific sonographic findings and usually require diagnostic biopsy. *Desmoid tumors* are benign neoplasms arising from fascio-aponeurotic structures. They are most commonly found in the abdominal wall. They tend to recur after local excision. They affect, most commonly, multiparous women between 20 and 40 years of age; they are often related to previous abdominal surgery and to Gardner's syndrome (familial polyposis syndrome). Sonographically, they usually appear as well-encapsulated homogeneous hypoechoic masses (24).

The abdominal wall may be locally invaded by malignancies arising from the pleura, peritoneum, or diaphragm (mesothelioma, rhabdomyosarcoma, fibrosarcoma) or from the bowel. It may also be the site of distant metastases arising from melanoma (most common), lymphoma, carcinoma of the breast, ovary, and colon (23). The metastasis may occur as an isolated finding (Fig. 2.23), but more frequently it is seen in patients with widespread metastatic disease elsewhere.

Diaphragmatic Pathology

Diaphragmatic Paralysis

Real-time sonography is replacing fluoroscopy in the study of diaphragmatic motion. Children can be safely examined this way without risk of radiation. Another major advantage is that the examination can be per-

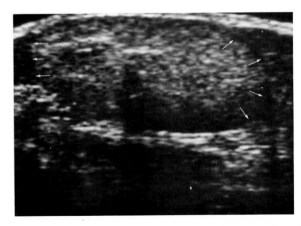

FIG. 2.22. Lipoma of abdominal wall. This fatty neoplasm is usually more echogenic than desmoid tumors. It is well demarcated (*arrows*) from surrounding normal tissues. This suggests that it is a benign neoplasm.

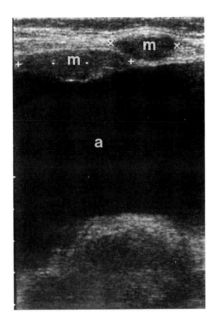

FIG. 2.23. Metastases in abdominal wall. Note hypoechoic masses (*m*) and large ascites (*a*). Patient with ovarian carcinoma.

formed at the patient's bedside. For patients on a respirator, unassisted ventilation can be evaluated with the respirator disconnected for a few seconds. The transverse scan over the xyphoid allows simultaneous views of both hemidiaphragms (25,26).

A frequent situation is the investigation of an elevated or obscured hemidiaphragm seen on chest radiograph. Is this due to eventration, paralysis, or peridiaphragmatic abnormalities? The answer can be readily obtained with real-time sonography. Normal excursion of the right hemidiaphragm in the newborn measures 2.6 (±0.1) cm for the anterior third, 3.6 (±0.2) cm for the middle third,

and 4.5 (±0.2) cm for the posterior third (27). Paralysis of one hemidiaphragm can be detected by showing absent or paradoxical motion on the affected side as compared with the normal or exaggerated excursion on the opposite side (25,26). Unlike fluoroscopy, however, ultrasound can demonstrate the diaphragm even in the presence of peridiaphragmatic mass or fluid collections (Fig. 2.24a,b).

Diaphragmatic Eventration

Traditionally, this is considered to be a developmental anomaly, resulting from incomplete muscularization of the membranous diaphragm. More recently, it has been suggested that it may be acquired, related to muscular weakness secondary to focal ischemia, infarct, or neuromuscular dysfunction (8).

The condition constitutes 5% of all diaphragmatic defects. It may be partial (segmental) or may be complete (total). Segmental eventration affects, most commonly, the anterior portion of the right hemidiaphragm. Complete eventration occurs more commonly in males and on the left side (9,28–30). Unilateral eventration is often associated with rib anomalies. Bilateral eventration is often associated with trisomies 13-15 and 18 and with Beckwith-Wiedemann syndrome (9,28,29).

Sonographically, the eventration produces a bulge or pouch in the contour of the diaphragm that moves normally with respiration. Normally, this is filled with the liver (Fig. 2.25a,b). In the presence of ascites, fluid may be seen filling the pouch separating the liver from the diaphragm. Prominent diaphragmatic slips are often associated with eventration. They have been discussed in the previous section of this chapter. Diaphragmatic eventration has been diagnosed antenatally by ultrasound (31).

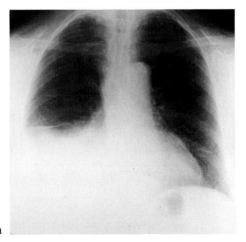 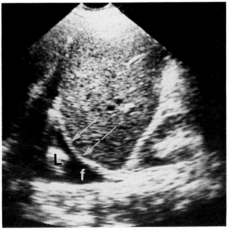

FIG. 2.24. Right pleural effusion. **a:** chest radiograph. Right hemidiaphragm cannot be seen. Is this due to fluid or tumor? Is it moving normally? **b:** parasagittal scan. Answers are readily provided by sonography. Right hemidiaphragm (*arrows*) is well outlined by pleural fluid (*f*), which surrounds collapsed lung (*L*). Its motion is well demonstrated on real-time sonography.

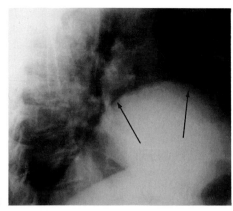
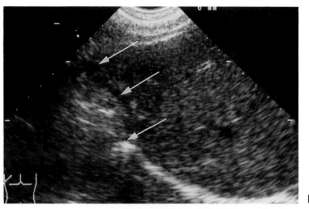

a   b

FIG. 2.25. Eventration: parasagittal scan. **a:** chest radiograph; **b:** corresponding parasagittal sonogram. Lateral chest radiograph shows elevation of anterior aspect of right hemidiaphragm (*black arrows*). Oblique sonogram shows that this is due to thinning of anterior leaflet (*white arrows*). Space adjacent to eventration is filled by liver.

Diaphragmatic Hernia

Defects in the diaphragm are usually congenital, caused by developmental anomaly, but may be acquired, related to previous trauma or surgery. Congenital diaphragmatic hernias occur in about one in 2,000 to 5,000 live births. More than 50% of cases are associated with other malformations (32,33).

Posterior Bochdalek hernia is the most common congenital diaphragmatic defect, caused by failure of fusion of the pleuroperitoneal canal during development. It is most often unilateral (97% of cases), affecting, more commonly, the left side. On the left side, omental fat, stomach, spleen, or kidney may herniate through the defect. On the right side, omental fat or part of the liver or right kidney may be found above the diaphragm (9,32–34). Chest radiographs usually show a focal hump in the posterior diaphragmatic contour that corresponds on sonography to the herniated organ.

Anterior Morgani hernia is less frequent and is usually seen in the anterior and medial right cardiophrenic angle. It is due to maldevelopment of the septum transversum and may be associated with a pericardial defect through which the heart may herniate into the upper abdomen or abdominal contents into the pericardial cavity. Because of its location, Morgani hernia is more difficult to detect by sonography than the Bochdalek type (9,32,33).

Antenatal detection of diaphragmatic hernia has been reported (32,33,35). The normal diaphragm may be seen in the fetus as a thin echo-poor band separating the thorax from the abdomen (Fig. 2.26). In CDH, sonography may show the herniated fluid-filled stomach or bowel in the lower thorax, displacing the fetal heart (Fig. 2.27). Compression of the fetal lung by the herniated abdominal viscera often results in pulmonary hypoplasia. More than 50% of infants with congenital diaphrag-

matic hernia die from respiratory failure. Differential diagnosis of CDH in the neonate should include cystic adenomatoid malformation of the lung, bronchogenic or neuroenteric cysts, or extralobar pulmonary sequestration (33,35,36).

Diaphragmatic Inversion

Diaphragmatic inversion is most commonly caused by a large pleural effusion and less commonly by a large thoracic neoplasm invading the diaphragm. The left side is more frequently affected. Only part of or the entire hemidiaphragm may be involved (37).

On sagittal scan, the inverted hemidiaphragm bulges inferiorly, with convexity toward the abdomen (Fig. 2.28). It shows little or asynchronous motion, resulting

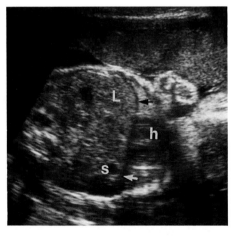

FIG. 2.26. Normal fetal diaphragm. This coronal view of a 32-week-old fetus shows diaphragm (*arrows*) as an echo-poor band separating thorax from abdomen. *h,* heart; *L,* liver; *s,* stomach.

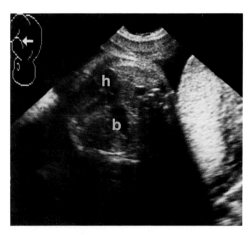

FIG. 2.27. Congenital diaphragmatic hernia: obstetrical scan (18 weeks menstrual age). Axial view of fetal thorax reveals herniated fluid-filled bowel (*b*) adjacent to and displacing heart (*h*). Differential diagnosis includes cystic adenomatoid malformation of lung and bronchogenic and neurenteric cysts.

in air exchange between the two lungs in inspiration and expiration and causing respiratory distress.

Because of its cone shape, an inverted right hemidiaphragm may simulate a mass in the dome of the liver on transverse CT scan. The mistake can be avoided by using sagittal and transverse sonographic scan planes.

Diaphragmatic Rupture

Diaphragmatic rupture may be due to a penetrating injury or blunt trauma. Rarely it is secondary to infection such as amebiasis. The left side is more commonly affected in blunt abdominal trauma (38,39).

The preoperative diagnosis is difficult, often obscured by other life-threatening conditions associated with multiple injuries and poor patient cooperation. It may be suspected on chest radiographs, fluoroscopy, liver–spleen scintigraphy, and peritoneal lavage. Other diagnostic modalities include contrast studies of the GI tract, CT, and MR imaging (38).

Sonography can occasionally detect diaphragmatic rupture, which is often extensive, measuring more than 10 cm long. Disruption of the diaphragmatic echoes and herniation of abdominal viscera through the rent have been described (40,41).

Posttraumatic rupture of the diaphragm should be closed surgically. Delayed diagnosis results in higher morbidity and mortality.

Diaphragmatic Neoplasms

The diaphragm is an uncommon site for neoplastic disease, either primary or secondary. Primary neoplasms usually are sarcomas. Secondary involvement is usually due to local invasion by adjacent pleural, peritoneal, or thoracic and abdominal wall malignancies. Distant metastases from bronchogenic or ovarian carcinoma, Wilm's tumor, and osteogenic sarcoma have been reported (42,43).

Sonography shows disruption or interruption of the diaphragmatic echoes at the site of metastatic implants. Partial or complete inversion of the hemidiaphragm may be seen, usually caused by neoplasms of enormous size (Fig. 2.29).

Peritoneal Pathology

Ascites

Ascites is fluid accumulated in the peritoneal cavity. Fluid may be a transudate such as seen in hypoalbumin-

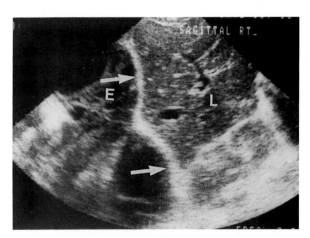

FIG. 2.28. Inverted right hemidiaphragm: parasagittal scan. Septated empyema (*E*) displaces the diaphragm, which appears concave toward abdomen (*arrows*). *L,* liver.

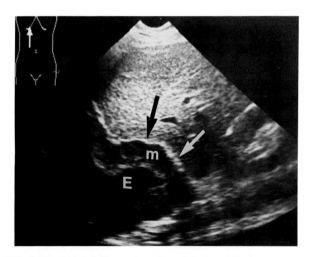

FIG. 2.29. Mesothelioma invading right hemidiaphragm: parasagittal scan. Note focal inversion (*arrows*) caused by thick tumor (*m*). Pleural fluid (*E*) is also present.

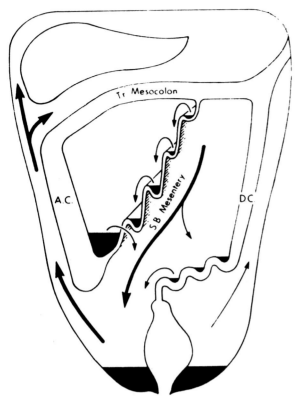

FIG. 2.30. Flow of ascitic fluid. *AC,* ascending colon; *DC,* descending colon; *SB,* small bowel. (From Siegel MJ. Spleen and peritoneal cavity. In: Siegel MJ, ed. *Pediatric sonography.* New York: Raven Press; 1991:161–178, with permission.)

emia and hepatic, cardiac, and renal failure; it may be an exudate, such as seen in inflammatory or neoplastic diseases; it may be blood, chyle, bile, or urine.

Because of the anatomical compartmentalization, the action of gravity, and variations in intra-abdominal pressures during respiration, ascitic fluid tends to collect in certain pooling sites: the pelvic cul-de-sac (pouch of Douglas), the lower end of the mesenteric root at the ileo-cecal junction, the sigmoid mesocolon, and the right

paracolic gutter (Fig. 2.30). The natural flow of peritoneal fluid occurs along the peritoneal reflections. In the erect position, by action of gravity, fluid collects in the recesses of the infra-mesocolic compartment. From there, it spills into the pelvic cul-de-sac and paravesical recesses. In the recumbent position, fluid flows preferentially upward along the right paracolic gutter to pool in the right subphrenic and right perihepatic spaces. In the left paracolic gutter, the flow is weak and limited superiorly by the phrenocolic ligament, which isolates the left subphrenic space (44–48).

With modern real-time transducers, as little as a few milliliters of fluid can be identified. The most sensitive and reliable sites for detection of minimal ascites in the abdomen are Morison's pouch and the right perihepatic spaces (Fig. 2.31a,b) (44–46). When this is seen, one should always look into the pelvis to identify fluid in the cul-de-sac. Superficial small fluid collections superior and anterior to the liver may be missed with a 3.5-MHz medium focus transducer, which is unable to visualize the near field. In this situation, a 7.5-MHz linear array transducer should be used. Fluid does not accumulate along the posterosuperior surface of the liver, which is the bare area not covered by peritoneum. When fluid is seen in this location, it is either pleural or subcapsular.

Localization of fluid collections may be at times difficult. A subphrenic collection may mimic a pleural effusion. Identification of the diaphragm is important, and this can be achieved in most cases. In the parasagittal scan, subphrenic fluid is inferior to the diaphragm, between it and the liver or spleen. On the right side, abdominal fluid does not extend posterior to the inferior vena cava, as a right pleural effusion often does.

It may be difficult to distinguish peritoneal fluid from a subcapsular collection. As a general rule, ascitic fluid follows the natural contour of the liver or spleen, whereas a large subcapsular collection often causes focal external indentation on the surface of the organ.

Massive ascites displaces the liver, spleen, and bowel

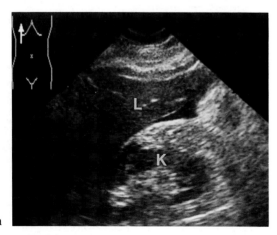

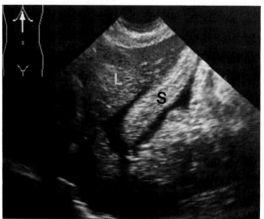

FIG. 2.31. Minimal ascites. **a:** in Morison's pouch (parasagittal scan); **b:** in right subhepatic space (parasagittal scan). *L,* liver; *K,* kidney; *S,* stomach.

loops medially and toward the center of the abdomen. The mesentery appears as strong linear echoes radiating in a fan-shaped manner from its posterior attachment. Bowel loops are arranged as round or tubular echogenic structures around the periphery of the fan-shaped mesentery. Adhesions may be identified when surrounded by fluid (Fig. 2.32).

Simple ascites or a transudate is usually echo-free. Septations and floating debris are usually found in exudates or in ascites complicated by hemorrhage or infection (49) (Fig. 2.33).

Loculated ascites as an isolated finding is difficult to distinguish from a mesenteric or omental cyst, lymphocele, abscess, or cystic neoplasm, especially when septations are present. It is, however, more commonly seen in the course of nonpyogenic inflammatory conditions such as pancreatitis, in which the exudate dissects along the mesenteric pathways and becomes walled off by surrounding peritoneal adhesions. Diagnosis often requires fine needle percutaneous aspiration, which is frequently performed under ultrasound guidance.

Intraperitoneal Abscesses

The causes of intraperitoneal abscesses include perforation of hollow viscera (such as seen in perforated ulcers, appendicitis, Crohn's disease), complication of recent abdominal trauma or surgery, or infection of a pseudocyst, hematoma, or ascitic fluid collection. About 70% of subphrenic and subhepatic abscesses are complications from previous surgery to the GI tract and biliary tree (10). The most common offending organisms are *Escherichia coli*, non–group A streptococci, staphylococci, and *Klebsiella*. Mixed infections are also common. Clinical findings typically include fever, leukocytosis, abdominal pain, and tenderness. Peritoneal

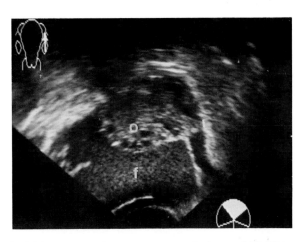

FIG. 2.33. Hemoperitoneum: transvaginal scan. Fluid (*f*) is so echogenic that it simulates a solid mass. This is seen in a patient with ruptured ectopic pregnancy. *O*, ovary.

infections tend to localize in the upper abdomen, between the transverse colon and diaphragm. Sixty percent occur on the right; 25% occur on the left; 15% are bilateral (50,51).

The subphrenic and perihepatic abscesses are well suited for sonographic detection, although the left upper quadrant may present some difficulties. A left anterior subphrenic abscess may be difficult to distinguish from a lesser sac abscess. It may also simulate an abscess in the left lobe of the liver (Figs. 2.34 and 2.35). In general, it often occurs after generalized peritonitis. It is seen in a higher plane than lesser sac collection, immediately inferior to the diaphragm extending on both sides of the midline, anterior to the stomach and left lobe of the liver. It is usually drained surgically via a transthoracic extrapleural approach, whereas a lesser sac abscess requires an abdominal transperitoneal route for drainage (52). In the mid and lower abdomen, the study is often severely lim-

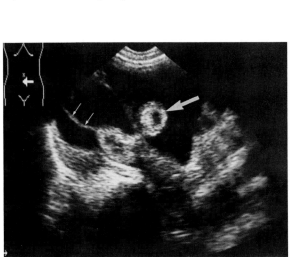

FIG. 2.32. Ascites and adhesions. Adhesions (*small arrow*) and bowel (*large arrow*) are well seen when surrounded by ascites.

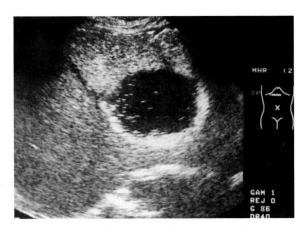

FIG. 2.34. Left anterior subphrenic abscess: transverse sonogram. In this projection, abscess appears to be in left lobe of the liver.

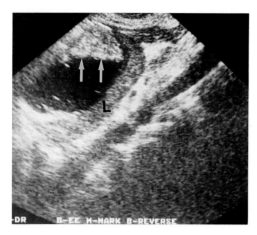

FIG. 2.35. Left anterior subphrenic abscess: parasagittal sonogram. Liver (*L*) is, in fact, displaced posteriorly by abscess. Note solid debris floating on top of fluid (*arrows*).

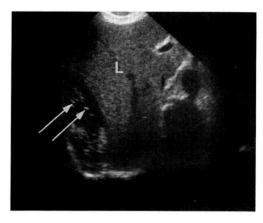

FIG. 2.36. Right subphrenic abscess: transverse scan. Note small echoes representing air and debris (*arrows*) in fluid collection. *L*, liver.

ited by the presence of open wounds, drainage tubes, large dressings, and bowel gas, which may hide a gas-containing abscess. Despite these difficulties, a few series still claim an accuracy rate ranging from 80% to more than 90% for the sonographic detection of intra-abdominal abscesses (50,51). Our own experience is more similar to the results published by Lundstedt et al. (53), who reported a detection rate of 44%. It is generally accepted that CT performs better than sonography in identifying abscesses, particularly in the lower abdomen. The choice of the initial imaging modality depends therefore on the patient's clinical status and the patient's size. For large or obese patients or in the recent postoperative period, CT scanning is the best screening technique. For thin patients or those in whom a specific site is suspected, sonography will be more beneficial. When both CT and ultrasound fail, then isotope scanning with Gallium or Indium 111 may be helpful. The best results are often obtained by the appropriate use of more than one imaging technique.

Typically, an abscess appears as a fluid collection with irregular borders, containing septation and floating debris. Occasionally, gas bubbles may be identified (Figs. 2.36 and 2.37). A fluid–fluid level may be detected. Sometimes, however, the abscess may appear entirely echo-free like a simple cystic lesion or entirely echogenic as a solid mass. Quite often, a complex mass is found containing solid and cystic materials. CT performs better in identifying small gas bubbles in the mass (50,51). Golding et al. (54) have shown that, to demonstrate an air–fluid level in an abscess cavity with the patient lying supine, one should scan the cavity from the posterior fluid-filled portion, aiming the sound beam anteromedially. Scanning from an anterior approach with the beam directed posteriorly will produce reverberation/ring-down artifacts caused by the presence of air in the nondependent portion of the cavity.

Most intraperitoneal abscesses can be safely aspirated and drained under ultrasound or CT guidance (55). Please refer to Chapter 13 for further details about the procedure.

Meconium Peritonitis

Meconium peritonitis is an aseptic chemical inflammation of the peritoneum secondary to prenatal bowel perforation. Sixty-five percent of the cases are due to intestinal stenosis or atresia and meconium ileus (cystic fibrosis). Less frequent causes include perforated Meckel's diverticulum or appendix and bowel perforation related to volvulus, internal hernia, and vascular thrombosis (56). Extravasation of sterile meconium from the perforation into the peritoneal cavity produces an intense foreign body reaction resulting in a fibroadhesive peritonitis, which may calcify over time. The mass of spilled meconium may be surrounded by a calcified fibrous wall, forming a pseudocyst (Fig. 2.38a,b).

Antenatal sonography often detects a focal mass in the

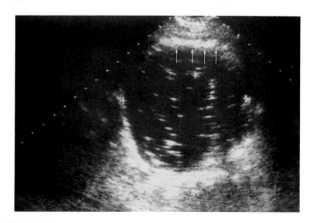

FIG. 2.37. Abscess. Pus was drained percutaneously from this fluid collection in lower abdomen. Gas bubbles appear as strong linear echoes (*arrows*) floating on top of abscess.

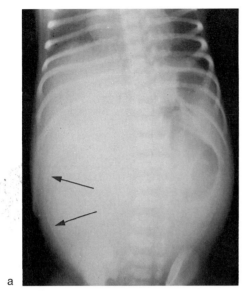

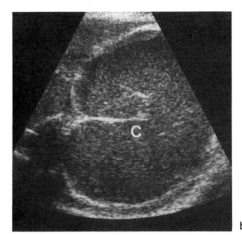

a   b

FIG. 2.38. Meconium pseudocyst. **a:** abdominal radiograph; **b:** sonogram. Curvilinear calcification (*arrows*) is seen along right side of abdomen. Note little gas in bowel, which is displaced to left. Sonogram showed a large septated echogenic mass (*c*), which at surgery proved to be a meconium pseudocyst. The infant had perforation during fetal life *in utero* caused by jejunal torsion.

fetal abdomen. The mass may be complex or may appear cystic, with echogenic wall. Calcified peritoneal thickening may be seen as scattered linear echoes with acoustic shadowing (56–58). Associated findings may include fetal ascites, dilated bowel loops, and polyhydraminos. After birth, radiography of the abdomen may show calcification in the liver and scrotum. Calcification in the abdomen may produce a diffuse echogenicity referred to as a "snowstorm" appearance. Prognosis for patients with meconium peritonitis has improved in recent years, in part because of early detection.

Peritoneal Tuberculosis

Peritoneal tuberculosis is now rarely seen in the Western world. This occurs either as direct spread of GI tuberculosis or as hematogenous dissemination from a lung focus. Ascites, enlarged necrotic mesenteric nodes, and echogenic epigastric masses corresponding to caseating granulomata have been reported in the ultrasound literature (59).

When the greater omentum is involved, it may be thickened by granulomatous infiltration and adhesions. Sonography performed with high transducer frequency shows the characteristic "omental cake" appearance (Fig. 2.39), simulating peritoneal carcinomatosis or mesothelioma (60). Diagnosis should be confirmed by peritoneoscopy and biopsy. Ultrasound may also be used to monitor response to antituberculous therapy.

Lymphoceles

Lymphoceles are lymph-containing collections that develop most commonly after previous surgery (e.g.,

lymphadenectomy, gynecological and urologic procedures, renal transplantation) and rarely after trauma. Leakage of lymph occurs from disrupted lymphatic vessels (61,62).

Lymphoceles are most commonly seen in the pelvis. In the abdomen, they can occur anywhere, in the retroperitoneum or in the peritoneal spaces. When large and under tension, they often cause displacement of the surrounding organs (63). They are usually small, but some may attain considerable size, measuring several centimeters and causing pressure symptoms or hydronephrosis of the transplanted kidney.

Sonographically, they are usually echo-free fluid collections indistinguishable from loculated simple ascites

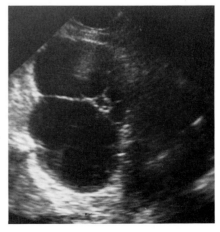

FIG. 2.39. Lymphocele: sagittal scan. There is a septated pelvo-abdominal fluid collection in this patient who had nodal dissection for lymphoma staging.

or mesenteric cysts or pancreatic pseudocysts. Occasionally, however, they may contain septations and floating debris most likely as a result of previous hemorrhage (Fig. 2.40). The diagnosis is established by clinical history or percutaneous aspiration. The fluid is serosanguinous or dark brown, containing fat globules.

Small lymphoceles usually resorb over time. Large and symptomatic lymphoceles should be drained either percutaneously or surgically (62). Some success has been obtained with sclerotherapy using instillation of tetracycline into the lymphoceles (64).

Peritoneal Mesothelioma

Peritoneal mesothelioma is a rare primary mesenchymal neoplasm arising from the serous membranes, related to previous asbestos exposure. It affects solely the pleura in 65% of cases, primarily the peritoneum in 33%, and the pleura and the peritoneum in about 2% (65). The latent period is usually long, with the disease frequently manifesting at 40 to 45 years after initial exposure to asbestos.

The typical sonographic finding seen in peritoneal mesothelioma is sheet-like thickening of the omentum described as omental "mantle" or "cake" (65–67). The anterior superficial surface of the mass follows the contour of the abdominal cavity; the posterior deeper surface is lobulated, following the contour of adjacent bowel loops. The thickness of the mass varies from a few millimeters to several centimeters. The texture is usually hypoechoic, with scattered focal small echoes representing entrapped fat (Fig. 2.41). The appearances correlate closely with those seen on CT. Ascites when present is minimal (65).

Computed tomography performs better than ultrasound in detecting small nodules attached to the perito-

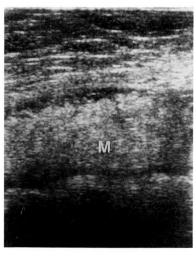

FIG. 2.41. Mesothelioma: transverse sonogram. A thick echogenic mass (*M*) is seen posterior to abdominal wall. Posterior contour is lobulated because of adjacent bowel. Note absence of ascites.

neal surface or buried in the mesenteric fat, peritoneal thickening, and calcified pleural plaques (66,67). Gallium uptake by pleural and peritoneal mesotheliomas has been reported (67). Diagnosis may be made by fine needle aspiration biopsies, which should be performed in different locations to obtain adequate samples (68). In most cases, peritoneoscopy or laparotomy is required.

Peritoneal Carcinomatosis

Peritoneal metastatic disease originates from a wide variety of primary malignancies, the most common being carcinoma of the ovary and the GI tract (69). It occurs by four mechanisms: invasion through mesenteric and ligamentous attachments, intraperitoneal seeding, lymphatic spread, and hematogenous dissemination.

Meyers et al. (10,69,70) illustrated well the mesenteric pathways for spread of GI cancers. The gastrocolic ligament may serve as a conduit for spread of carcinoma of the stomach and of the transverse colon. Carcinoma of the pancreas may grow along the transverse mesocolon to affect the posteroinferior border of the transverse colon. Carcinoma of the hepatic flexure may also extend along the transverse mesocolon to involve the paraduodenal area.

Intraperitoneal seeding follows the natural flow of ascitic fluid, which has been discussed previously. Malignant cells shed in the fluid grow at specific locations where fluid tends to pool, namely, the pelvic cul-de-sac, the root of the mesentery at the ileo-cecal junction, the sigmoid mesocolon, and the right paracolic gutter. At these sites, metastatic masses often produce characteristic nodular indentations and displacement of the bowel on barium studies (71,72). They may be detected by sonography. Large superficial omental masses are readily

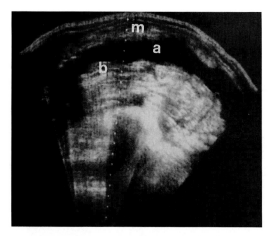

FIG. 2.40. Peritoneal tuberculosis. Greater omentum is thickened (*m*), resulting in classical omental "mantle" or "cake" appearance. Note ascites (*a*) separating thickened omentum from bowel (*b*).

identified by high-frequency transducers, appearing as omental mantle or cake not unlike that described in peritoneal mesothelioma or tuberculosis. Small nodules (2–3 mm) attached to the abdominal wall or omentum are particularly well seen in the presence of large ascites (Fig. 2.42) (73).

Metastatic emboli, carried by the mesenteric arteries to the vasa recta on the antimesenteric border of the bowel, occur most commonly with melanoma and carcinoma of the breast and lung (72). They grow as submucosal nodules, which may be detected by ultrasound.

Pseudomyxoma Peritonei

This condition is characterized by mucinous peritoneal implants and gelatinous ascites, most often caused by metastases from mucin-producing adenocarcinoma of the ovary, appendix, colon, or rectum. Some benign neoplasms of the ovary and appendix may also be the cause (74).

Only a few reports describe the sonographic appearance of pseudomyxoma peritonei (75–77). These include multiple hypoechoic masses throughout the peritoneum and mesentery, and strongly echogenic nodular lesions in the hepatorenal recess. They may show abnormal uptake on a technetium 99m-MDP scan, and they correspond to calcified masses seen on the abdominal radiograph. Ascites when present is usually massive. It may be echogenic, reflecting the gelatinous content of the fluid (Fig. 2.43).

Retained Surgical Sponges

Retained surgical sponges in the abdomen are rare occurrences. Without opaque markers, they cannot be seen on the abdominal radiographs. They may or may not be associated with a surrounding abscess.

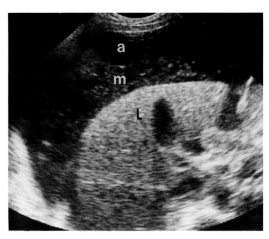

FIG. 2.43. Pseudomyxoma peritonei. Hypoechoic masses (*m*) are seen floating in ascites (*a*) surrounding liver (*L*). Patient had intraperitoneal spread from mucinous carcinoma of ovary, proven at autopsy.

The ones surrounded by an abscess appear sonographically as infected collections with irregular borders and internal echoes (78). The ones not associated with abscess show a clean, clear-cut acoustic shadow in relation to a palpable mass (79). The findings should be correlated with a radiograph of the abdomen to rule out residual barium in the bowel or a calcified neoplasm.

2.4 PITFALLS, ARTIFACTS, AND PRACTICAL TIPS

Artifactual Disruption and Displacement of Diaphragmatic Echoes

Disruption of the diaphragmatic echoes is often a sign of diaphragmatic disease such as traumatic rupture or infiltration by neoplasms (42).

In certain conditions, however, the interruption is artifactual. This is seen in the presence of a cystic lesion or fatty mass in the liver or right adrenal gland. This artifact

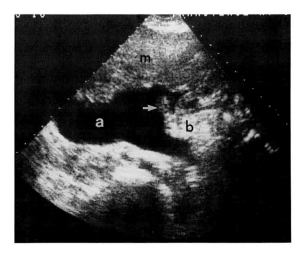

FIG. 2.42. Peritoneal seedings. Note omental cake (*m*), ascites (*a*), and small nodule (*arrow*) attached to bowel (*b*).

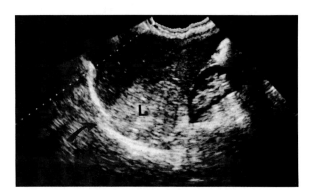

FIG. 2.44. Propagation speed artifact. Note apparent disruption and posterior displacement of diaphragm (*arrow*) in relation to fatty mass (lipoma) in liver (*L*).

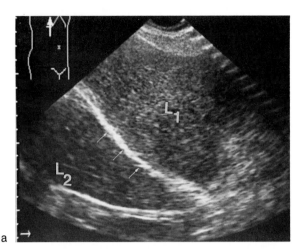 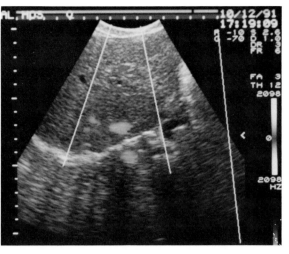

a   b

FIG. 2.45. Mirror image artifact. *(See color image of part **b** in the color plate section, which follows page 50)* **a:** liver *(L₁)* is reproduced as a mirror image *(L₂)* on thoracic side of diaphragm *(arrows)*. **b:** True IVC *(in blue)* is reproduced as a mirror artifact *(in red)* across diaphragm. *Blue color* indicates flow toward transducer. *Red color* indicates flow away from transducer.

results from the altered velocity of the sound beam through the lesion, as well as the refraction of the sound beam at the edge of the lesion. This has been termed the "propagation speed artifact," which causes apparent disruption and displacement of the diaphragmatic echoes posterior to the cystic or fatty mass (Fig. 2.44). The apparent diaphragmatic displacement may be away or toward the lesion, depending on the speed of sound in the mass lesion (80,81).

Mirror Image Artifact

The lung–right hemidiaphragm interface is a common source of mirror image artifact because of the presence of air-containing lung adjacent to the diaphragm. An echogenic mass in the liver or a subphrenic fluid collection may be reproduced cephalad to the diaphragm on the sagittal view or posterior to the diaphragm on the transverse view (Fig. 2.45a,b). The mechanism producing this artifact is as follows (Fig. 2.46): the incident beam hitting the diaphragm–lung interface is reflected toward the liver. The reflected beam, when hitting the echogenic mass in the liver, is returned by scattered reflection to the diaphragm, which in turn reflects it back to the transducer. It takes longer for these scattered reflected echoes to reach the transducer; they therefore appear to originate from the other side of the diaphragm. They are thus displayed as a phantom mass or fluid collection at the base of the lung (82–84).

This artifact can be used to advantage. When a phantom mass is seen above the diaphragm, one should carefully scan the liver to look for the real lesion that is the source of the artifact.

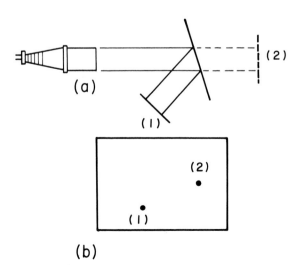

FIG. 2.46. Mechanism of mirror image production. See text for explanation. (From Kremkau, ref. 84, with permission.)

REFERENCES

Scanning Techniques

1. Tornaga BD, Torichi DH, Rifkin MD. Small parts real time sonography: a new "water path." *J Ultrasound Med* 1984;3:355–357.
2. Pozniak MA, Crass JR, Zagzebski J, et al. Clinical efficacy of Kitecko ultrasonic conductor. *Invest Radiol* 1989;24:128–132.
3. Claes HP, Reygaerts DO, Boven FA, et al. An echo-free silicone elastomer block for ultrasonography. *Radiology* 1984;150:596.
4. Fataar S, Goodman H, Tuft R, et al. Postoperative abdominal sonography using a transonic sealing membrane. *AJR* 1983; 141:565–566.

Normal Anatomy

5. Shafir R, Itzchak Y, Heymen Z, Azizi E, Tsur H, Hiss J. Postoperative ultrasonic measurements of the thickness of cutaneous malignant melanomas. *J Ultrasound Med* 1984;3:205–208.

6. Engel JM, Deitch EE. Sonography of the anterior abdominal wall. *AJR* 1981;137:73–77.
7. Lewandowski BJ, Winsberg F. Echographic appearance of the right hemidiaphragm. *J Ultrasound Med* 1983;2:243–249.
8. Yeh H-C, Halton KP, Gray CE. Anatomic variations and abnormalities in the diaphragm seen with ultrasound. *Radiographics* 1990;10:1019–1030.
9. Panicek DM, Benson CB, Gotlieb RH, Heitzman ER. The diaphragm: anatomic, pathologic and radiologic considerations. *Radiographics* 1988;8:385–425.
10. Meyers MA, ed. *Dynamic radiology of the abdomen. Normal and pathologic anatomy.* 3rd ed. New York: Springer-Verlag; 1988.
11. Heiken JP. Abdominal wall and peritoneal cavity. In: Lee TL, Sagel SS, Stanley RJ, eds. *Computed body tomography with MRI correlation.* New York: Raven Press; 1988:661–705.

Pathology

12. Fornage BD, Lorigan JG. Sonographic detection and fine needle aspiration biopsy of nonpalpable recurrent or metastatic melanoma in subcutaneous tissues. *J Ultrasound Med* 1989;8:421–424.
13. Sauerbrei EE, Nguyen KT, Nolan RL. The fetus. In: Sauerbrei EE, ed. *A practical guide to ultrasound in obstetrics and gynecology.* New York: Raven Press; 1987:111–159.
14. Thomas JL, Cunningham JJ. Ultrasonic evaluation of ventral hernias disguised as intra-abdominal neoplasms. *Arch Surg* 1978;113:589–590.
15. Fried AM, Meeker WR. Incarcerated Spigelian hernia: ultrasonic differential diagnosis. *AJR* 1979;133:107–110.
16. Siffring PA, Forrest TS, Frick MP. Hernias of the inferior lumbar space. Diagnosis with US. *Radiology* 1989;170:190.
17. Fornaga BD, Nerot C. Sonographic diagnosis of rhabdomyolysis. *JCU* 1986;14:389–392.
18. Bree RL, Silver TM. Sonography of bladder and perivesical abnormalities. *AJR* 1981;136:1101–1103.
19. Kwok-Liu JF, Zikman JM, Cockshott WP. Carcinoma of the urachus: the role of computed tomography. *Radiology* 1980;137:731–734.
20. Kaftori JK, Rosenbergen A, Pollack S, Fish JH. Rectus sheath hematoma: ultrasonographic diagnosis. *AJR* 1977;128:283–285.
21. Spitz HB, Wyatt GM. Rectus sheath hematoma. *JCU* 1977;5:413–416.
22. Savage PE, Joseph AEA, Adam EJ. Massive abdominal wall hematoma: real time ultrasound localization of bleeding. *J Ultrasound Med* 1985;4:157–158.
23. Diakoumakis EE, Weinberg B, Seife B. Unusual case studies of anterior wall mass as diagnosed by ultrasonography. *JCU* 1984;12:351–354.
24. Hanson RD, Hunter TB, Haber K. Ultrasonographic appearance of anterior abdominal wall desmoid tumours. *J Ultrasound Med* 1983;2:141–142.
25. Haber K, Asher WM, Freimann AK. Echographic evaluation of diaphragmatic motion in intra-abdominal disease. *Radiology* 1975;114:141–144.
26. Diament MJ, Boechat MI, Kangarloo H. Real time sector ultrasound in the evaluation of suspected abnormalities of diaphragmatic motion. *JCU* 1985;13:539–543.
27. Laing IA, Teele RL, Stark AR. Diaphragmatic movements in newborn infants. *J Pediatr* 1988;112:638–643.
28. Symbas PN, Hatcher CR Jr, Waldo W. Diaphragmatic eventration in infancy and childhood. *Ann Thorac Surg* 1977;24:113–119.
29. Weller MH. Bilateral eventration of the diaphragm. *West J Med* 1976;124:415–419.
30. Pery M, Kaftori JK, Rosenberger A. Causes of abnormal right diaphragmatic position diagnosed by ultrasound. *JCU* 1983;11:269–275.
31. Jurcak-Zaleski S, Comstock C, Kirk JS. Eventration of the diaphragm—prenatal diagnosis. *J Ultrasound Med* 1990;9:351–354.
32. Comstock CH. The antenatal diagnosis of diaphragmatic anomalies. *J Ultrasound Med* 1986;5:391–396.
33. Nakayama DK, Harrison MR, Chinn DH, et al. Prenatal diagnosis and natural history of the fetus with a congenital diaphragmatic hernia: initial clinical experience. *J Pediatr Surg* 1985;20:118–124.

34. Khan AN, Gould DA. Sonographic diagnosis of right renal herniation through the canal of Bochdalek. *JCU* 1984;12:237–238.
35. Chinn DH, Tilly RA, Callen PW, Nakayama DK, Harrison MR. Congenital diaphragmatic hernia diagnosed prenatally by ultrasound. *Radiology* 1983;148:119–123.
36. Stiller RJ, Roberts NS, Weiner S, Vaughn B. Congenital diaphragmatic hernia: antenatal diagnosis and obstetrical management. *JCU* 1985;13:212–215.
37. Subramanyam BR, Raghavendra BN, LeFleur RS. Sonography of the inverted right hemidiaphragm. *AJR* 1981;136:1004–1006.
38. Landay MJ, Setiawan H, Hirsch G, et al. Hepatic and thoracic amebiasis. *AJR* 1980;135:449–454.
39. Gelman R, Mirvis SE, Gens D. Diaphragmatic rupture due to blunt trauma: sensitivity on plain chest radiographs. *AJR* 1991;156:51–57.
40. Rao KG, Woodlief RM. Grey-scale ultrasonic documentation of ruptured right hemi-diaphragm. *Br J Radiol* 1980;53:812–814.
41. Ammann AM, Brewer WH, Mauhl KI, Walsh JW. Traumatic rupture of the diaphragm: real-time sonographic diagnosis. *AJR* 1983;140:915–916.
42. Worthen NJ, Worthen WF II. Disruption of the diaphragmatic echoes: a sonographic sign of diaphragmatic disease. *JCU* 1982;10:43–45.
43. Kangarloo H, Sukov R, Sample WF, et al. Ultrasonographic evaluation of juxtadiaphragmatic masses in children. *Radiology* 1977;125:785–787.
44. Proto AV, Lane EJ, Marangola JP. A new concept of ascitic fluid distribution. *AJR* 1976;126:974–977.
45. Goldberg BB, Harris R, Clearfield HR, et al. Ultrasonic determination of ascites. *Arch Intern Med* 1973;131:217–220.
46. Meyers MA. The spread and localization of acute intraperitoneal effusions. *Radiology* 1970;95:547–554.
47. Yeh HC, Wolf BS. Ultrasonography in ascites. *Radiology* 1977;124:783–790.
48. Gooding GAW, Cummings SR. Sonographic detection of ascites in liver disease. *J Ultrasound Med* 1984;3:169–172.
49. Edell SL, Gefter WB. Ultrasonic differentiation of types of ascitic fluid. *AJR* 1979;133:111–114.
50. Taylor KJ, Wasson JF, De Graaff C, Rosenfield AT, Andriole VT. Accuracy of grey-scale ultrasound in the diagnosis of abdominal and pelvic abscesses in 220 patients. *Lancet* 1978;1:83–84.
51. Mueller PR, Simeone JF. Intra abdominal abscesses: diagnosis by sonography and computed tomography. *Radiol Clin North Am* 1983;21:425–443.
52. Halvorsen RA, Jones MA, Rice RP, Thompson WM. Anterior left subphrenic abscess: characteristic plain films and CT appearance. *AJR* 1982;139:283–289.
53. Lundstedt C, Hederström E, Holmin T, Lunderquist A, Navne T, Owman T. Radiological diagnosis in proven intra-abdominal abscesses formation: a comparison between plain films of the abdomen, ultrasonography and computed tomography. *Gastrointest Radiol* 1983;8:261–266.
54. Golding RH, Li DKB, Cooperberg PL. Sonographic demonstration of air–fluid levels in abdominal abscesses. *J Ultrasound Med* 1982;1:151–155.
55. Van Sonnenberg E, Mueller PR, Ferrucci JT. Percutaneous drainage of 250 abdominal abscesses and fluid collections. Part I: results, failures and complications. *Radiology* 1984;151:337–341.
56. Brugman SM, Bjelland JJ, Thomasson JE, Anderson SF, Giles HR. Sonographic findings with radiographic correlation in meconium peritonitis. *JCU* 1979;7:305–306.
57. Blumenthal D, Rushovich AM, Williams RK, Rochester D. Prenatal sonographic findings of meconium peritonitis with pathologic correlation. *JCU* 1982;10:350–352.
58. Lauer JD, Cradock TV. Meconium pseudocyst: prenatal sonographic and antenatal radiologic correlation. *J Ultrasound Med* 1982;1:333–335.
59. Borgia G, Ciampi R, Nappa S, Vallone G, Marano I, Crowell J. Tuberculous mesenteric lymphadenitis clinically presenting as abdominal mass: CT and sonographic findings. *JCU* 1985;13:491–493.
60. Wu C-C, Chow K-S, Lü T-N, Huang F-T. Sonographic features of tuberculous omental cakes in peritoneal tuberculosis. *JCU* 1988;16:195–198.
61. Spring DB, Schroeder D, Babu S, Agee R, Gooding GAW. Ultra-

sonic evaluation of lymphocele formation after staging lymphadenectomy for prostatic carcinoma. *Radiology* 1981;141:479–483.

62. Lessner AM, Lempert N, Pietrocola DM, MacDowell RT, Haisch CE, Cerilli J. Diagnosis and treatment of pelvic lymphoceles in the renal transplant recipient. *NY State J Med* 1984;84:491–494.

63. Doust BD, Thompson R. Ultrasonography of abdominal fluid collections. *Gastrointest Radiol* 1978;3:273–279.

64. White M, Mueller PR, Ferrucci JT Jr., et al. Percutaneous drainage of postoperative abdominal and pelvic lymphoceles. *AJR* 1985;145:1065–1069.

65. Moertel CG. Peritoneal mesothelioma. *Gastroenterology* 1972;63: 346–350.

66. Yeh H-C, Chahinian AP. Ultrasonography and computed tomography of peritoneal mesothelioma. *Radiology* 1980;135:705–712.

67. Dach J, Patel N, Patel S, Petassnick J. Peritoneal mesothelioma: CT, sonography and gallium 67 scan. *AJR* 1980;135:614–616.

68. Reuter K, Raptopoulos V, Reale F, et al. Diagnosis of peritoneal mesothelioma: computed tomography, sonography and fine needle aspiration biopsy. *AJR* 1983;140:1189–1194.

69. Meyers MA. Metastatic disease along the small bowel mesentery: roentgen features. *AJR* 1975;123:67–73.

70. Meyers MA. Distribution of intraabdominal malignant seeding: dependency on dynamics of flow and ascitic fluid. *AJR* 1973;119:198–206.

71. Meyers MA, McSweeney J. Secondary neoplasms of the bowel. *Radiology* 1979;133:419–424.

72. Levitt RG, Koehler RE, Sagel SS, Lee JKT. Metastatic disease of the mesentery and omentum. *Radiol Clin North Am* 1982;20:501–510.

73. Goerg C, Schwerk W-B. Peritoneal carcinomatosis with ascites. *AJR* 1991;156:1185–1187.

74. Fernandez R, Daly JM. Pseudomyxoma peritonei. *Arch Surg* 1980;115:409–414.

75. Merritt CB, Williams SM. Ultrasound findings in a patient with pseudomyxoma peritonei. *JCU* 1978;6:417–418.

76. Seshill MB, Coulam CM. Pseudomyxoma peritonei: computed tomography and sonography. *AJR* 1981;136:803–806.

77. Seale WB. Sonographic findings in a patient with pseudomyxoma peritonei. *JCU* 1982;10:441–443.

78. Sekiba K, Akamatsu N, Niwa K. Ultrasound characteristics of abdominal abscesses involving foreign bodies (gauze). *JCU* 1979;7:284–285.

79. Barriga P, Garcia C. Ultrasonography in the detection of intra-abdominal retained surgical sponges. *J Ultrasound Med* 1984;3:173–176.

Pitfalls, Artifacts, and Practical Tips

80. Richman TS, Taylor KJW, Kremkau FW. Propagation speed artifact in a fatty tumour (myelolipoma): significance for tissue differential diagnosis. *J Ultrasound Med* 1983;2:45–47.

81. Mayo J, Cooperberg PL. Displacement of the diaphragmatic echo by hepatic cysts: a new explanation with computer simulation. *J Ultrasound Med* 1984;3:337–340.

82. Laing FC. Commonly encountered artifacts in clinical ultrasound. *Semin Ultrasound* 1983;4:27–43.

83. Zagzebski JA. Images and artifacts. In: Hagen-Ansert SL, ed. *Textbook of diagnostic ultrasonography*. St. Louis: C.V. Mosby; 1983:44–60.

84. Kremkau FW. Imaging artifacts. In: Kremkau FW, ed. *Diagnostic ultrasound—principles, instruments and exercises*. Philadelphia: WB Saunders; 1989:147–176.

CHAPTER 3

The Gallbladder

INTRODUCTION

Ultrasound is the imaging method of choice for examining the gallbladder. By far the most common indications for gallbladder ultrasound are possible cholelithiasis and cholecystitis. Many other abnormalities affect the gallbladder, but they are all uncommon in clinical practice compared with gallstones and cholecystitis. Some of these uncommon but important entities are also discussed in this chapter.

3.1 SCANNING TECHNIQUES

Scans of the gallbladder are performed after 4 to 6 hr fasting with a real-time sector probe of the highest frequency possible. This is usually a 5-MHz or 3.5-MHz probe. The gallbladder examination includes long-axis (sagittal or coronal) and transverse scans with the patient in the supine position. The left lateral decubitus position is often necessary for complete evaluation, and erect positions may also be helpful. Scans are obtained with the probe placed in the right subcostal area and in various right intercostal spaces. The following is a technique that

reliably locates the gallbladder: locate the main portal vein and common bile duct in transverse scans of the porta hepatis; the gallbladder neck lies immediately to the right of the main portal vein and common bile duct (Fig. 3.1).

In a normal study, the minimum hard copy images required are a long-axis scan of the gallbladder neck, body, and fundus and transverse scans of the neck and body (Figs. 3.1 and 3.2).

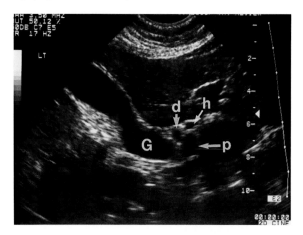

FIG. 3.1. Normal gallbladder and porta hepatis. Transverse scan of porta hepatis demonstrates gallbladder (*G*) lateral to portal vein (*p*) and common bile duct (*d*). *h*, proper hepatic artery.

Abbreviations: **CT,** computed tomography; **ESWL,** extracorporeal shock wave lithotripsy; **IDA scans,** iminodiacetic acid scans; **WES triad,** *w*all *e*cho *s*hadow triad.

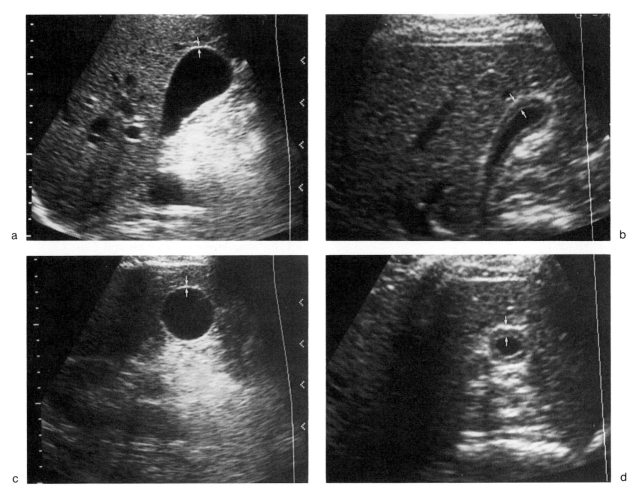

FIG. 3.2. Normal gallbladder, pre- and postprandial. **a:** Sagittal scan of gallbladder after 12 hr fasting. Volume = 38.6 cc. Note normal thin echogenic wall (*arrows*). **b:** Sagittal scan of same gallbladder 45 min after a meal. Volume = 0.8 cc. Ejection fraction 98%. Note normal thickening of gallbladder wall (*arrows*) when gallbladder is contracted. Total thickness of anterior gallbladder wall was 3.5 mm. Contracted wall has a thick middle hypoechoic band, bounded by an inner and outer thin hyperechoic line. **c:** Transverse scan of distal gallbladder body in same person after 12 hr fasting. *Arrows,* anterior gallbladder wall. **d:** Transverse scan in same position 45 min after a meal. *Arrows,* anterior gallbladder wall. (Scans are courtesy of Dr. Steve Valentine, Radiology Resident, Kingston General Hospital, Queen's University, Kingston, Ontario, Canada.)

3.2 NORMAL ANATOMY AND PHYSIOLOGY

The gallbladder is an elongated sac whose length is approximately two times the maximum transverse diameter in the adult. The narrowest portion is the neck and the widest portion is the mid to distal body (Fig. 3.2). The gallbladder is attached to the posterior caudal surface of the liver, and it separates the liver into left and right hepatic lobes. The neck of the gallbladder bears a constant relation to the portal triad: it lies along the right lateral aspect of the common bile duct and main portal vein and thus is well visualized in transverse scans of the porta hepatis (Fig. 3.1).

The distal cystic duct can be visualized by ultrasound in about 50% of normal adults and more frequently in patients with dilated bile ducts and in those with pre-

vious cholecystectomy (1). The cystic duct is 3 to 4 cm long, but ultrasound usually visualizes the distal 1 to 2 cm near its insertion into the common bile duct (Fig. 3.3). When the cystic duct is observed at ultrasound, 95% insert along the posterior aspect of the common bile duct. With a normal common bile duct and gallbladder, the cystic duct measures 1 to 3 mm in internal diameter, whereas postcholecystectomy, the cystic duct remnant may be significantly larger (1).

The gallbladder wall contains smooth muscle that contracts after a fatty meal. Fat in the duodenum and jejunum releases cholecystokinin from intestinal mucosal cells into the bloodstream. This contracts the gallbladder. In normal adults, a fatty meal containing 25 g of fat causes a reduction of gallbladder volume from about 28 ml (mean) to 11 ml (mean), which represents an ejection

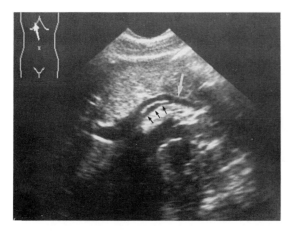

FIG. 3.3. Normal cystic duct. Oblique scan in right upper quadrant demonstrates distal cystic duct (*small arrows*) as it inserts into common bile duct (*large arrow*).

fraction of 62% (Fig. 3.2) (2,3). Maximum emptying is observed between 45 and 60 min after the fatty meal. A fatty meal or intravenous injection of cholecystokinin is occasionally useful in patients with enlarged gallbladders without other evidence of acute cholecystitis or obstruction. If there is normal fractional emptying of the gallbladder in 45 to 60 min, this is strongly suggestive of a normal gallbladder. It is very important to note, however, that in fasting hospitalized patients, lack of contraction of the gallbladder after injection of cholecystokinin may not signify pathology. Post laparotomy, only 25% of patients will have a normal ejection fraction (4).

**Gallbladder Size and Wall Thickness
(Summary in Table 3.1)**

One may assess gallbladder size by measuring the transverse diameter, length, or volume. Although ranges of normal have been described in adults and children, there is considerable variation in gallbladder size and shape, and this makes gallbladder size somewhat limited for practical purposes. The most commonly used parameter is the cross-sectional diameter taken through the wid-

TABLE 3.1. *Normal fasting gallbladder measurements*[a]

Measurement	Adult (range)		Newborn (mean)	
Length (cm)	4–11	(7,8)	3	(5)
Width (cm)	1.5–4	(5,6)	1	(5)
Volume (cc)	11–51	(2,3)	1.6	(3,5)
	(mean = 28)			
Fractional emptying after fatty meal (%)	62–67	(2,3)	—	
Wall thickness (mm)	1–3	(5,9)	—	

[a] Volume of gallbladder = $\pi/6$ ($L \times W \times H$); L is length, W is width, and H is height or anteroposterior diameter (3).

est part of the gallbladder (Fig. 3.2). Some use 4 cm as the upper limit of normal (5) and others use 5 cm (6). In our practice for adults, a diameter of 4 to 5 cm is taken to be borderline enlarged, and the significance must be correlated with other sonographic and clinical findings. If the diameter is greater than 5 cm, the gallbladder *is* enlarged, and there is a high probability of significant pathology in the gallbladder, cystic duct, and/or common bile duct. In adults, the length is less than 11 cm in 97% of normals (7). In newborns, the length is approximately 3 cm and the width is one-third of the length (5).

The lower limit for gallbladder length in the adult is poorly defined but may be 4 to 5 cm (8). The lower limit for width may be 1.5 to 2.0 cm. Twenty (20) cc is the approximate lower limit of normal fasting gallbladder volume in the adult. Gallbladder volume is calculated using the following formula:

$$\left[\text{Volume} = \frac{\pi}{6} (L \times W \times H) \right]$$

where L is the length, W is the width, and H is the height. Volume determination is useful for determining post–fatty meal ejection fractions (3).

The anterior gallbladder wall is measured in long-axis or transverse scans (Fig. 3.2). Three millimeter is the upper limit of normal in the fasting state (5,9). In a postprandial gallbladder, the gallbladder wall will appear thicker but should still measure 3 mm or less in thickness.

Normal Variants

Early in embryological development, the gallbladder is a hollow organ, but epithelial cell proliferation causes it to become temporarily solid. The lumen then develops by recanalization of the epithelial tissue. Failure of this process leads to a tiny atretic gallbladder that cannot be visualized with imaging techniques (10). Other developmental abnormalities include duplication, partial subdivision, and diverticula of the gallbladder.

Double gallbladder (duplication) has been described many times in the surgical literature (11), but few cases have been described in the ultrasound literature (12). Although the diagnosis of double gallbladder depends on the demonstration of two distinct cystic ducts, ultrasound can strongly suggest the diagnosis even though the cystic ducts may not be visualized (Fig. 3.4).

A bicameral gallbladder has a partition that divides the lumen into fundal and proximal compartments that are approximately equal in size. The partition may be complete or almost complete, and it may represent a congenital fold, a kink in the gallbladder, or a stricture caused by adenomyomatosis (Fig. 3.5) (13). Some literature suggests that the incidence of bicameral gallbladder may be as high as 5% (14). When the partition is almost

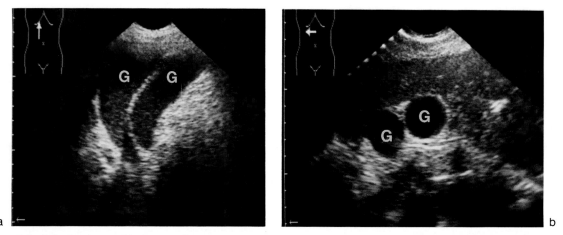

FIG. 3.4. Double gallbladder. **a:** Sagittal scan demonstrates two gallbladders (*G*) separated by a common wall. Echogenic material in gallbladders is sludge secondary to biliary stasis. The patient had a carcinoma of pancreatic head obstructing distal common bile duct. **b:** Transverse scan demonstrates two gallbladders (*G*) in their short axis.

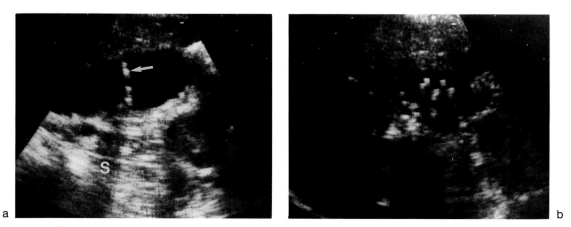

FIG. 3.5. Bicameral gallbladder caused by adenomyomatosis. **a:** Long-axis scan demonstrates a septum (*arrow*) in body of the gallbladder. *s,* acoustic shadowing posterior to septum. **b:** Transverse scan through septum demonstrates multiple hyperechoic foci in septum associated with comet-tail artifacts behind them. These are reverberation echoes from cholesterol crystals in septum.

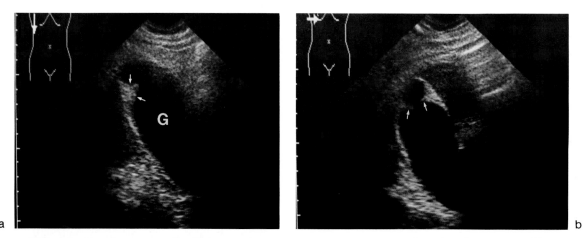

FIG. 3.6. Phrygian cap. **a:** Sagittal scan demonstrates an anteverted gallbladder (*G*) with a wedge-shaped structure (*arrows*) impinging into fundus. **b:** Transverse scan demonstrates an incomplete septum (*arrows*) in gallbladder fundus.

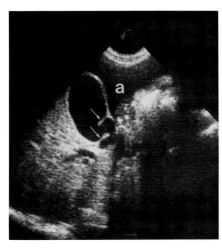

FIG. 3.7. Folds in neck of gallbladder. Transverse scan demonstrates normal thin folds (*arrows*) in neck of gallbladder. Note ascites (*a*) medial to gallbladder.

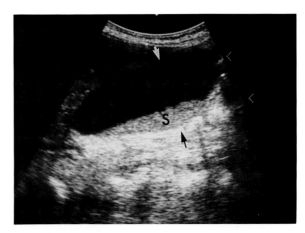

FIG. 3.9. Enlarged gallbladder: fasting. Sagittal scan demonstrates an enlarged gallbladder. Anteroposterior diameter (*arrows*) measured 4.8 cm. Note sludge (*s*) in gallbladder. This patient had been fasting for 30 hr. After a meal, the gallbladder contracted normally.

complete, biliary stasis, stone formation, and cholecystitis are more common.

When there is a sharp kink near the distal end of the gallbladder, a partial thick septum is evident in the ultrasound scan (Fig. 3.6). This is called a Phrygian cap, and it is not clinically significant. This name arose because of the similarity to the "cap of liberty" bestowed on freed slaves in ancient Phrygia (15). More commonly one sees a fold in the neck of the gallbladder, and this also is insignificant clinically (Fig. 3.7).

A multiseptate gallbladder is very rare, and it manifests as multiple fine septa that bridge the gallbladder lumen. The septa are composed of two epithelial layers and a muscle layer. Some reported cases were asymptomatic and others had biliary colic (16).

The position of the gallbladder may be abnormal because of a long gallbladder mesentery. The gallbladder may be located in the lower abdomen, the left side of the abdomen, and between the liver and the diaphragm (Fig. 3.8) (17,18), and it may herniate into the foramen of

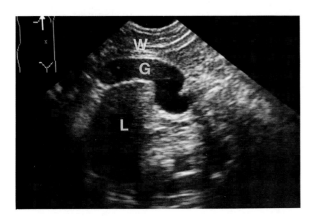

FIG. 3.8. Antedisplaced gallbladder. Sagittal scan of right upper quadrant demonstrates gallbladder (G) interposed between liver (L) and anterior abdominal wall (w).

Winslow (19). Other ectopic locations include intrahepatic, retroperitoneal, within the falciform ligament, and in the anterior abdominal wall (20).

3.3 PATHOLOGY

Abnormal Size

Gallbladder size is evaluated after 4 or more hr of fasting. An abnormally small gallbladder can result from chronic cholecystitis with concomitant fibrosis, which prevents normal gallbladder distension. Other causes of a small gallbladder in a fasting patient include acute hepatic dysfunction (e.g., secondary to hepatitis), bile duct obstruction proximal to the cystic duct, and a microgallbladder associated with cystic fibrosis (21,22).

An enlarged gallbladder can be caused by prolonged fasting (Fig. 3.9), obstruction of the common bile duct distal to the cystic duct insertion (Fig. 3.10), obstruction of the cystic duct, or acute cholecystitis. A rare cause of enlargement is hydrops of the gallbladder (see below). Occasionally, the gallbladder may be quite large yet normal, in which case a fatty meal demonstrates significant contraction.

Gallstones

Prevalence of Gallstones

In North American adults, the prevalence of gallstones is approximately 14% (23). In asymptomatic adults, the prevalence is 11%, and in those with right upper quadrant pain syndromes it is 33% (23). In Crohn's disease the prevalence of gallstones is 20% to 30% (24) because the reabsorption of bile salts in the diseased terminal ileum is disrupted. The prevalence of

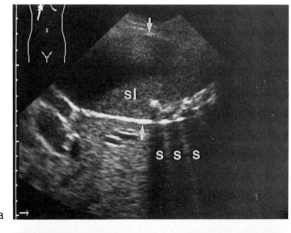

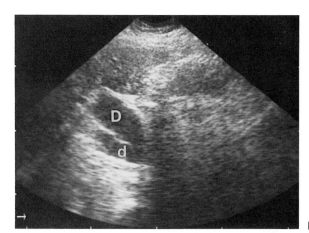

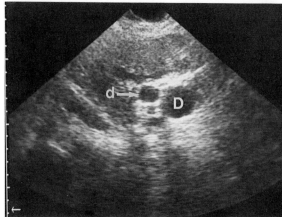

FIG. 3.10. Courvoisier gallbladder. Pancreatic carcinoma. **a:** Sagittal scan demonstrates enlarged gallbladder whose anteroposterior diameter is 5.7 cm. Note multiple small calculi and sludge (*sl*) within gallbladder lumen. *s*, shadows behind calculi. **b:** Enlarged cystic duct. Oblique scan in right upper quadrant demonstrates a dilated common hepatic duct (*D*) and a dilated cystic duct (*d*) inserting into posterior aspect of common hepatic duct. **c:** Enlarged cystic duct. Transverse scan of same patient as (b) demonstrates enlarged common hepatic duct (*D*) and enlarged cystic duct (*d*) lateral to bile duct.

gallstones increases with age, and gallstones are more common in women (F:M = 2:1). It is noteworthy that most people with gallstones are asymptomatic.

Ultrasound Characteristics of Gallbladder Calculi

The ultrasonic diagnosis of cholelithiasis rests on two main signs: echogenic focus in the gallbladder lumen and an acoustic shadow posterior to the echogenic focus (Fig. 3.11). The mobility of an intraluminal focus is a sign that is useful in equivocal cases (i.e., where a definite acoustic shadow is not demonstrated). It may be difficult to elicit a shadow behind small calculi (e.g., ≤5 mm), depending on the ultrasound beam characteristics. To optimize the study, one attempts to use the highest frequency possible and to position the calculus in the narrowest part of the beam (i.e., at the focal spot of the beam). The production of the shadow depends on the size of the calculus, the orientation of the calculus, the surface characteristics of the calculus (smooth vs. rough), and the beam geometry.

In 1985, Cover et al. (25) demonstrated that small crystalline cholesterol calculi produced short comet-tail or reverberatory echoes posterior to them (Fig. 3.12) but no distal shadowing. These crystalline calculi were ap-

proximately 1 to 2 mm thick and they were flat crystals. The comet-tail artifacts were most evident when the beam struck the flat crystal surface at right angles. This effect is created from multiple internal reflections between parallel surfaces of the crystals. In contrast, noncholesterol stones reflect about one quarter of the sound back to the probe. The clear posterior shadow is produced by absorption of sound by these calculi.

Calculi are usually denser than bile and thus sink to the dependent portion of the gallbladder (Fig. 3.11). However, in some cases the calculus may float within the fluid (Fig. 3.13). This can occur when the bile contains contrast material from an oral cholecystogram or when echogenic sludge is present. Stones impacted in the cystic duct or gallbladder neck are important to identify but may be easily overlooked (Fig. 3.14) (1). Impacted calculi usually cause abdominal pain and acute cholecystitis. To routinely detect these calculi, one must trace the gallbladder neck back to the portal vein by scanning the gallbladder in its short and long axes.

When the patient has not fasted before the exam, the gallbladder will be less distended and perhaps less suitable for ultrasound examination. However, Birnholz (23) suggested that most (98%) gallbladders can be satisfactorily scanned without any preparation (Figs. 3.2 and

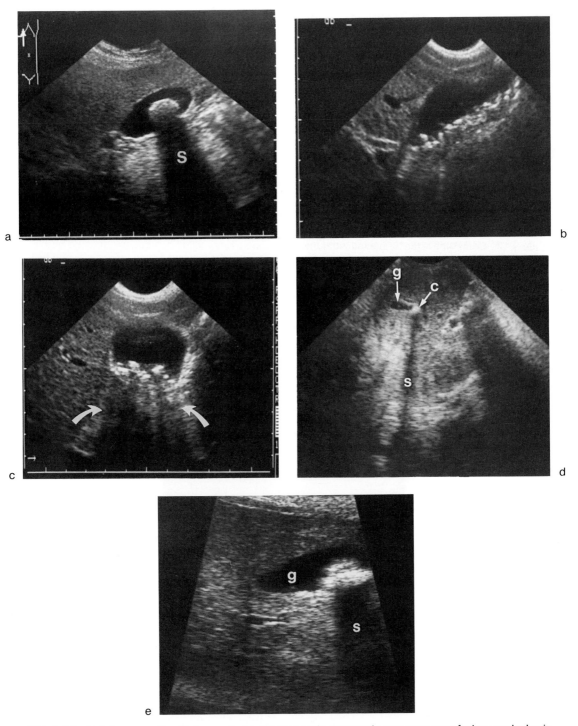

FIG. 3.11. Gallstones. **a:** Sagittal scan demonstrates pathognomonic appearances of a large calculus in gallbladder associated with a posterior acoustic shadow (S). **b,c:** Sagittal and transverse scans of another gallbladder containing multiple small calculi. In sagittal scan it is difficult to perceive posterior acoustic shadows behind intraluminal calculi. However, in transverse scan, posterior shadows (*arrow*) can be perceived. **d:** Transverse scan of a *fetal abdomen* at 38 weeks gestation demonstrates a calculus (c) in neck of gallbladder (g). *s,* acoustic shadow. **e:** Sagittal scan 1 day after birth [same patient as (d)] demonstrates a hyperechoic calculus in gallbladder (g) with a posterior acoustic shadow (s).

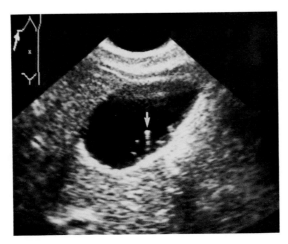

FIG. 3.12. Comet-tail artifacts behind intraluminal calculus. Tiny mobile hyperechoic foci are visible in gallbladder lumen. One calculus has a comet-tail artifact behind it (*arrow*). These were small crystalline cholesterol calculi.

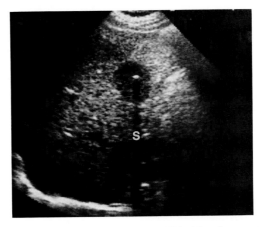

FIG. 3.13. Floating gallstone. Transverse scan through gallbladder demonstrates a small calculus suspended in mid portion of gallbladder lumen. Echogenic bile is denser than normal bile and about the same density as this small calculus. Thus calculus "floats." *s*, acoustic shadow.

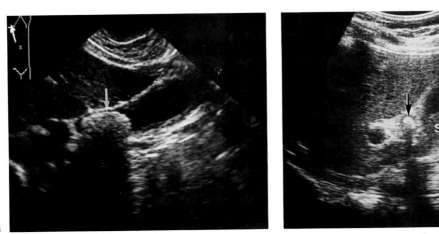

a   b

FIG. 3.14. Impacted gallstones. **a:** A large calculus (*arrow*) is impacted in gallbladder neck. Note thickening of gallbladder wall, which measured 5 mm in thickness. With this size of calculus and location, diagnosis was not difficult. **b:** A smaller calculus (*arrow*) is impacted in gallbladder neck causing obstruction of gallbladder. Sludge (*s*) is secondary to resulting stasis of fluid in the gallbladder. This diagnosis is more difficult because obstructing calculus appears to lie outside of lumen of gallbladder.

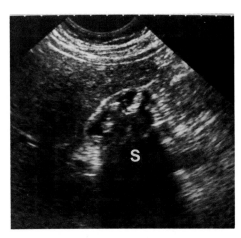

FIG. 3.15. Cholelithiasis. Partly contracted gallbladder. Diagnosis of cholelithiasis may be more difficult when very little fluid is in the gallbladder. However, with this amount of fluid in the gallbladder, diagnosis of cholelithiasis is usually still straightforward. *s,* acoustic shadow behind calculi.

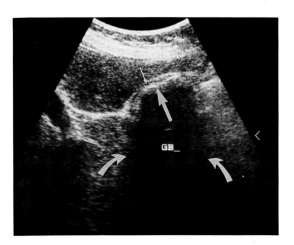

FIG. 3.16. WES triad (W, wall; E, echo; S, shadow). Gallbladder is totally contracted, and sagittal scan demonstrates an echogenic line (*large arrow*) representing calculi in gallbladder. Thin hypoechoic band (*small arrows*) anterior to calculi represents anterior wall of gallbladder. Broad shadow (*curved arrows*) posterior to calculi is acoustic shadow.

3.15). In most cases of a contracted gallbladder containing calculi, one may diagnose calculi with confidence by using the WES triad (26), although other entities may mimic the WES triad (see *Pitfalls, Artifacts, and Practical Tips*). The WES triad stands for the *w*all, the *e*cho (the calculus), and the *s*hadow (the acoustic shadow posterior to the calculus) (Fig. 3.16).

Accuracy of Ultrasound

Despite some limitations of ultrasound in evaluating gallbladder stones, ultrasound is the most accurate technique for this purpose (the diagnostic accuracy is about 96%) (27). In the study by Cooperberg and Burhenne (27), the sensitivity (i.e., the frequency the test detects the presence of calculi) was 98% and the specificity (i.e., the frequency the test is normal in truly normal gallbladders) was between 93.5% and 97.7%. In practice one wishes to minimize false-positive exams to minimize unnecessary surgery.

A more recent study examined ultrasound and oral cholecystography in assessing the gallbladder in morbidly obese patients (28). This study was particularly interesting because all patients had surgery, and thus a negative study could be tested against surgical results. The sensitivity of ultrasound in detecting gallstones was 75%, and the sensitivity of oral cholecystography was 43%. The specificity of ultrasound and oral cholecystography was 100%. The calculi missed by ultrasound were 1 to 2 mm in diameter.

Lithotripsy of Gallstones

Extracorporeal shock wave lithotripsy has been used recently to fragment stones inside the gallbladder. Shock

waves are focused on the calculi and cause the calculi to fragment into small pieces (<4-mm diameter), which pass spontaneously through the cystic duct and common bile duct. Some treatment protocols require that the number of stones be three or less and that the stone diameters be 0.5 to 3.0 cm (29). It is possible for ultrasound to accurately count the number of stones and measure their maximum diameters when six or fewer are present (30).

After ESWL, ultrasound can detect fragments larger than 1.5 mm diameter, and it is more accurate than fluoroscopy or spot radiography in assessing the number and diameter of post-ESWL fragments (31). Khouri et al. (32) have shown that fragments will clump together after ESWL and mimic a larger stone. However, by rolling the patient over, one can observe the fragments dispersing through the gallbladder fluid and thus distinguish between multiple small fragments and large calculi.

In some post-ESWL patients, small echogenic foci may have a V-shaped artifact or comet-tail artifact posterior to them (Fig. 3.12). This is caused by reverberation of the sound beam within small cholesterol crystal fragments ranging in maximum diameter from 0.5 to 1.5 mm (33). This finding is identical to the V-shaped artifact from small crystalline calculi inside Rokitansky-Aschoff sinuses in adenomyomatosis and chronic cholecystitis (34). The same short comet-tail reverberations were observed by Cover et al. (23) posterior to small crystalline cholesterol calculi in the gallbladder lumen.

Cholecystitis

Chronic Cholecystitis

Chronic cholecystitis is characterized clinically by long-standing recurrent vague abdominal discomfort and other symptoms such as nausea, belching, and fatty food intolerance. Pathologically it is characterized by the presence of gallstones (90% of cases), low-grade inflammatory changes in the gallbladder wall, a variable amount of fibrotic changes, and Rokitansky-Aschoff sinuses (90% of cases) (35). The sinuses arise when inflammation causes focal weakness in the wall with subsequent herniation of the epithelium. The gallbladder wall may be mildly to moderately thickened, and the gallbladder size can range from totally contracted to enlarged. On ultrasound the main finding is the presence of calculi. Focal or diffuse thickening of the gallbladder wall may be identified.

Acute Calculous Cholecystitis

Acute cholecystitis is characterized clinically by a high white cell count (leukocytosis), fever, and general toxicity (the patient is sick!). Pathologically, acute cholecystitis is characterized by one or more of the following:

1. transmural inflammation (neutrophils)
2. foci of hemorrhagic necrosis in the wall
3. significant neutrophilic infiltration in the muscle layer or mucosa (usually multifocal)

The etiology of most cases of acute cholecystitis is obstruction of the cystic duct or neck of the gallbladder by a calculus (about 90% of cases). About 10% of cases are acute acalculous cholecystitis (36). When a calculus obstructs the gallbladder, acute right upper quadrant pain (biliary colic) results. If the obstruction persists, acute inflammatory changes will develop in the gallbladder wall, and the above clinical signs and pathological changes will ensue. If acute cholecystitis is present, surgery is indicated within 24 to 48 hr to prevent complications and possible death.

In those patients with clinically suspected acute cholecystitis, ultrasound is a very useful test (high positive predictive value and high negative predictive value). The primary ultrasound finding in acute cholecystitis is gallstones. When a calculus is impacted in the gallbladder neck or cystic duct, the calculus is immobile and not surrounded by fluid (Fig. 3.14) and thus more difficult to detect. However, gallstones in general do not provide a specific diagnosis for acute cholecystitis: gallstones are common in asymptomatic people, and the clinical symptoms may be due to something else (e.g., liver disease or bowel disease). Ralls et al. (37) demonstrated that the use of two secondary ultrasound signs makes the ultrasound exam the method of choice in assessing for acute cholecystitis:

1. sonographic Murphy sign
2. thickened gallbladder wall (>3 mm) (Fig. 3.17)

The different combinations of ultrasound findings give the following positive predictive values:

1. stones + positive sonographic Murphy sign—92.2%
2. stones + thickened gallbladder wall—95.0%

The following negative predictive values were derived:

1. no stones, negative sonographic Murphy sign—95.0%
2. no stones, normal gallbladder wall—96.7%.

Note that a positive sonographic Murphy sign is present *only* when tenderness is maximum at the site of the sonographically localized gallbladder. Patients can have a positive clinical Murphy sign but a negative sonographic Murphy sign (e.g., tenderness at a location that does not correspond to the sonographically localized gallbladder). In practice, a positive sonographic Murphy sign can be misleading. Similar tenderness may be caused by a tender liver, a tender bowel loop adjacent to the gallbladder,

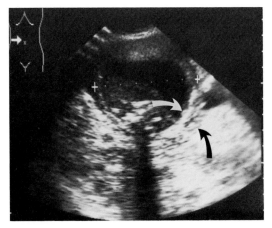
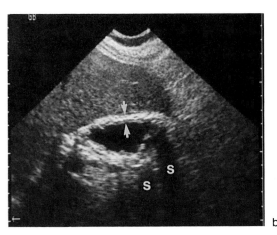

a   b

FIG. 3.17. Acute calculous cholecystitis. **a:** Transverse scan demonstrates an enlarged gallbladder (+) containing multiple small hyperechoic calculi within layering sludge. Gallbladder wall is grossly thickened (*curved arrows*). **b:** Another patient with acute calculous cholecystitis with a partially contracted gallbladder. Gallbladder wall is thickened (*arrows*), and small calculi are present in fundus of gallbladder associated with posterior acoustic shadowing (*s*).

or other right upper quadrant inflammatory foci. Therefore, the sonographic Murphy sign must be evaluated with great caution.

Nuclear medicine cholescintigraphy is also accurate in assessing for acute cholecystitis. Depending on local expertise in nuclear medicine and ultrasound, cholescintigraphy or ultrasound could be used as the initial test in assessing for acute cholecystitis. In our practice we use ultrasound as the initial modality and reserve nuclear medicine for the following situations:

1. normal ultrasound but very strong clinical suspicion of acute cholecystitis
2. only one of three ultrasound findings present

Gallbladder wall thickening can be caused by other intrinsic gallbladder abnormalities (e.g., chronic cholecystitis, adenomyomatosis, and tumor) and extrinsic causes (see below). Cohan et al. (38) contended that a thickened wall containing striated lucencies is probably acute cholecystitis (Fig. 3.18). A uniformly hypoechoic wall probably is due to extrinsic causes (38). More recently, Teefey et al. (39) found that striated lucencies within a thickened wall is a nonspecific finding that may be seen in acute cholecystitis or other noninflammatory conditions. Therefore, the internal characteristics of gallbladder wall thickening do not appear very useful in distinguishing between acute cholecystitis and other noninflammatory conditions.

Acute Acalculous Cholecystitis

Acute acalculous cholecystitis accounts for about 10% of cases of acute cholecystitis (36) but 47% of postoperative cholecystitis (40). The cause is unknown, but it usually occurs in very ill patients (e.g., after major trauma, burns, surgery, sepsis, shock, hyperalimentation, and prolonged fasting). Mortality is very high (incidence 33–75%). Gallbladder necrosis, perforation, and gangrene occur more frequently (about 50% of cases) than with acute calculous cholecystitis (41). It is more common in men than women (M:F = 3.5:1) (4).

This is a difficult entity to diagnose with ultrasound or isotope scans (IDA scans). These patients often have multiorgan abnormalities, and signs and symptoms could be due to many causes. Ultrasound diagnosis is difficult because two of the major signs of acute calculous cholecystitis are missing: (a) no calculi present; and (b) because the patient is often unconscious or taking pain medication, the sonographic Murphy sign often cannot be used. Gallbladder wall thickening (>3 mm) and gallbladder enlargement (>4-cm transverse diameter) are the remaining ultrasound signs that suggest acute acalculous cholecystitis (Fig. 3.18). However, gallbladder wall thickening may be related to many extrinsic causes in someone with multiple organ abnormalities, and gallbladder enlargement can be seen in fasting patients without cholecystitis (see below). Other abnormalities that favor acute cholecystitis include:

1. a loculated pericholecystic fluid collection
2. intraluminal membranes (sloughed mucosa)
3. gas in gallbladder wall (emphysematous cholecystitis) (see next section) Intraluminal sludge is not a useful sign of acute acalculous cholecystitis because many fasting patients have echogenic bile in the gallbladder in the absence of acute cholecystitis (see below).

Shuman et al. (42) demonstrated fairly low sensitivities for sonography (67%) and cholescintigraphy (68%) in assessing 33 patients with proven acalculous cholecystitis. Raduns et al. (4) demonstrated that administration of cholecystokinin in the postoperative patient is not useful in the assessment for cholecystitis because many patients without cholecystitis have very little or no gallbladder contraction in the postoperative period.

Complications of Acute Cholecystitis

The major complications of acute cholecystitis include gangrene (43,44), emphysematous cholecystitis (45,46), gallbladder perforation (47), hemorrhagic cholecystitis (48), and pericholecystic abscess.

Gangrenous cholecystitis is characterized by wall necrosis, microabscess formation, and hemorrhage. Other features include pus inside the lumen (empyema), fibrinous strands in the lumen, and mucosal ulcers (43,44,49). The mortality rate is about 20% compared with 1% for acute nongangrenous cholecystitis (50). Perforation, which occurs in 10% of cases, is usually a sequela of acute gangrenous cholecystitis. On ultrasound,

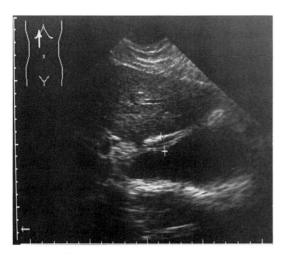

FIG. 3.18. Acute acalculous cholecystitis. Sagittal scan demonstrates focal thickening in anterior wall of gallbladder (+). Note linear echoes within thickened wall. This patient had acute acalculous cholecystitis associated with focal gangrene in gallbladder wall.

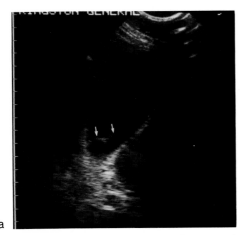
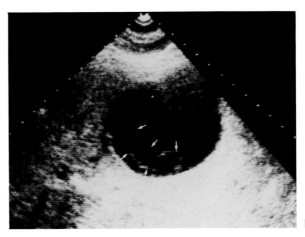

a

b

FIG. 3.19. Acute cholecystitis associated with intraluminal membranes. **a:** Scan demonstrates intraluminal thin membranes (*arrows*). At surgery mucosal lining was separated from walls of gallbladder. Patient had acute gangrenous cholecystitis. **b:** Transverse scan of another patient demonstrates complete separation of mucosal lining (*arrows*) from the rest of gallbladder wall.

58% of cases have findings suggestive of gangrenous cholecystitis: intraluminal membranes and coarse echoes (strands of fibrinous exudate or necrotic mucosa) (Fig. 3.19) and marked focal irregularities of the gallbladder wall (e.g., ulcers, intramural hemorrhage, or abscess formation) (Fig. 3.17). In uncomplicated acute cholecystitis, the sonographic Murphy sign is positive in 95% of cases, whereas in gangrenous cholecystitis, it is positive in only 33% (44).

Emphysematous cholecystitis is a rare form of acute cholecystitis caused by gas-forming organisms leading to collections of gas in the lumen and wall of the gallbladder. This can lead rapidly to gangrene, perforation, and pericholecystic abscess, and therefore prompt diagnosis is essential. Diabetics are susceptible to emphysematous cholecystitis, and the symptoms may be quite mild. Ultrasound demonstrates gas completely or partially filling the gallbladder lumen or bubbles of gas in the wall. The

gas manifests as hyperechoic foci that may have a posterior shadow or a posterior ring-down artifact. Plain radiographs or CT should be performed for further confirmation (Fig. 3.20).

Hemorrhagic cholecystitis is a severe form of acute cholecystitis characterized pathologically by significant intramural hemorrhage. Hemorrhagic cholecystitis probably represents a stage in the development toward gangrenous cholecystitis (48). In 19 patients with hemorrhagic cholecystitis, gangrene was found in 47%. In 74%, ultrasound displayed sonographic features not commonly seen with acute cholecystitis: focal wall irregularity (7/19), intraluminal membrane (3/19), and coarse nonshadowing nonlayering intraluminal echoes. It is not possible by ultrasound to distinguish between hemorrhagic cholecystitis without gangrene and hemorrhagic cholecystitis with gangrene.

Gallbladder perforation is a sequela of gangrenous

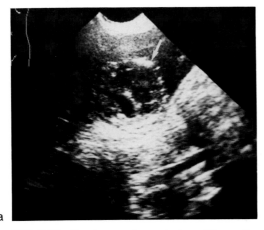
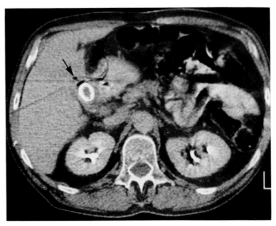

a

b

FIG. 3.20. Emphysematous cholecystitis. **a:** Transverse scan demonstrates multiple hyperechoic foci (*arrow*) in wall of gallbladder. **b:** CT scan at a different level in gallbladder demonstrates bubbles of gas (*arrow*) in anterior wall of gallbladder.

cholecystitis and the associated mortality is 19% to 24% (51). Perforation usually occurs in the fundus, and most commonly a localized pericholecystic abscess forms (occasionally perforation causes acute bile peritonitis). Perforation with abscess formation occurs more frequently in acute acalculous cholecystitis than acute calculous cholecystitis. The ultrasound exam may demonstrate a well-defined fluid collection adjacent to or surrounding the gallbladder, usually containing internal echoes (Fig. 3.21) or a poorly defined hypoechoic mass that obscures the gallbladder margins.

Wall Abnormalities

Diffuse Thickening

Diffuse wall thickening may be simulated by a contracted gallbladder (Fig. 3.22). True wall thickening is most commonly caused by noninflammatory edema (extrinsic causes) and inflammation (intrinsic gallbladder disease). Uncommon causes include tumor infiltration, varices secondary to portal hypertension, and adenomyomatosis (often focal or segmental).

Noninflammatory edema is the most common pathology causing thickened gallbladder wall (63% of cases) (38), and many etiologies can lead to this: hypoproteinemia or hypoalbuminemia (liver disease, renal disease), hepatitis, and ascites. The pathophysiology in most cases of nonmalignant ascites involves liver disease such as cirrhosis with portal venous or lymphatic congestion with or without hypoalbuminemia. Kaftori et al. (52) demonstrated that patients with only hypoalbuminemia and chronic renal failure do not develop a thickened gallbladder wall. Other causes include obstruction of lymph drainage by tumor replacement in portal lymph nodes

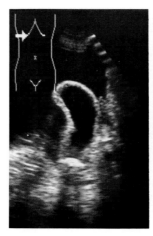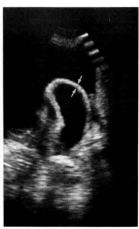

FIG. 3.22. Gallbladder wall thickness in presence of ascites. Gallbladder wall is mildly thickened (*arrows*). Note uniform hyperechoic nature of gallbladder wall. Gallbladder is surrounded by ascites, and gallbladder is partly contracted.

and increased venous pressure in the gallbladder veins caused by portal hypertension or congestive heart failure (Fig. 3.23).

Diffuse wall thickening can be seen in chronic cholecystitis, but most cases of chronic cholecystitis with cholelithiasis have normal-appearing walls on ultrasound. Many cases of acute cholecystitis are associated with thickening of the gallbladder wall, but this is not a constant finding. We have seen many patients with proven acute cholecystitis where gallbladder wall thickening could not be perceived. As noted previously, the internal characteristics of the thickened wall are not very useful in distinguishing between acute cholecystitis and noninflammatory conditions (39).

A study by Huang et al. (53) suggested that gallbladder wall thickness may help distinguish between malignant

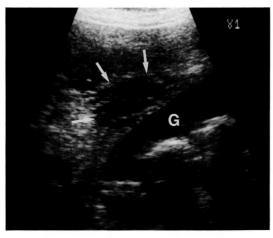

FIG. 3.21. Pericholecystic abscess. Sagittal scan of neck of gallbladder (G) demonstrates a focal pericholecystic fluid collection (*arrows*), which represents a focal pericholecystic abscess.

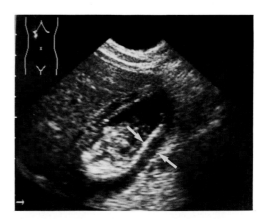

FIG. 3.23. Thickened gallbladder wall caused by noninflammatory edema. Sagittal scan of gallbladder demonstrates acute thickening (*arrows*) of gallbladder wall associated with chronic liver disease. There was no sign of acute cholecystitis. Echogenic material within lumen of gallbladder is sludge secondary to fasting.

and cirrhotic ascites. If the wall was nonthickened (≤3 mm) and single layered, the ascites was usually malignant. If the wall was thickened (>3 mm) and double layered, the ascites was usually cirrhotic.

Adenomyomatosis

Adenomyomatosis is thought to be a noninflammatory intrinsic disease of the gallbladder wall, characterized by hyperplasia and thickening of the mucosa and muscular layer and by intramural diverticula (Rokitansky-Aschoff sinuses) (54,55). The mucosa herniates through weak spots in the muscularis mucosa into the deeper layers of the gallbladder wall. The diverticula may communicate with the gallbladder lumen, but when they become occluded, they become isolated intramural cavities. The diverticula may contain clear bile, sludge, cellular debris, or small calculi. The etiology for this condition is not known. There is no propensity toward malignant transformation. Note that Rokitansky-Aschoff sinuses are also common in chronic cholecystitis (35).

The abnormality may be focal (usually in the gallbladder fundus), segmental (usually an annular thickening of the body of the gallbladder), or diffuse. The focal variety is the most common. The abnormality is seen in up to 25% of gallbladders removed at surgery, but the incidence of detection with oral cholecystography and ultrasound is much less (55). There is controversy as to whether adenomyomatosis alone gives clinical symptoms. In those cases with coexisting gallstones, most think that clinical symptoms arise because of the calculi and associated chronic cholecystitis and not the adenomyomatosis.

On ultrasound, the focal variety of adenomyomatosis will appear as a focal fundal mass protruding into the lumen (Fig. 3.24). In the segmental and diffuse forms,

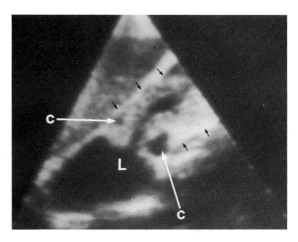

FIG. 3.25. Segmental adenomyomatosis. Sagittal scan demonstrates segmental thickening of gallbladder wall along anterior and posterior aspects (arrows). Note lack of wall thickening in proximal gallbladder and fluid within lumen of proximal gallbladder (L). Lumen between thickened anterior and posterior walls is very thin, and it communicates with lumen of proximal gallbladder. Note also cysts (c) within thickened wall. These are Rokitansky-Aschoff sinuses.

the wall is thickened (>3 mm), and there may or may not be fluid-filled diverticula or sinuses visible within the thickened wall (Fig. 3.25) (55–58). When the diverticula contain small calculi (cholesterol calculi), ultrasound demonstrates small hyperechoic intramural foci with V-shaped artifacts posterior to the foci (Fig. 3.26) (34). In milder forms of adenomyomatosis, only mild wall thickening is present, and this may not be detected with ultrasound (57).

Polyps (Cholesterolosis)

A polyp is a fixed solid mass arising from the gallbladder wall and protruding into the lumen. The most common etiology of a polyp is cholesterolosis (55), but other pathologies may present with single or multiple polyps: focal adenomyomatosis, adenoma, papilloma, carcinoid tumor, carcinoma, metastases, epithelial and mucous retention cysts, and inflammatory polyps.

Cholesterolosis is a noninflammatory condition of the gallbladder characterized by deposits of cholesterol esters, cholesterol precursors, and triglycerides within macrophages found in the epithelium and lamina propria of the gallbladder wall. About 10% of gallbladders removed at surgery have cholesterolosis, but cholesterolosis is diagnosed with imaging less commonly. The reason for this is that most cases have multiple small (<1 mm) mucosal nodules, whereas relatively few develop "macroscopic" polyps large enough to be detected with ultrasound (2–10-mm diameter). It is noteworthy that cholesterolosis has no relationship with systemic cholesterol or triglyceride abnormalities, vascular disease, diabetes, etc., but the exact etiology of cholesterolosis is not

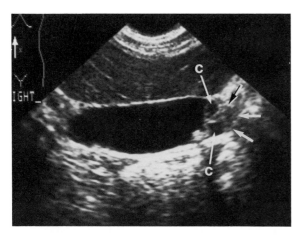

FIG. 3.24. Focal adenomyomatosis. Sagittal scan demonstrates a focal mass in fundus of gallbladder (arrows). Note two cystic components (c) within this mass (Rokitansky-Aschoff sinuses).

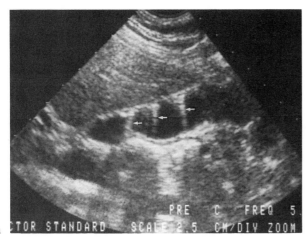 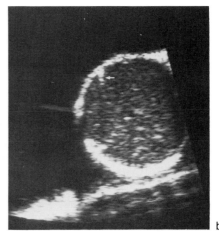

FIG. 3.26. Cholesterol crystals in gallbladder wall (in Rokitansky-Aschoff sinuses). **a:** Sagittal scan demonstrates three hyperechoic foci in anterior gallbladder wall with posterior comet-tail artifacts (*arrows*). Artifact arises from small cholesterol crystals within anterior wall of gallbladder caused by reverberation within crystals. **b:** Transverse scan of gallbladder *in vitro*. A small comet-tail artifact (*arrow*) is present posterior to a small intramural cholesterol crystal.

known. Cholesterolosis is only symptomatic if a large polyp detaches and causes obstructive symptoms (e.g., biliary colic) or if calculi coexist with the condition (10–15% of cases) (55). A detached polyp may be a nidus for the formation of a calculus. On ultrasound (and oral cholecystography), most cases are not detectable. However, larger polyps (e.g., ≥2 mm) are usually detected with ultrasound. They are often uniformly hyperechoic and small (<5-mm diameter) (Fig. 3.27).

Carcinoma

Gallbladder carcinoma accounts for 1% to 4.4% of all malignancies in different parts of the world: it is more common in India than North America (59). It is the fifth most common malignancy of the gastrointestinal tract (after colon, pancreas, stomach, and esophagus) (60).

Seventy percent to 80% of gallbladder carcinomas coexist with gallstones and chronic cholecystitis; the sex ratio is F:M = 3:1; and the incidence is highest in older people (sixth and seventh decades of life). About 25% of porcelain gallbladders (i.e., gallbladders with calcification in the walls) have carcinoma present. Most cases of gallbladder carcinoma are adenocarcinoma.

In the early stages of carcinoma, the patient is asymptomatic. As the tumor invades neighboring structures, the patients develop symptoms that mimic benign gallbladder disease (e.g., pain, anorexia). As the disease spreads, other signs and symptoms develop: weight loss, jaundice, hepatomegaly, palpable mass. Much less than 50% of patients with gallbladder carcinoma (as low as 4%) (59,61) are suspected clinically of having carcinoma. Therefore, most patients are diagnosed primarily by an ultrasound scan performed for nonspecific symptoms. Unfortunately, most gallbladder carcinomas (50–70%)

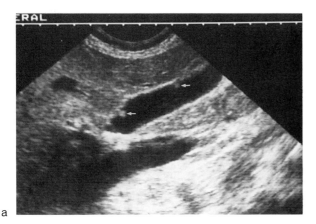 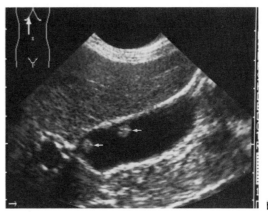

FIG. 3.27. Cholesterolosis (polyps). **a:** Sagittal scan demonstrates two small hyperechoic foci arising from anterior gallbladder wall. These are small cholesterol polyps (*arrows*). **b:** Sagittal scan of another gallbladder demonstrates two medium-sized hyperechoic polyps (*arrows*). These are cholesterol polyps.

(60) have invaded neighboring structures or metastasized to other sites at the time of initial scanning.

The tumor arises from the mucosa (epithelium and lamina propria) and invades the single muscle layer (analogous to muscularis mucosa of bowel), the perimuscular connective tissue, and the serosa (note that the serosa is absent where gallbladder interfaces with liver). Tumor extension into neighboring liver is very common (Fig. 3.28). The submucosa and double-layered muscularis propria (which are present in gut) are lacking in the gallbladder (60). Invasion through the single muscle layer then allows invasion of the lymphatics and blood vessels in the perimuscular connective tissue. Lymph node metastases occur along the cystic duct, common bile duct, and peripancreatic area. Blood-borne metastases are usually to liver and lung.

The following are the most common ultrasound manifestations at initial scan:

1. solid tumor totally replacing the gallbladder (40–65%) (59,60)
2. focal polypoid mass protruding into gallbladder lumen (15–30%) (59,60). A polyp greater than 1-cm diameter is suspicious for carcinoma (62)
3. focal or diffuse wall thickening (infiltrative pattern) (5–30%) (59,60) (Fig. 3.29)

In the study by Kuo et al. (62), the authors reviewed 29 cases of gallbladder carcinoma missed by ultrasound (i.e., false negatives) and 22 cases mistakenly diagnosed as carcinoma (i.e., false positives). In the false-negative cases, 62% were diagnosed as cholelithiasis only, 21% as cholecystitis, 7% as bile sludge, 7% as benign polyps, and 3% as liver tumor. In the false-positive cases, 18% were benign polyps, 23% were sludge, 36% were cholecystitis, and 23% were empyema.

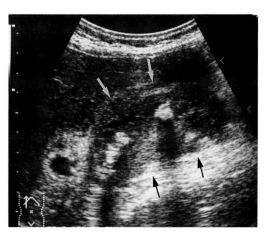

FIG. 3.29. Gallbladder carcinoma. Anterior wall (*white arrows*) and posterior wall (*black arrows*) of gallbladder are very thick because of gallbladder carcinoma. Note three hyperechoic calculi within small residual lumen of gallbladder. Anterior margin of gallbladder is poorly defined. Tumor had invaded into liver parenchyma.

In a series of 80 patients with gallbladder carcinoma (36), the following were other abnormalities observed at ultrasound: calculi 76%, direct invasion of liver 73%, dilated intrahepatic bile ducts 48%, distant liver metastases 70%, portal lymphadenopathy 28%, peripancreatic lymphadenopathy 23%, ascites 6%.

Metastases to Gallbladder

Metastatic deposits may develop in the gallbladder wall (via blood-borne cells) from the pancreas, liver, colon, ovary, kidney, and skin (melanoma). With gallbladder metastases, calculi are usually absent (whereas in primary gallbladder carcinoma, calculi are often present), and other sites are commonly involved (e.g., liver, lungs, bone). The ultrasound patterns include focal wall thickening, an intraluminal mass, and loss of definition of the gallbladder wall (Fig. 3.30) (63,64).

Hyperechoic Mural Foci

Hyperechoic mural foci may arise from calcification (porcelain gallbladder), small intramural calculi (calculi within Rokitansky-Aschoff sinuses), calculi adherent to the mucosa (Fig. 3.31), calcified cholesterol polyps, and gas within the wall (emphysematous cholecystitis).

In a porcelain gallbladder, the calcification may be continuous in the muscle layer or it may represent multiple tiny microliths in the mucosa and in Rokitansky-Aschoff sinuses. About 25% of cases are associated with gallbladder carcinoma and 95% with gallstones. If the calcification is heavy and continuous, the ultrasound scan will demonstrate a hyperechoic area with distal

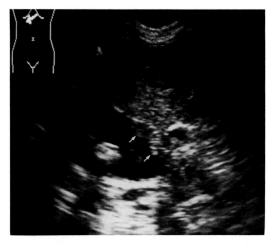

FIG. 3.28. Gallbladder carcinoma. Transverse scan demonstrates a small mural tumor (*arrows*) arising from gallbladder wall. At surgery, this tumor had invaded through gallbladder wall into liver parenchyma.

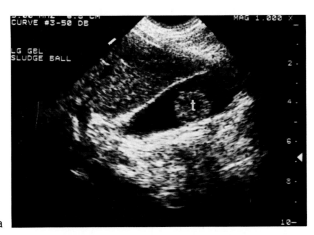 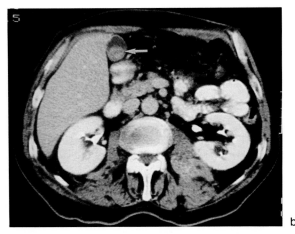

a   b

FIG. 3.30. Metastatic tumor to gallbladder wall. **a:** Sagittal scan of gallbladder demonstrates a round tumor (*t*) arising from posterior wall. **b:** CT scan demonstrates tumor (*arrow*) arising from posterior gallbladder wall. This represented a metastatic focus of malignant melanoma. (Scans are courtesy of Dr. Howard Greenberg, Department of Radiology, Health Sciences Center, Winnipeg, Canada.)

shadowing, mimicking a contracted gallbladder with calculi (Fig. 3.32). If the calcification is less dense, the gallbladder wall will be uniformly or focally more echogenic than usual without distal shadowing.

Small calculi within Rokitansky-Aschoff sinuses (in adenomyomatosis or chronic cholecystitis) will also manifest as small hyperechoic foci. Many of these have a small V-shaped artifact posterior to them, and this finding is characteristic (Fig. 3.26) (34). Some of the foci have no posterior V-shaped artifact.

Intramural gas causes focal or diffuse bright echoes. These may have no posterior shadowing or artifact, or there may be posterior shadowing, or there may be a long posterior ring-down artifact (Fig. 3.20) (65). Only the latter finding is characteristic of gas in the wall.

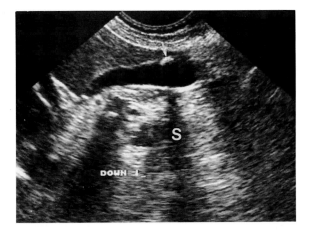

FIG. 3.31. Adherent calculus. Sagittal scan of gallbladder demonstrates a small calculus (*arrow*) stuck to anterior wall of gallbladder. Note posterior acoustic shadow (*s*) behind gallbladder.

Other Intraluminal Entities

Sludge

Biliary "sludge," in ultrasound parlance, has come to mean echogenic bile caused by calcium bilirubinate or cholesterol crystals in suspension (66). Any form of stasis of bile leads to the formation of these crystals. The most common cause of stasis is prolonged fasting. The next most common cause is obstruction of bile flow (e.g., cystic duct obstruction, common bile duct obstruction).

On ultrasound, sludge usually manifests as echogenic material that layers in the dependent portion of the gallbladder (Fig. 3.33). The echogenicity may be lower than or equal to normal liver parenchyma. If the sludge completely fills the gallbladder, the gallbladder may be difficult to distinguish from liver. This is called "hepatization" of the gallbladder. Occasionally, sludge may clump together to form masses or balls within the gallbladder lumen (Fig. 3.33). This has been called "tumefactive" sludge and sludge balls.

Blood

In clinical practice, blood in the gallbladder is rare. Possible causes include acute hemorrhagic cholecystitis, blunt abdominal trauma (e.g., postbiopsy), surgical trauma (e.g., needle biopsy), anticoagulation, and biliary neoplasms. Blood in the gallbladder may be identical to sludge sonographically: one may see layering echogenic material in the dependent portion of the gallbladder or clumps of echogenic material simulating tumefactive sludge (Fig. 3.34) (67). In the acute phase of hemobilia, CT scanning may demonstrate hyperdense material in the gallbladder and thus differentiate blood or milk of

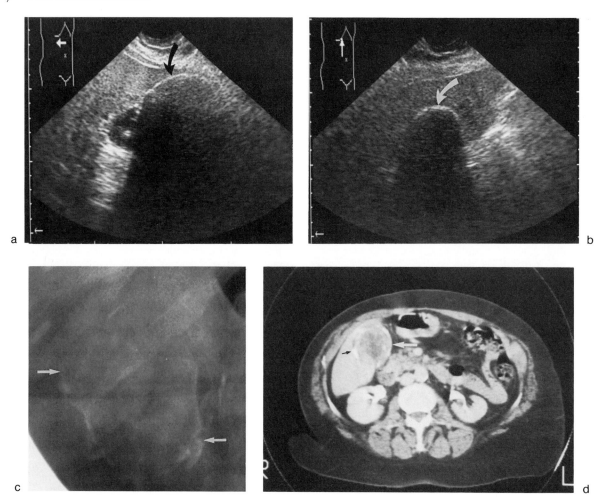

FIG. 3.32. Porcelain gallbladder and carcinoma of gallbladder. **a:** Sagittal scan of gallbladder demonstrates a linear hyperechoic focus (*arrow*) in anterior gallbladder wall, associated with a broad posterior acoustic shadow. **b:** Transverse scan of gallbladder body demonstrates a thin hyperechoic arc (*arrow*) in anterior gallbladder wall associated with a broad posterior acoustic shadow. **c:** Radiograph of right upper quadrant demonstrates irregular and thick curvilinear calcifications (*arrows*) arising in gallbladder wall. **d:** CT scan demonstrates thick mural calcifications (*arrows*) associated with irregular soft tissue density within gallbladder lumen.

calcium from sludge (as long as no contrast material is in the gallbladder) (68).

Pus (Empyema of the Gallbladder)

Intraluminal pus manifests as low- to mid-level irregular echoes throughout the lumen. Usually the echogenic material does not layer like sludge. Other signs of acute cholecystitis are usually present to help distinguish between empyema and other forms of echogenic bile (Fig. 3.35) (43,69).

Milk of Calcium

Milk of calcium represents bile containing a high concentration of calcium carbonate, which forms a solution of viscous fluid layering in the dependent portion of the gallbladder. The cystic duct is usually obstructed, there is chronic cholecystitis, and the gallbladder mucosa has lost its normal absorptive and secretory functions. On ultrasound, the supernatant is echo-free fluid and the dependent fluid is very echogenic material, causing distal shadowing. This can be difficult to distinguish from multiple tiny calculi in the gallbladder (70,71).

Rare Abnormalities

Mirizzi Syndrome

Mirizzi syndrome is characterized by a calculus impacted in the cystic duct, partial obstruction of the common hepatic duct because of the calculus and surround-

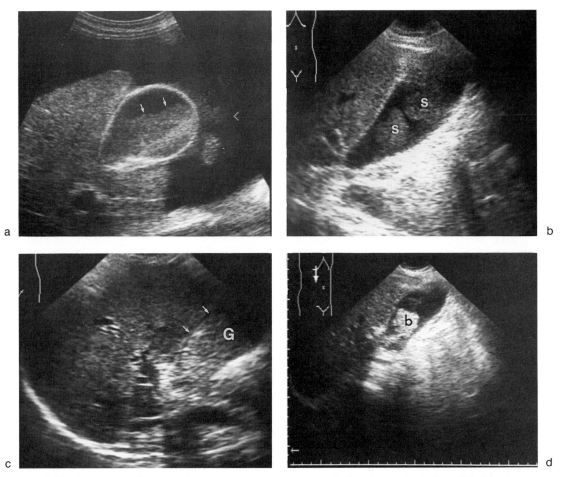

FIG. 3.33. Sludge. **a:** Sagittal scan demonstrates layering sludge (*arrows*) within gallbladder lumen. Note ascites around gallbladder. **b:** Sagittal scan demonstrates tumefactive sludge or sludge balls (*s*) within lumen. **c:** Hepatization of gallbladder. Gallbladder (*G*) is filled with echogenic sludge, whose appearance is similar to neighboring liver parenchyma. *Arrows* demarcate anterior gallbladder wall. **d:** Sagittal scan of another patient demonstrates bright echoes (*b*) caused by barium, which had refluxed through common bile duct after a barium meal. Patient had previous sphincterotomy performed.

ing inflammation, and jaundice (72). In most cases the anatomy of the cystic duct is congenitally abnormal: it runs parallel and adjacent to the common bile duct and thus allows a cystic duct stone to partially compress the common bile duct. On ultrasound, one visualizes an impacted stone in the cystic duct or neck of the gallbladder, dilated bile ducts proximal to the calculus, and a normal-sized common bile duct distal to the calculus.

Ascariasis

Ascaris lumbricoides is a round worm that may infest the human gut. It is quite common in some parts of the world but rare in North America. The worms, which are 2 to 5 mm thick and 15 to 20 cm long, reside in the jejunum. Occasionally the worms migrate into the common bile duct and gallbladder, where they can lead to

obstruction and cholangitis. On ultrasound, one may see single or multiple linear echoes, coils, or amorphous fragments (73,74).

Chlonorchiasis

Chlonorchis sinensis is a small leaf-like worm that measures 8 to 15 mm long, 1.5 to 4 mm wide, and 1 mm thick (75). Humans become infested by eating raw fish that contain encysted cercariae (metamorphosed eggs). These cercariae migrate into the bile ducts and reside in small- to medium-sized intrahepatic bile ducts. Although this is mainly a disease of the intrahepatic bile ducts, about one-third of cases have worms in the gallbladder (75). On ultrasound, the worms appear as floating or dependent, discrete, nonshadowing echogenic foci in the lumen.

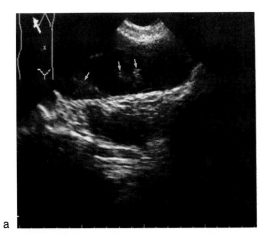
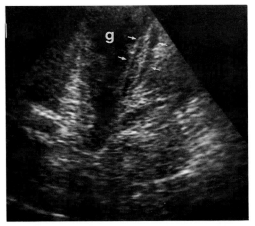

FIG. 3.34. Blood in gallbladder. **a:** This patient had a previous transhepatic cholangiogram, complicated by bleeding into biliary system. Note low-level echoes (*arrows*) within gallbladder lumen, representing blood. **b:** This 24-year-old patient was recently kicked in right upper quadrant. Note low-level echoes (blood) in gallbladder lumen (*g*) and hemorrhagic-edematous thickening of wall (*arrows*).

Cystic Fibrosis

Complications of cystic fibrosis in early adulthood include cholelithiasis, microgallbladder, and bile duct dilatation. In a series of 23 patients, 17% had cholelithiasis, 30% had microgallbladder, and in one patient the gallbladder was not visualized (76). In this series, 36% of gallbladders were abnormal.

Hydrops of the Gallbladder

With long-standing total obstruction of the cystic duct, the gallbladder may become distended and thin-walled. The bile is resorbed, and the mucosa secretes a clear mucinous fluid that distends the gallbladder. Hydrops is often asymptomatic, although some patients may have pain or nausea, or both.

Hydrops may develop in children and infants with other diseases such as mucocutaneous lymph node syndrome, scarlet fever, leptospirosis, streptococcal infection, and familial Mediterranean fever (77). In these cases there is no obstruction and no evidence of cholecystitis. The gallbladder usually returns to normal when the systemic disease subsides. The gallbladder abnormality may be related to mural vasculitis.

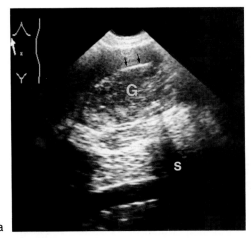
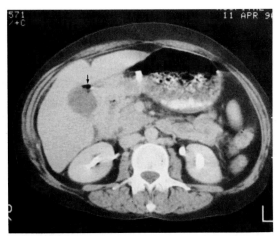

FIG. 3.35. Empyema of gallbladder. **a:** Sagittal scan demonstrates irregularly echogenic material filling gallbladder lumen (*G*). Note shadow (*s*) posterior to small calculus in lumen of gallbladder and gas in anterior wall of gallbladder (*arrows*). **b:** CT scan [same patient as (a)] demonstrates collection of gas in anterior gallbladder wall (*arrow*). Density of fluid is higher than normal bile, and this was due to pus in gallbladder lumen.

3.4 PITFALLS, ARTIFACTS, AND PRACTICAL TIPS

Nonshadowing Calculi

If a calculus is small with respect to the ultrasound beam width, an acoustic shadow may not be visible. For example, a 2-mm calculus scanned with a 3.5-MHz mechanical sector probe may not yield a shadow. One must use the highest frequency possible and place the scan in the focal zone of the transducer to optimize acoustic shadowing. However, there still will be occasions when even larger calculi (4–8 mm) do not shadow with optimal preoperative and intraoperative techniques (78) (Fig. 3.36).

Some very small calculi are known to have comet-tail artifacts or V-shaped artifacts behind them (Fig. 3.12). These crystalline calculi are approximately 0.5 to 1.5 mm in diameter and may be found in the gallbladder lumen especially after ESWL (33) and in Rokitansky-Aschoff sinuses in the gallbladder wall with adenomyomatosis and chronic cholecystitis (34).

Nonmobile Calculi

Mobility of an intraluminal echogenic focus can distinguish between a calculus and a polyp in many cases. However, smaller calculi may stick to the gallbladder wall especially in cases of cholecystitis (Fig. 3.31). Rarely a small calculus may be nonshadowing and nonmobile (78). In these circumstances, it is impossible to diagnose a calculus.

Impacted Calculi

Calculi free in the gallbladder lumen may be asymptomatic for years. If a calculus becomes impacted in the cystic duct or gallbladder neck, abdominal pain and acute cholecystitis ensue. On ultrasound, the free intraluminal calculi are seen, but the impacted calculus is often overlooked for the following reasons: the calculus is not in the gallbladder lumen, which is often enlarged; the calculus is often small; there is no fluid surrounding the calculus; and the scanner does not specifically look for an impacted calculus. One must trace the gallbladder neck back to the portal vein and specifically search for a stone adjacent to the portal vein and common bile duct (Fig. 3.14).

Stones with "Dirty" Shadows

The quality of the acoustic shadow behind a stone depends on the surface characteristics of the stone, the curvature of the stone, the orientation of the stone in the ultrasound beam, and the size of the stone with respect to the cross-sectional area of the beam. A calculus with a flat smooth surface may produce a "dirty" shadow and thus mimic gas in neighboring bowel. Calculi with a curved rough surface, however, tend to produce "clean" shadows (15). Rubin et al. (79) demonstrated the quality of the shadow (dirty vs. clean) provides little information about the structure of the echogenic focus (e.g., stones vs. gas). Independent of the reflecting material, cleaner shadows are produced by rougher surfaces and a smaller radius of curvature of the interface being insonated (79).

Shadowing Polyps

Cholesterol polyps may have a posterior acoustic shadow if there is calcification in the polyp. In this case it is impossible to distinguish between an adherent calculus and a polyp. This is a rare occurrence (80,81).

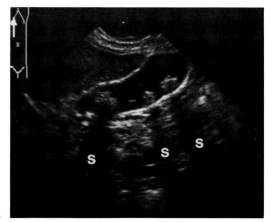
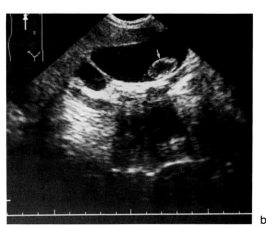

FIG. 3.36. Calculi versus sludge balls. **a:** Only faint shadows (*s*) are present posterior to three echogenic foci in gallbladder lumen. **b:** A similar oval-shaped structure (*arrow*) lies within gallbladder lumen in another patient. No posterior acoustic shadowing is present. In this case it is very difficult to distinguish between a calculus and a sludge ball.

Bowel Gas with "Clean" Shadows (Pseudo WES Triad)

Bowel gas may produce a clean shadow or a dirty shadow. If a bowel loop indents the gallbladder and produces a "clean" posterior shadow, this will closely mimic a gallbladder stone. One must watch for peristalsis or move the patient (and thus the gallbladder) to demonstrate that the echogenic focus is extrinsic to the gallbladder.

One can usually distinguish between a gas-distended loop of bowel and a contracted gallbladder containing a calculus by using the WES triad (Fig. 3.16) (26). In a distended loop of normal bowel, the wall is thin and difficult to perceive with ultrasound. However, in diseased bowel (e.g., inflamed or edematous bowel), the wall is thickened and will appear as a hypoechoic band. Gas in this bowel can exactly mimic a contracted gallbladder with calculus (Fig. 3.37). This is a pseudo WES sign. One can have the patient drink water and watch for bowel peristalsis to help distinguish. In occasional cases of a contracted gallbladder containing calculi, one may not identify the W of the WES triad (Fig. 3.38) despite excellent visualization of the gallbladder. The persistence of the echo and distal shadowing in the gallbladder fossa, however, would be very suspicious for cholelithiasis.

Pseudo Sludge

Low-level echoes in the gallbladder may be caused by two types of artifacts: slice thickness artifact, and side

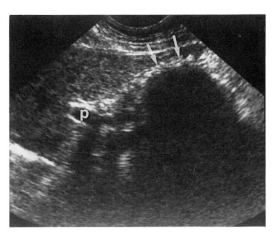

FIG. 3.38. Calculi simulating a porcelain gallbladder. Multiple hyperechoic foci are present in gallbladder fossa (*arrows*). It is very difficult to perceive hypoechoic anterior wall of gallbladder in this case. Sonographically this could represent calcification in gallbladder wall. However, this patient had calculi in a contracted gallbladder.

lobe artifacts. In slice thickness artifact, the finite-width ultrasound beam intersects the curvature of the fluid-filled gallbladder. At a given distance from the transducer, some of the sound beam is in the gallbladder lumen and some in neighboring soft tissue such as liver. The ultrasound machine records liver echoes as coming from the center of the beam and thus prints low-level echoes in the gallbladder lumen (Fig. 3.39) (82,83). To minimize this effect, scan at the center of the fluid-filled structure (i.e., where there is very little curvature) and scan with a focused narrow beam. To distinguish between real sludge and pseudo sludge, change the patient's position: real sludge will move, whereas pseudo sludge will not move.

Pseudo sludge may also be caused by low-intensity side lobes that lie adjacent to the main ultrasound beam. Side lobes interact with reflectors outside the gallbladder lumen, and these echoes are interpreted by the machine as originating inside the lumen. This effect also generates pseudo sludge inside the gallbladder (84).

Noise in the Near Field of the Gallbladder

Reverberation of sound between the ultrasound probe and near-field structures gives rise to multiple parallel echoes that occupy the proximal gallbladder lumen (Fig. 3.39). This will obscure the detail of the anterior wall, and these echoes can be mistaken for real intraluminal structures. This effect may be minimized by using a higher frequency probe with a closer focal zone and by repositioning the patient to change the relationship of probe and gallbladder.

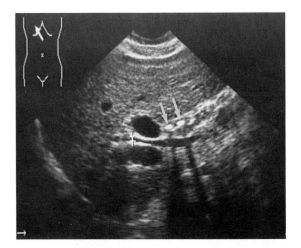

FIG. 3.37. Duodenal gas simulating gallstones. Oblique scan through right upper quadrant demonstrates two hyperechoic foci (*arrows*) associated with posterior acoustic shadows. Note thin hypoechoic band of tissue anterior to hyperechoic foci. This could be mistaken for a contracted gallbladder (WES triad). However, this represents gas within duodenum, and hypoechoic band represents duodenal wall.

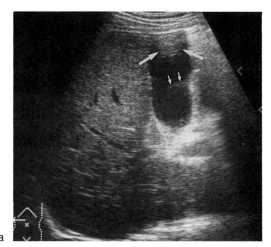 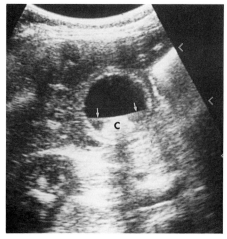

FIG. 3.39. Pseudo sludge in gallbladder. **a:** Transverse scan demonstrates echogenic material in medial aspect of gallbladder (*small arrows*). This simulates layering sludge, but it represents side-lobe artifacts or beam-width artifact caused by sound interaction with medial wall of gallbladder. Note that echoes only extend half way across lumen of gallbladder. *Large arrows* indicate pseudo sludge caused by a reverberation artifact from structures anterior to gallbladder wall. **b:** Transverse scan demonstrates a calculus (*c*) within lumen of gallbladder. Note linear artifacts on either side of calculus (*arrows*), which simulate sludge in gallbladder. However, this represents a beam-width artifact arising from sound interaction with calculus.

The Nonvisualized Gallbladder

Several conditions cause nonvisualization of the gallbladder: agenesis (very rare); ectopic location (rare); contraction of gallbladder without stones; abnormalities of the anterior gallbladder wall that cause total reflection or absorption of sound (e.g., porcelain gallbladder, gas in gallbladder wall); hepatization of gallbladder (i.e., gallbladder filled with sludge that mimics the liver parenchyma) (Fig. 3.33c) (85).

REFERENCES

Normal Anatomy

1. Parulekar SG. Sonography of the distal cystic duct. *J Ultrasound Med* 1989;8:367–373.
2. Nino-Murcia M, Burton D, Chang P, Stone J, Perkash I. Gallbladder contractility in patients with spinal cord injuries: a sonographic investigation. *AJR* 1990;154:521–524.
3. Kishk SMA, Darweesh RMA, Dodds WJ, et al. Sonographic evaluation of resting gallbladder volume and postprandial emptying in patients with gallstones. *AJR* 1987;148:875–879.
4. Raduns K, McGahan JP, Beal S. Cholecystokinin sonography: lack of utility in diagnosis of acute acalculous cholecystitis. *Radiology* 1990;175:463–466.
5. Wolson AH. Ultrasound measurements of the gallbladder. In: Goldberg BB, Kurtz A, eds. *Normal values in ultrasound*. New York: Raven Press; 1989:108–112.
6. Kane RA. Ultrasonographic evaluation of the gallbladder. *CRC Crit Rev Diag Imaging* 1982;17:107–159.
7. Hopman WPM, Rosenbusch G, Jansen JBMJ, de Jong AJ, Lamers CB. Gallbladder contraction: effects of fatty meals and cholecystokinin. *Radiology* 1985;157:37–39.

8. Hatfield PM, Wise RE. Anatomic variation in the gallbladder and bile ducts. *Semin Roentgenol* 1976;10:157–164.
9. Ralls PW, Quinn MF, Juttner HU, Halls JM, Boswell WD. Gallbladder wall thickening: patients without intrinsic gallbladder disease. *AJR* 1981;137:65–68.
10. Sadler TW, ed. *Langman's medical embryology*. 6th ed. Toronto: Williams & Wilkins; 1990:245.
11. Guyer PB, McLoughlin M. Congenital double gallbladder: a review and report of two cases. *Br J Radiol* 1967;40:214–219.
12. Garfield HD, Lyons EA, Levi CS. Sonographic findings in double gallbladder with cholelithiasis of both lobes. *J Ultrasound Med* 1988;7:589–591.
13. Muragama S, Mizushima A, Russel WJ, Higashi Y. Sonographic diagnosis of bicameral gallbladders: a report of three cases. *J Ultrasound Med* 1985;4:539–543.
14. Lichtenstein ME. Significance of the "folded fundus" gallbladder. *Surg Gynecol Obstet* 1937;64:684–688.
15. Rosenthal SJ, Cox GG, Wetzel LH, Batnitzky S. Pitfalls and differential diagnosis in biliary sonography. *Radiographics* 1990; 10:285–311.
16. Lev-Toaff AS, Friedman AC, Rindsberg SN, Caroline DF, Maurer AH, Radecki PD. Multiseptate gallbladder: incidental diagnosis on sonography. *AJR* 1987;148:1119–1120.
17. Greaves F, Nguyen KT, Sauerbrei EE. Retrohepatic gallbladder diagnosed by ultrasound and scintigraphy. *J Can Assoc Radiol* 1983;34:319–320.
18. Youngwirth LD, Peters JC, Perry MC. The suprahepatic gallbladder. An unusual anatomical variant. *Radiology* 1983;149:57–58.
19. Bach DB, Satin R, Palayew M, Lisbona R, Tessler F. Herniation and strangulation of the gallbladder through the foramen of Winslow. *AJR* 1984;142:541–542.
20. Blanton DE, Bream CA, Mandel SR. Gallbladder ectopia. A review of anomalies of position. *AJR* 1974;121:396–400.

Pathology

21. Wilson-Sharp RC, Irving HC, Brown RC, Chalmers DM, Littlewood JM. Ultrasonography of the pancreas, liver and biliary system in cystic fibrosis. *Arch Dis Child* 1984;59:923–926.

22. Kramer NR, Karasick D, Karasick S. Microgallbladder—a clue to cystic fibrosis. *J Can Assoc Radiol* 1983;34:271–272.
23. Birnholz JC. Population survey: ultrasonic cholecystography. *Gastrointest Radiol* 1982;7:165–167.
24. Whorwell PJ, Hawkins R, Dewbury K, Wright R. Ultrasound survey of gallstones and other hepatobiliary disorders in patients with Crohn's disease. *Dig Dis Sci* 1984; 29:930–933.
25. Cover KL, Slasky BS, Skolnick ML. Sonography of cholesterol in the biliary system. *J Ultrasound Med* 1985;4:647–653.
26. MacDonald FR, Cooperberg PL, Cohen M. The WES triad—a specific sonographic sign of gallstones in the contracted gallbladder. *Gastrointest Radiol* 1981;6:39–41.
27. Cooperberg PL, Burhenne HJ. Real time ultrasonography. Diagnostic technique of choice in calculous gallbladder disease. *N Engl J Med* 1980;302:1277–1279.
28. Klingensmith WC III, Eckhout GV. Cholelithiasis in the morbidly obese: diagnosis by ultrasound and oral cholecystography. *Radiology* 1986;160:27–28.
29. Brink JA, Simeone JF, Mueller PR, et al. Routine sonographic techniques fail to quantify gallstone size and number: a retrospective study of 111 surgically proved cases. *AJR* 1989;153:503–506.
30. Mathieson JR, So CB, Malone DE, Becker CD, Burhenne HJ. Accuracy of sonography for determining the number and size of gallbladder stones before and after lithotripsy. *AJR* 1989;153; 977–980.
31. Garra BS, Davros WJ, Lack EE, Horii SC, Silverman PM, Zeman RK. Visibility of gallstone fragments at ultrasound and fluoroscopy: implications for monitoring gallstone lithotripsy. *Radiology* 1990;174:343–347.
32. Khouri MR, Goldszmidt JB, Lauter I, et al. Intact stones or fragments? Potential pitfalls in the imaging of patients after biliary extracorporeal shock wave lithotripsy. *Radiology* 1990;177: 147–151.
33. Shapiro RS, Winsberg F. Comet-tail artifact from cholesterol crystals: observations in the post lithotripsy gallbladder and an *in vitro* model. *Radiology* 1990;177:153–156.
34. Lafortune M, Gariépy G, Dumont A, Breton G, Lapointe R. The V-shaped artifact of the gallbladder wall. *AJR* 1986;147:505–508.
35. O'Brien MJ, Gottlieb LS. The liver and biliary tract. In: Robbins SL, Cotran RS, eds. *Pathological basis of disease*. Philadelphia: WB Saunders; 1979.
36. Glenn F, Becker CG. Acute acalculous cholecystitis: an increasing entity. *Ann Surg* 1982;195:131–136.
37. Ralls PW, Colletti PM, Lapin SA, et al. Real-time sonography in suspected acute cholecystitis. Prospective evaluation of primary and secondary signs. *Radiology* 1985;155:767–771.
38. Cohan RH, Mahoney BS, Bowie JD, Cooper C, Baker ME, Illescas FF. Striated intraluminal gallbladder lucencies on ultrasound studies: predictors of acute cholecystitis. *Radiology* 1987;164:31–35.
39. Teefey SA, Baron RL, Bigler SA. Sonography of the gallbladder: significance of striated (layered) thickening of the gallbladder wall. *AJR* 1991;156:945–947.
40. Jönsson PE, Andersson A. Postoperative acute acalculous cholecystitis. *Arch Surg* 1976;111:1097–1101.
41. Howard RJ. Acute acalculous cholecystitis. *Am J Surg* 1981; 141:194–198.
42. Shuman WP, Rogers JV, Rudd TG, Mack LA, Plumley T, Larson EB. Low sensitivity of sonography and cholescintigraphy in acalculous cholecystitis. *AJR* 1984;142:531–534.
43. Jeffrey RB, Laing FC, Wong W, Callen PW. Gangrenous cholecystitis: diagnosis by ultrasound. *Radiology* 1983;148:219–221.
44. Simeone JF, Brink JA, Mueller PR, et al. The sonographic diagnosis of acute cholecystitis: importance of the Murphy sign. *AJR* 1989;152:289–290.
45. Bloom RM, Libson E, Lebensart PD, et al. The ultrasound spectrum of emphysematous cholecystitis. *JCU* 1989;17:251–256.
46. Nemcek AA, Gore RM, Vogelzang RL, Grant M. The effervescent gallbladder: a sonographic sign of emphysematous cholecystitis. *AJR* 1988;150:575–577.
47. Takada T, Yasuda H, Uchiyama K, Hasegawa H, Asagoe T, Skikata J. Pericholecystic abscess: classification of ultrasound findings to determine the proper therapy. *Radiology* 1989;172:693–697.
48. Chinn DH, Miller E, Piper N. Hemorrhagic cholecystitis. Sono-
graphic appearance and clinical presentation. *J Ultrasound Med* 1987;6:313–317.
49. Kane RA. Ultrasonographic diagnosis of gangrenous cholecystitis and empyema of the gallbladder. *Radiology* 1980;134:191–194.
50. Ralls PW, Halls J, Lapin SA, Quinn MF, Morris UL, Boswell W. Prospective evaluation of the sonographic Murphy sign in suspected acute cholecystitis. *JCU* 1982;10:113–115.
51. Fleischer AC, Muhletaler CA, Jones TB. Sonographic detection of gallbladder perforation. *South Med J* 1982;75:606–607.
52. Kaftori JK, Pery M, Green J, Gaitini D. Thickness of the gallbladder wall in patients with hypoalbuminemia: a sonographic study of patients on peritoneal dialysis. *AJR* 1987;148:1117–1118.
53. Huang Y-S, Lee S-D, Wu J-C, Wang S-S, Lin H-C, Tsai Y-T. Utility of sonographic gallbladder wall patterns in differentiating malignant from cirrhotic ascites. *JCU* 1989;17:187–192.
54. Jutras JA, Longtin JM, Levesque MD. Hyperplastic cholecystoses. Hickey Lecture, *AJR* 1960;83:795–827.
55. Berk RN, Van der Vegt JG, Lichtenstein JE. The hyperplastic cholecystoses: cholesterolosis and adenomyomatosis. *Radiology* 1983;146:593–601.
56. Rice J, Sauerbrei EE, Semogas P, Cooperberg PL, Burhenne HJ. Ultrasound appearances of adenomyomatosis of the gallbladder. *JCU* 1981;9:336–337.
57. Raghavendra BN, Subramanyam BR, Balthazar EJ, Horii SC, Megibow AJ, Hilton S. Sonography of adenomyomatosis of the gallbladder: radiologic–pathologic correlation. *Radiology* 1983; 146:747–752.
58. Kidney M, Goiney R, Cooperberg PL. Adenomyomatosis of the gallbladder: a pictorial exhibit. *J Ultrasound Med* 1986;5:331–333.
59. Kumar A, Aggarwal S, Berry M, Shawney S, Kapur BML, Bhargava S. Ultrasonography of the gallbladder: an analysis of 80 cases. *JCU* 1990;18:715–720.
60. Lane J, Buck J, Zeman RK. Primary carcinoma of the gallbladder: a pictorial essay. *Radiographics* 1989;9:209–228.
61. Shieh CJ, Dunn E, Standard JE. Primary carcinoma of the gallbladder: a review of a 16 year experience at the Waterbury Hospital Health Centre. *Cancer* 1981;47:996–1004.
62. Kuo Y-C, Liu J-W, Sheen I-S, Yang C-Y, Lin D-Y, Chang Chein C-S. Ultrasonographic difficulties and pitfalls in diagnosing primary carcinoma of the gallbladder. *JCU* 1990;18:639–647.
63. Phillips G, Pochaczevsky R, Goodman J, Kumari S. Ultrasound patterns of metastatic tumors in the gallbladder. *JCU* 1982;10: 379–383.
64. Stutte H, Müller PH, di Hoedt B, Stroebel W. Ultrasonographic diagnosis of melanoma metastases in liver, gallbladder and spleen. *J Ultrasound Med* 1989;8:541–547.
65. Avruch L, Cooperberg PL. The ring down artifact. *J Ultrasound Med* 1985;4:24–28.
66. Filly RA, Allen B, Minton MJ, Berhoft R, Way LW. *In vitro* investigation of the origin of echoes within biliary sludge. *JCU* 1980;8:193–200.
67. Grant EG, Smirniotopoulas JG. Intraluminal gallbladder hematoma: sonographic evidence of hemobilia. *JCU* 1983;11:507–509.
68. Krudy AG, Doppman JL, Bissonette MB, Girton M. Hemobilia: computed tomographic diagnosis. *Radiology* 1983;148:785–789.
69. Kane RA. Ultrasonographic diagnosis of gangrenous cholecystitis and empyema of the gallbladder. *Radiology* 1980;134:191–194.
70. Love MB. Sonographic features of milk of calcium bile. *J Ultrasound Med* 1982;1:325–327.
71. Chun GH, Deutsch AL, Scheible W. Sonographic findings in milk of calcium bile. *Gastrointest Radiol* 1982;7:371–373.
72. Becker CD, Hassler H, Terrier F. Preoperative diagnosis of the Mirizzi syndrome: limitations of sonography and computed tomography. *AJR* 1984;143:591–596.
73. Cerri GG, Leite GJ, Simoes JB, et al. Ultrasonographic evaluation of ascaris in the biliary tract. *Radiology* 1983;146:753–754.
74. Schulman A, Loxton AJ, Heydenrych JJ, Abdurahman KE. Sonographic diagnosis of biliary ascariasis. *AJR* 1982;139:485–489.
75. Lim JH, Ko YT, Lee DH, Kim SY. Clonorchiasis: sonographic findings in 59 proved cases. *AJR* 1989;152:761–764.
76. Dobson RL, Johnson MA, Hennig RC, Brown NE. Sonography of

the gallbladder, biliary tree and pancreas in adults with cystic fibrosis. *J Can Assoc Radiol* 1988;39:257–259.

77. Bradford BF, Reid BS, Weinstein BJ, Oh KS, Girdany BR. Ultrasonographic evaluation of the gallbladder in mucocutaneous lymph node syndrome. *Radiology* 1982;142:381–384.

Pitfalls, Artifacts, and Practical Tips

78. Machi J, Iwanaga D, Tanaka M, et al. Gallstones simulating polyps sonographically: a report of two cases. *J Ultrasound Med* 1986;5:597–600.
79. Rubin JM, Adler RS, Bude RO, Fowlkes JB, Carson PL. Clean and dirty shadowing at ultrasound: a reappraisal. *Radiology* 1991; 181:231–236.
80. Ruhe AH, Zachman JP, Mulder BD, Rime AE. Cholesterol polyps of the gallbladder: ultrasound demonstration. *JCU* 1979;7: 386–388.
81. Price RJ, Stewart ET, Foley WD, Dodds WJ. Sonography of polypoid cholesterolosis. *AJR* 1982;139:1197–1198.
82. Fiske CE, Filly RA. Pseudosludge. A spurious ultrasound appearance within the gallbladder. *Radiology* 1982;144:631–632.
83. Goldstein A, Madrazo BL. Slice-thickness artifacts in gray-scale ultrasound. *JCU* 1981;9:365–375.
84. Laing FC, Kurtz AB. The importance of ultrasonic side-lobe artifacts. *Radiology* 1982;145:763–768.
85. Hammond DI. Unusual causes of sonographic nonvisualization or nonrecognition of the gallbladder: a review. *JCU* 1988;16:77–85.

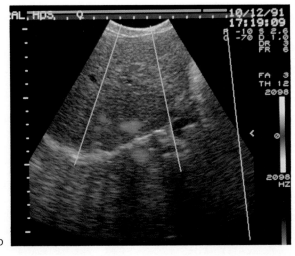

b

FIG. 2.45. Mirror image artifact. (*See page 22 for part a*.) **a:** liver (*L₁*) is reproduced as a mirror image (*L₂*) on thoracic side of diaphragm (*arrows*). **b: True IVC (*in blue*) is reproduced as a mirror artifact (*in red*) across diaphragm. *Blue color* indicates flow toward transducer. *Red color* indicates flow away from transducer.**

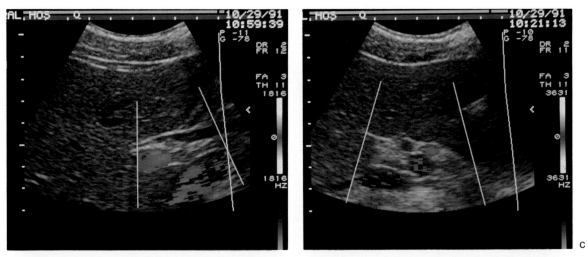

b

c

FIG. 4.5. Position of right hepatic artery. (*See page 55 for part a*.) **a:** Longitudinal scan demonstrates right hepatic artery (*straight arrow*) anterior to bile duct (*curved arrow*). Usually right hepatic artery lies posterior to bile duct. **b: Sagittal color Doppler scan demonstrates blood flow (*blue*—away from probe) in inferior vena cava, portal vein, and right hepatic artery (*small blue circle* anterior to portal vein). Bile duct lies anterior to right hepatic artery, and bile duct has no color within it. c: Transverse color Doppler scan of porta hepatis demonstrates blood flow in proper hepatic artery (*blue*) and some blood flow in main portal vein (*red*). Common bile duct lies lateral to proper hepatic artery and has no flow within it.**

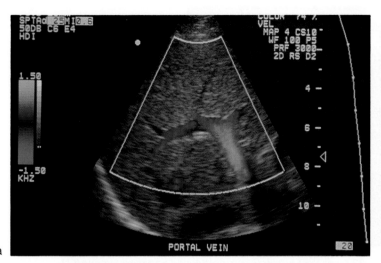
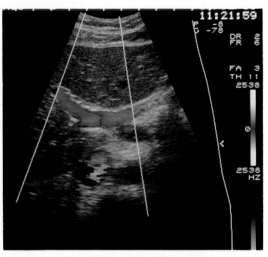

a

PORTAL VEIN

b

FIG. 5.3. Doppler ultrasound of portal veins. (*See page 78 for part c*.) **a: Blood flow in main portal vein is toward liver (hepatopedal). It is coded red because flow is toward the ultrasound probe. Flow in right portal vein is away from the probe and thus coded blue. [Scan is courtesy of Advanced Technology Laboratories (ATL).] b: Color Doppler of portal vein bifurcation. Blood flow in right portal vein is coded red because its net flow is toward the ultrasound probe. Flow in left portal vein is coded red because net flow is slightly away from the probe. c:** Pulsed wave spectrum. Sagittal scan of right upper quadrant demonstrates pulsed wave Doppler cursor in main portal vein. *v,* inferior vena cava. Doppler spectrum (*arrows*) demonstrates blood flow toward the liver. Blood flow is low velocity and continuous, with mild temporal fluctuations in peak velocity caused by cardiac pulsations. Note increase in the velocity toward right of the graph with patient inspiration.

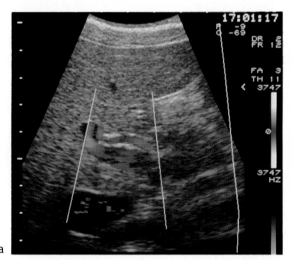
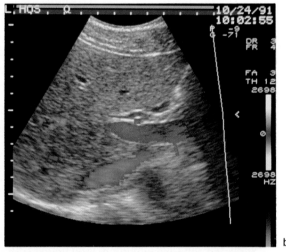

a

b

FIG. 5.4. Doppler ultrasound of hepatic artery. (*See page 79 for part c*.) **a: Color Doppler of hepatic artery. Oblique scan of right upper quadrant demonstrates proper hepatic artery anterior to portal vein. Flow in proximal portion of the artery is red (toward probe) and in distal portion blue (away from probe). This represents blood flow toward the liver. (Scan is courtesy of Mr. Tyler Sauerbrei.) b: Color Doppler of right hepatic artery. Right hepatic artery is a small circle with red in it (flow toward probe). It lies posterior to common duct (no color flow) and anterior to portal vein (red). Note blue color in the inferior vena cava (flow away from probe). c:** Pulsed wave spectrum of hepatic artery. Note forward flow in diastole (*arrows*). This indicates relatively low resistance to hepatic artery flow.

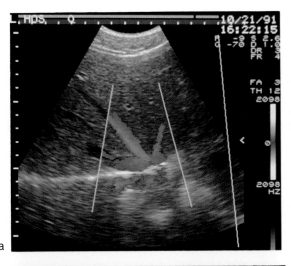

a

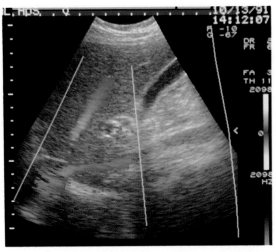

c

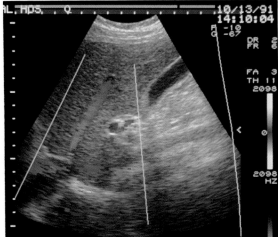

d

FIG. 5.5. Doppler ultrasound of hepatic veins. (*See page 80 for part b.*) **a: Color Doppler ultrasound—transverse. Blood flow in right, middle, and left hepatic veins is toward inferior vena cava. Flow in middle and left hepatic veins is coded blue (flow away from probe). (Scan is courtesy of Mr. Peter Sauerbrei.) b:** Pulsed wave ultrasound spectrum. Transverse scan demonstrates PW spectrum of blood flow in middle hepatic vein. Most of the time, flow is toward the inferior vena cava and thus away from the probe: the spectrum demonstrates flow below baseline (*A,V*). For short time intervals, flow is away from inferior vena cava and thus toward the probe: the spectrum demonstrates flow above baseline (*s*). *A*, atrial diastole; *V*, ventricular diastole; *S*, atrial systole. **c: Color Doppler ultrasound—sagittal. Blood flow throughout middle hepatic vein is toward** the inferior vena cava at this time. Flow in hepatic vein is coded blue (flow away from probe). Flow in inferior vena cava is toward right atrium. **d: Color Doppler—sagittal. Same patient as (c), slightly later in same cardiac cycle. Cine loop function allows color depiction of flow a fraction of a second later when there is momentary reversal of flow in hepatic vein. This corresponds to "S" component of spectrum in (b).**

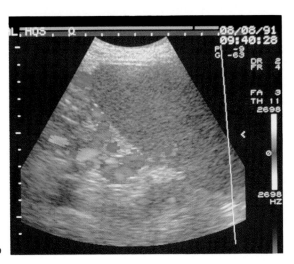

b

FIG. 5.29. (*See page 100 for part a.*) **a:** Dilated coronary vein. Sagittal scan demonstrates a slightly dilated coronary vein (i.e., left gastric vein) arising from splenic vein (*s*) and passing over splenic artery (*a*). Note pancreatic duct (*d*) in body of pancreas. *L*, left hepatic lobe; *arrows*, linea alba; ++, inner diameter of left gastric vein is slightly dilated (7 mm). **b: Short gastric veins—color Doppler ultrasound. Transverse scan through spleen in another patient demonstrates multiple tortuous enlarged veins medial to spleen. Blood flow is coded red and blue in these veins because some loops have flow toward the probe (*red*) and some away from the probe (*blue*).**

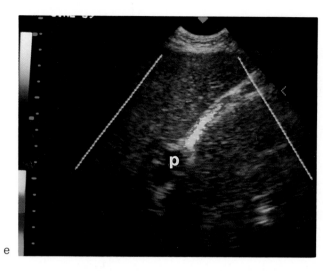
e

FIG. 5.30. Recanalized paraumbilical veins. (*See page 101 for parts a–d.*) **a,b:** Sagittal and transverse scans through left hepatic lobe demonstrate a recanalized paraumbilical vein (PW Doppler *cursor*). Doppler spectrum analysis (*small arrows*) demonstrates blood flow from left portal vein (*p*) toward the umbilicus. *Large arrow*, paraumbilical vein. **c,d:** Sagittal and transverse scans of another patient with an enlarged paraumbilical vein (*arrow*). Note echogenic material filling paraumbilical vein in this patient. Doppler examination demonstrated no blood flow within the vein. This represented thrombosis within a previously patent recanalized paraumbilical vein. **e: Color Doppler flow study in another patient demonstrates blood flow (*yellow* and *red*) in recanalized paraumbilical vein from left portal vein (*p*) toward umbilicus.**

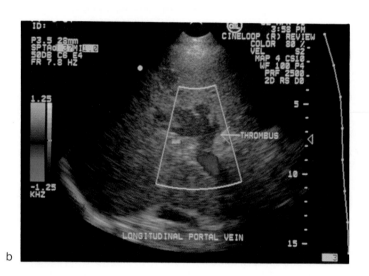
b

FIG. 5.33. (*See page 103 for part a.*) Portal vein thrombosis. **a:** Scan through long axis of portal vein (*p*) demonstrates echogenic material filling lumen of portal vein. Note PW Doppler cursor within proximal portion of portal vein. Corresponding Doppler study on right side of the picture demonstrates no evidence of blood flow within the portal vein. **b: Color Doppler ultrasound. Oblique scan demonstrates some slow flow in main portal vein toward the probe and thus toward the liver (*dark red color*). Intrahepatic portal vein branches are filled with echogenic thrombus. There is no flow detected in these branches. (Scan is courtesy of Advanced Technology Laboratories [ATL].)**

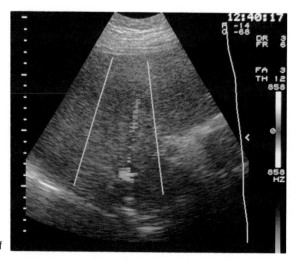
f

FIG. 5.36. Budd-Chiari syndrome. (*See page 106 for parts a–e.*) **a,b:** Sagittal and transverse scans through left hepatic lobe demonstrate marked narrowing of left and middle hepatic veins (*arrows*). *a*, right atrium; *v*, inferior vena cava. This patient had myelofibrosis. **c:** Transverse scan through right hepatic lobe of another patient demonstrates multiple ill-defined hypoechoic areas (*!*) within liver parenchyma in a patient with Budd-Chiari syndrome. These changes may occur secondary to hepatic vein occlusion. **d:** CT scan through same area as (c) demonstrating multiple ill-defined hypodense areas(*!*). **e:** Isotope liver scan of same patient as (c) and (d) demonstrates multiple ill-defined areas of decreased photon emission corresponding to hypoechoic areas on ultrasound and hypodense areas on CT. Liver parenchyma will return to normal appearances after successful treatment of Budd-Chiari syndrome. **f: Color Doppler ultrasound. Sagittal scan demonstrates slow blood flow (*dark blue*) in a very small hepatic vein. This vessel was not visible on 2-D real-time imaging. Blood flow is coded *blue* (away from the probe) and thus toward inferior vena cava.**

CHAPTER 4

The Bile Ducts

INTRODUCTION

Ultrasound is an accurate and reliable technique for assessing the size of the bile ducts and the status of the neighboring soft tissues such as the liver, other structures in the porta hepatis, gallbladder, and pancreas. In some circumstances, CT is needed for further evaluation of the biliary system, and in some instances nuclear medicine scanning is required to further assess biliary dynamics. This chapter will discuss the sonographic techniques for assessing the bile ducts, the normal anatomy and physiology, the common pathologies affecting the bile ducts, and various pitfalls and artifacts.

4.1 SCANNING TECHNIQUES

A sector probe with a small contact area is the best probe for right upper quadrant structures because of the small access sometimes afforded by the patient's anatomy. Curved and linear array probes can also be used; these are most useful when scanning in the subcostal area.

One of the best scanning techniques for examination of the bile ducts is described by Laing et al. (1,2). The

Abbreviations: **CT**, computed tomography; **ERCP**, endoscopic retrograde cholangioportography.

first part of the examination visualizes the distal common duct (i.e., the retroduodenal and intrapancreatic portion of the duct). For this part of the examination, the patient is semierect and right posterior oblique, and transverse scan planes are used. If bowel contents obscure the anatomy, the patient drinks 6 to 12 oz of water and lies in the right lateral decubitus position for 2 to 3 min. The patient then assumes the semierect oblique position, and transverse and sagittal scans of the distal bile duct are obtained.

The second part of the study examines the common duct proximal to the duodenum with the patient in a supine left posterior oblique position. Scans are usually optimized in deep inspiration. Transverse and longitudinal scans are obtained of the proximal common duct, the right and left hepatic ducts, and more proximal intrahepatic bile duct branches. The diameter of the extrahepatic bile duct is measured as follows: the probe is placed along the anterior abdominal wall or the right lateral-anterior abdominal wall, and the long axis of the proximal common duct is obtained. The *internal* diameter of the proximal common duct is measured from this view. This is the anteroposterior diameter or the oblique diameter of the bile duct lumen. Occasionally the right hepatic duct is the structure anterior to the right portal vein, and in this case, one should measure the duct caudal to the right portal vein.

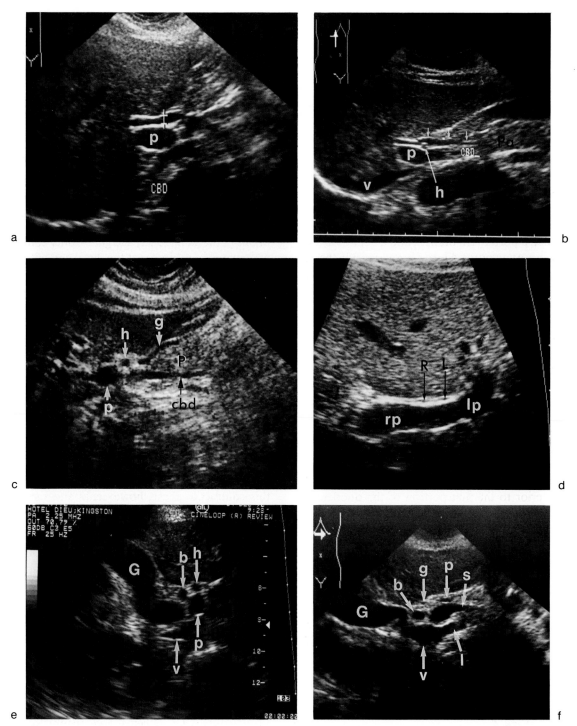

FIG. 4.1. Normal bile ducts. **a:** Sagittal scan demonstrates proximal extrahepatic bile duct (common hepatic duct) anterior to portal vein (*p*). Cursors indicate internal diameter of the duct, which measures 4 mm. **b:** Sagittal scan demonstrates extrahepatic bile duct (*arrows*) extending into pancreatic head (*Pa*). Bile duct measures less than 5-mm internal diameter. *v*, inferior vena cava; *h*, right hepatic artery; *p*, portal vein. **c:** Longitudinal scan demonstrates normal-sized common bile duct (*cbd*) along posterior aspect of pancreatic head (*P*). Gastroduodenal artery (*g*) defines anterior aspect of pancreatic head. *p*, portal vein; *h*, proper hepatic artery. **d:** Transverse scan demonstrates a tiny left hepatic duct (*L*) and right hepatic duct (*R*) anterior to left portal vein (*lp*) and right portal vein (*rp*), respectively. **e:** Transverse scan through portal vein (*p*) demonstrates extrahepatic bile duct (*b*) and proper hepatic artery (*h*) anterior to portal vein. Gallbladder (*G*) lies immediately lateral to main portal vein. *v*, inferior vena cava. **f:** Transverse scan through pancreatic neck demonstrates distal common bile duct (b) in superior portion of pancreatic head. Gallbladder (*G*) lies immediately lateral to bile duct, and gastroduodenal artery (*g*) lies along anterior aspect of pancreatic head. Note slightly prominent pancreatic duct (*p*) in pancreatic neck. *s*, splenic vein; *v*, inferior vena cava; *l*, left renal vein.

The hard copy films on each patient should include the following scans (Fig. 4.1):

1. longitudinal scan of the proximal common duct
2. longitudinal scan of the intrapancreatic bile duct
3. transverse scan of the portal vein bifurcation
4. transverse scan of the proximal extrahepatic bile duct
5. transverse scan of the intrapancreatic bile duct.

4.2 NORMAL ANATOMY

Usual Normal Anatomy and Physiology

Inside the liver, the portal triad consists of an intrahepatic bile duct, a portal vein branch, and a hepatic artery branch; these are surrounded by a fibrous capsule (hepatobiliary capsule of Glisson). The intrahepatic bile ducts drain into the right and left hepatic ducts, which in turn converge to form the common hepatic duct (Fig. 4.2). The intrahepatic bile ducts do not have a constant relationship with the portal vein branches (3,4). In other words, an intrahepatic bile duct may be anterior, posterior, caudal, or cranial to the accompanying portal vein branch.

The left and right hepatic ducts, which exit the liver, are located anterior to the left and right portal veins, respectively (Fig. 4.1d). The common hepatic duct courses caudally and slightly medially in the porta hepatis. The cystic duct joins the common hepatic duct at a variable location to form the common bile duct, which courses posterior to the first portion of the duodenum and proximal transverse colon and then into the posterior parenchyma of the pancreatic head. In its distal course, the common bile duct courses slightly laterally and posteriorly (Fig. 4.2). The pancreatic duct joins the common bile duct in the posterolateral aspect of the pancreatic head in the ampulla of Vater.

The proximal end of the common duct is fixed to the liver, and the distal end is fixed in the pancreatic head. The intervening portion of the common duct is relatively mobile in the lateral edge of the hepatoduodenal ligament (lesser omentum) along with the main portal vein and proper hepatic artery. The common duct lies anterior to the main portal vein and to the right of the proper hepatic artery (Figs. 4.1e and 4.2) (5).

The bile ducts transport bile from the liver cells to the duodenal lumen. The pressure within the bile ducts is less than the hepatic secretory pressure, and this allows bile to flow from the liver into the duodenum. The intrabiliary pressure is less than 100 to 150 mm of water. The volume and pressure within the ductal system at any given time is governed by three main factors: (a) rate of bile flow from the liver into the bile ducts; (b) gallbladder function including rate of gallbladder filling, resorption of bile in the gallbladder, and gallbladder contraction; (c) activity of the sphincter at the distal end of the common bile duct (the sphincter of Oddi). The contractility of the distal sphincter causes the most variability of the intraductal pressure. There is a cycle of approximately ten contractions and relaxations per minute of the distal sphincter, resulting in episodic release of bile into the duodenum (6). The extrahepatic bile duct lacks smooth muscle fibers in its wall, and therefore there is no active contraction of the common bile duct itself. The common duct wall is composed mainly of elastic and fibrous tissue, which expands when the intraductal pressure increases and retracts when the pressure is reduced. Contraction of the sphincter of Oddi will increase the intraductal pressure to 120 to 160 mm of water, at which point bile will flow into a normal gallbladder. During this contractile phase, however, bile will still flow into the duodenum but at a reduced rate.

Bile Ducts After a Fatty Meal

Studies in normal adults have shown that a fatty meal (7) or intravenous cholecystokinin (8) will cause the bile duct to remain the same or decrease slightly in caliber (Fig. 4.3). This is true whether the gallbladder is in place

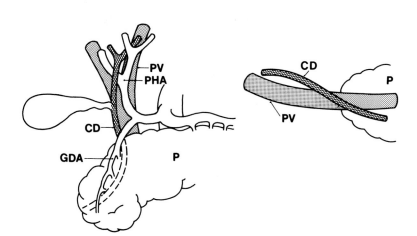

FIG. 4.2. Schematic drawings of porta hepatis in frontal and lateral projections (5). Frontal projection demonstrates position of common duct (CD) along anterolateral aspect of portal vein. Proximal common duct passes anterior to right hepatic artery and junction of right portal vein and main portal vein. Distal common bile duct veers laterally as it passes along posterior aspect of pancreatic head. Gastroduodenal artery (GDA) passes along anterior aspect of pancreatic head. **PV,** portal vein; **Pha,** proper hepatic artery; **p,** pancreas. Lateral projection demonstrates that common duct passes more posteriorly as it approaches pancreatic head.

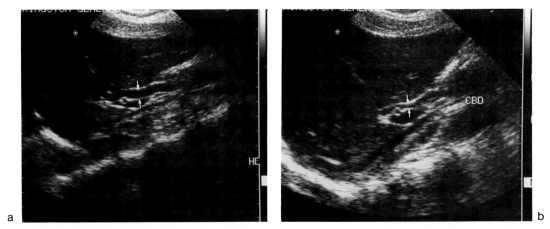

a

b

FIG. 4.3. Bile duct response to fatty meal. **a:** Sagittal scan of common duct demonstrates interior diameter to be 6–7 mm (*arrows*). This is at the upper limit of normal. **b:** Forty-five minutes after a fatty meal, extrahepatic bile duct diameter has decreased to 2–3 mm (*arrows*). This confirms absence of obstruction in bile duct.

or not. In the normal patient, these maneuvers increase bile production by the liver but also relax the sphincter of Oddi and therefore leave the bile ducts unaltered or decreased in diameter. The optimal time to assess the bile duct is 45 to 60 min after the meal.

Raptopoulos et al. (9) demonstrated in a group of 20 adults that there was no significant variation in the bile duct diameter during the day. This implies that choleresis (i.e., increased production of bile) associated with meals is balanced by relaxation of the sphincter of Oddi to maintain an equilibrium of fluid within the bile ducts. Occasionally, however, one does note a significant change in caliber of the extrahepatic bile duct within a short time frame (30–60 min) in normal adults (Fig. 4.4).

Normal Variants

Several anatomic variants may cause difficulty in the evaluation of the extrahepatic bile duct: hepatic artery variants, the transverse extrahepatic bile duct, accessory hepatic ducts, and a redundant neck of the gallbladder.

In most patients the right hepatic artery lies posterior to the right hepatic duct or proximal common hepatic duct, but in 30% the right hepatic artery lies anterior to the bile duct (Fig. 4.5). The left hepatic artery lies anterior to the left hepatic duct in most cases. The proper hepatic artery may become tortuous and enlarged, and this may cause confusion in the evaluation of the extrahepatic bile duct. To distinguish between bile duct and he-

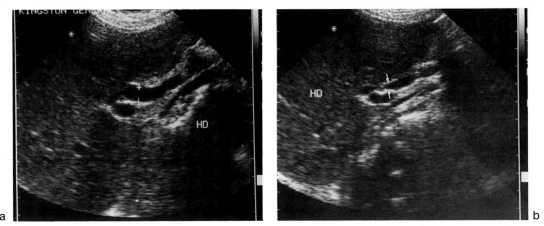

a

b

FIG. 4.4. Normal variation in bile duct diameter during a scan. **a:** At beginning of scan, bile duct (+) was mildly dilated, measuring 8 mm. **b:** Later in scan, bile duct spontaneously decreased in diameter to 3 mm (*arrows*). Occasionally during course of a scan, bile duct diameter is observed to change significantly in size. Spontaneous decrease in diameter is good evidence against biliary obstruction.

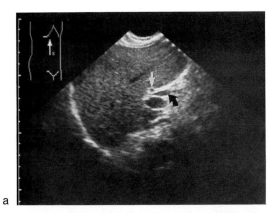

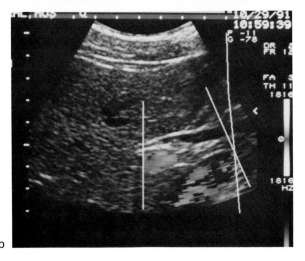
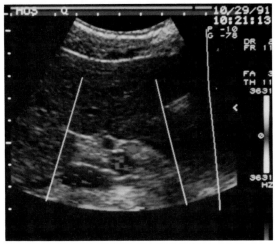

FIG. 4.5. Position of right hepatic artery. (*See color image of parts b and c in the color plate section, which follows page 50.*) **a:** Longitudinal scan demonstrates right hepatic artery (*straight arrow*) anterior to bile duct (*curved arrow*). Usually right hepatic artery lies posterior to bile duct. **b:** Sagittal color Doppler scan demonstrates blood flow (*blue*—away from probe) in inferior vena cava, portal vein, and right hepatic artery (*small blue circle* anterior to portal vein). Bile duct lies anterior to right hepatic artery, and bile duct has no color within it. **c:** Transverse color Doppler scan of porta hepatis demonstrates blood flow in proper hepatic artery (*blue*) and some blood flow in main portal vein (*red*). Common bile duct lies lateral to proper hepatic artery and has no flow within it.

patic artery, one traces the vessels to their origin, observes pulsations in the hepatic artery, or uses Doppler to assess for blood flow. Sensitive color Doppler affords a quick, reliable method to assess for blood flow and thus distinguish between the bile duct and hepatic artery (Fig. 4.5).

About 6% of nonobstructed bile ducts will have a long transverse segment that will course toward the midline.

If the bile duct is obstructed, it will be more tortuous, and as many as 18% of obstructed ducts will have a long transverse segment (10).

An accessory or aberrant hepatic duct may exit the liver and insert into the common hepatic duct, the cystic duct, or the common bile duct beyond the insertion of the cystic duct. Occasionally two accessory ducts may be present, and occasionally a small accessory duct may

TABLE 4.1. *Bile duct diameter with the gallbladder in place*

Source	No. of people in study[a]	Upper limit of normal range (mm)	No. of ducts above normal range
Sample, 1978 (13a)	57[b]	5	2 (4%)
Dewbury, 1980 (12)	126[c]	5	0
Cooperberg, 1978 (11)	98	4	0
Bruneton et al., 1981 (13)	750	4	40 (5%)
Niederau et al., 1983 (14)	830	4	41 (5%)

From Sauerbrei, ref. 5, with permission.
[a] All subjects were adults with no evidence of biliary obstruction.
[b] Fifty-seven patients with medical jaundice but no evidence of biliary obstruction. These patients had no previous biliary surgery.
[c] Author did not specify how many patients had gallbladder in place.

TABLE 4.2. *Upper limit of normal bile duct diameters (gallbladder in place)*

Age	Common duct (mm)	Right and left hepatic ducts (mm)	Branches of left and right hepatic ducts (mm)
Infants (0–1 year)	2	—	—
Children (1–10 years)	4	—	—
Adolescents (11–20 years)	6	3	2
Adults (<60 years)	6	3	2
Adults (>60 years)	8	3	2

empty from the liver parenchyma directly into the gallbladder.

Normal Bile Duct Sizes

Gallbladder in Place (See Tables 4.1 and 4.2)

Various studies have demonstrated that the internal diameter of the proximal common duct is 4 mm or less in 95% of the population (11–14). We consider diameters greater than 6 mm to be dilated (15). The left and right hepatic ducts are often visualized, and the upper limit of normal is taken to be 3 mm (16). Bile ducts proximal to the left and right hepatic ducts can also be visualized, and they are normally 2 mm or less in diameter (16).

In pregnancy, the gallbladder volume is increased. However, Mintz et al. (17) demonstrated that the upper limit of normal for bile duct diameter is 5 mm in the pregnant population and thus the common duct size during pregnancy is the same as the general population.

Wu et al. (18) demonstrated that the extrahepatic bile duct will increase slightly with age. They measured the maximum anteroposterior diameter of the extrahepatic bile duct at whatever level the caliber was maximum (18). The mean diameter increased from 4 to 5 mm for 30 to 50 years of age to 7 to 8 mm for older than 60 years

of age. Therefore the upper limit of normal for older than 60 years of age is 8 mm instead of 6 mm.

In infants younger than 1 year of age, the common duct should not exceed 2-mm internal diameter. In children between 1 year and 10 years of age, 4 mm is the upper limit of normal; in adolescence and young adulthood, the upper limit of normal is 6 mm (19) (Table 4.2).

After Cholecystectomy

Most people after a cholecystectomy have a normal caliber bile duct (i.e., 6 mm or less in internal anteroposterior diameter). Some patients (10–32%) have a mildly dilated bile duct postcholecystectomy (7–11-mm diameter) (Table 4.3) (23,24). In these patients a fatty meal may detect partial bile duct obstruction (7,20,21). If the bile duct diameter increases by 2 mm or more after a fatty meal (45–60 min postmeal), partial obstruction of the bile duct is likely. If the bile duct diameter stays the same or decreases in diameter, there is probably no obstruction present. Wedmann et al. (22) studied 64 patients before and after cholecystectomy (27–39 months after the operation). In some patients the bile duct diameters increased slightly and in others it decreased. It was their conclusion that either increases or decreases in the bile duct diameters may occur postcholecystectomy and that the postoperative evolution is governed by the exact

TABLE 4.3. *Bile duct diameter in asymptomatic people after cholecystectomy*

Source	No. in study	Defined upper limit of normal (mm)	Mean diameter (mm)	Range of diameters (mm)	Percentage with enlarged caliber (%)
Niederau et al., 1983 (14)[a]	55	4	5.2[b]	1–11	58
		5			32
Bruneton et al., 1981 (13)	77		4.5		
Graham et al., 1980 (23)[a]	67	4	3.7	2–10	16
		5			10
Mueller et al., 1981 (24)[a]	40	5	3.5	2–7	5

From Sauerbrei, ref. 5, with permission.

[a] These authors measured the proximal portion of the common duct just caudal to the confluence of the left and right hepatic ducts.

[b] Niederau et al. (14) found the mean duct diameter increased to 6.2 cm when measured more caudally at the widest point of the duct.

nature of the underlying biliary disease at the time of the cholecystectomy.

Discrepancies Between Radiographic and Sonographic Bile Duct Measurements

The bile duct measurements obtained after retrograde cholangiography or percutaneous transhepatic cholangiography are higher than the values obtained at ultrasound. With injection of contrast material into the biliary system, the bile ducts distend. This is most noticeable in patients postcholecystectomy (25). Radiographs overestimate the diameter of the bile duct because of radiographic magnification, which is a factor of approximately 1.3. In addition, the *width* of the bile duct is measured on radiographs, whereas the *anteroposterior diameter* is measured on ultrasound. This leads to a discrepancy if the bile duct is oval in cross-sectional shape. In radiographs, one measures the width of the lumen where the bile duct is largest. However, on ultrasound, the bile duct is measured at its proximal end. If there is a variation in bile duct diameter throughout its length, this causes a discrepancy in the measured values (26).

4.3 PATHOLOGY

Physiology of Bile Duct Obstruction

The walls of the extrahepatic bile ducts contain elastic tissue that allows passive distention of the duct secondary to distal obstruction. When the obstruction is relieved, the bile duct recoils to normal size if the elasticity of the wall is normal.

After acute complete obstruction of the bile duct, scintigraphy shows delayed clearance with no activity in the bowel (27–29). Dilatation of the ducts occurs several hours later, starting at the obstruction and proceeding proximally, involving first the distal common duct, then the proximal common duct, and finally the intrahepatic bile ducts (Fig. 4.6) (30,31). Some time later, the serum bilirubin becomes elevated and subsequently clinical jaundice ensues. After relief of complete obstruction, the intrahepatic ducts return to normal first, followed by the extrahepatic ducts.

Partial or intermittent obstruction of the common duct has not been elucidated as fully as acute complete obstruction, and it may present with a more varied clini-

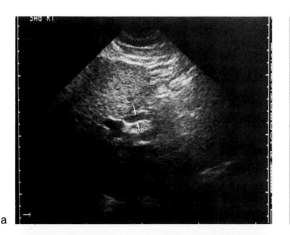

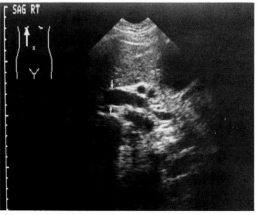

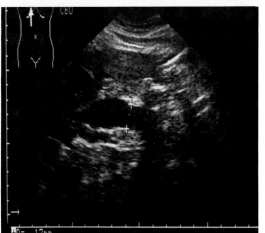

FIG. 4.6. Developing bile duct obstruction–carcinoma of pancreas. **a:** Initial scan of proximal common duct demonstrates diameter to be 5 mm (*arrows*), which is within normal. Serum alkaline phosphatase was raised, and there was a clinical suspicion of biliary obstruction. **b:** One week later, bile duct diameter is variable, but proximal common duct is dilated, now measuring 12 mm (*arrows*). **c:** Two weeks after initial scan, common duct is very dilated. Proximal duct measures 20 mm in diameter (measured proximal to cursors).

cal picture in terms of biochemical findings, the size of the bile ducts at ultrasound, and the biliary dynamics at scintigraphy.

Obstruction Without Dilatation

In early complete obstruction (within 24 hr of the acute episode) and in incomplete or intermittent obstruction, the bile duct may be normal. In 131 patients referred because of right upper quadrant symptoms or abnormal liver function tests, 8% had obstructing lesions but normal-sized bile ducts (20). The commonest cause of biliary obstruction associated with nondilated bile ducts is choledocholithiasis. Fat stimulation will help in detecting a higher percentage of patients with choledocholithiasis (see below) with or without dilated bile ducts.

Dilatation Without Obstruction

The extrahepatic bile duct may be dilated without obstruction. This is most commonly seen in elderly people and in postcholecystectomy patients. Ultrasound examination in the fasting state may lead to measurements above the normal range. A fatty meal can detect those patients with a nonobstructed enlarged bile duct, and this eliminates the need for further investigations (Fig. 4.7) (see below).

Bile Duct Size in Biliary Obstruction

Gallbladder in Place

In adults younger than 60 years of age with obstruction, most common ducts will be greater than 6-mm di-

ameter (Figs. 4.8 and 4.9). However, as noted previously, some patients with biliary obstruction have common duct sizes less than or equal to 6 mm. The latter leads to a significant number of false-negative examinations in clinical practice (i.e., normal bile duct sizes with biliary obstruction).

Direct measurement of the common duct therefore provides a good but not perfect screening method in distinguishing between an obstructed and nonobstructed biliary system. Note, however, that most of the false-negative and false-positive scans arise in the nonjaundiced patient (i.e., those with early, partial or intermittent obstruction). If there is raised serum bilirubin or clinical jaundice, the ultrasonic bile duct diameter is a very accurate test in distinguishing between obstruction versus nonobstruction.

After Cholecystectomy

The ultrasonic bile duct diameter remains a good test in detecting obstruction postcholecystectomy, but the sensitivity and specificity are less than the precholecystectomy state (32). If the patient is jaundiced, the test is very good in distinguishing between obstruction versus nonobstruction.

Use of the Fatty Meal

Several studies have shown that the fatty meal significantly improves on the diagnostic accuracy of ultrasonic bile duct measurement in the evaluation of biliary obstruction (7,20,21). Darweesh et al. (7) demonstrated that in nonobstructed bile ducts, the bile duct diameter remains unchanged, shows an insignificant change of ±1 mm, or decreases by greater than or equal to 2 mm (Fig.

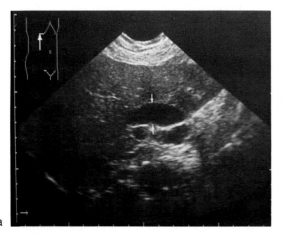
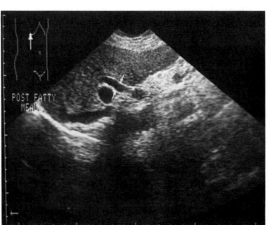

a   b

FIG. 4.7. Fatty meal in a dilated, not obstructed bile duct. **a:** Initial scan of proximal common duct demonstrates it to be quite dilated (*arrows*). Diameter was 16 mm. **b:** Forty-five minutes after a fatty meal, proximal duct (*arrows*) has decreased in diameter to 5 mm. This confirms absence of bile duct obstruction.

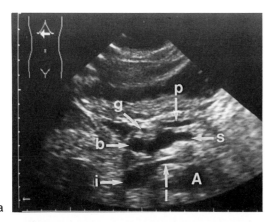

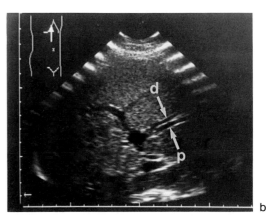

a

b

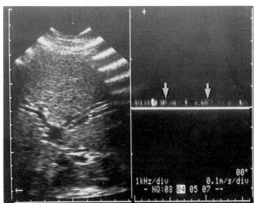

FIG. 4.8. Obstructive jaundice with mild to moderate biliary dilatation. **a:** Transverse scan through pancreatic head demonstrates mild dilatation of common bile duct (*b*), measuring 10 mm in diameter. Pancreatic duct (*p*) is also mildly dilated, measuring 4-mm maximum diameter. *s*, splenic vein; *l*, left renal vein; *i*, inferior vena cava; *g*, gastroduodenal artery; *A*, aorta. **b:** Scans in liver parenchyma demonstrate mild dilatation of intrahepatic bile ducts (*d*). *p*, portal vein branch. **c:** Duplex Doppler examination confirms that posterior tubular structure (cursor) is a portal vein branch. *Arrows*, velocity spectrum of blood flow in portal vein.

c

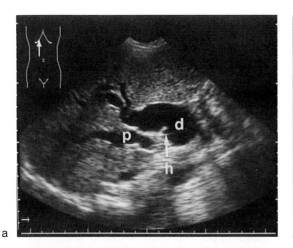

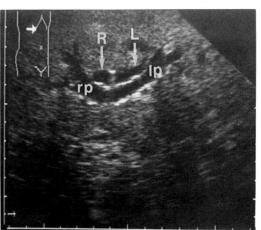

a

b

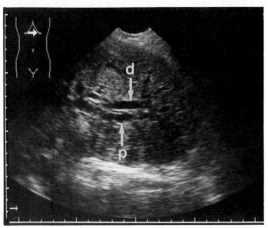

FIG. 4.9. Obstructive jaundice with massive dilatation of bile ducts. **a:** Sagittal scan demonstrates gross dilatation of the extrahepatic bile duct (*d*), measuring 35-mm maximum diameter. *p*, portal vein branch; *h*, right hepatic artery. **b:** Transverse scan demonstrates dilatation of right (*R*) and left (*L*) hepatic ducts. *rp*, right portal vein; *lp*, left portal vein. **c:** Moderately severe dilatation of intrahepatic hepatic bile ducts is present (*d*). This intrahepatic bile duct measures 8 mm in diameter. *p*, portal vein branch.

c

TABLE 4.4. *Causes of bile duct obstruction*

Source	No. of patients	Stones (%)	Neoplasm (%)	Pancreatitis (%)	Other (%)
Koenigsberg et al., 1979 (36)	32	25	59	9	7
Salem and Vas, 1981 (39)	66	42	49	3	6
Haubek et al., 1981 (35)	44	27	57	7	9
Baron et al., 1982 (34)	47	19	56	4	21
Laing et al., 1986 (2)	110	37	18	27	18
Gibson et al., 1986 (38)	65	5	86	2	7

4.7). A positive test (i.e., common duct increased by ≥2 mm) always indicated partial common duct obstruction (7). The test sensitivity was 74% in partial obstruction, and the specificity was 100%.

Simeone et al. (20) recommended the use of a fatty meal in the following circumstances:

1. mildly dilated common duct (7–11 mm), asymptomatic, normal chemistry
2. ultrasound normal, asymptomatic, chemistry abnormal (e.g., raised alkaline phosphatase)
3. ultrasound normal, right upper quadrant symptoms suggestive of biliary obstruction (especially postcholecystectomy), normal chemistry.

Obstructing Lesions

The commonest causes of biliary obstruction are choledocholithiasis and neoplasms of the pancreas and porta hepatis (Table 4.4) (2,34–39). In most published series, neoplasms are the most common etiology, whereas in one series (2), choledocholithiasis was the most common etiology.

Ultrasound Accuracy in Assessing the Presence, Level, and Cause of Obstruction

Because ultrasound can visualize the intrahepatic bile ducts and the extrahepatic bile duct in virtually every patient, the accuracy in detecting biliary dilatation is very high. In the jaundiced patient, the accuracy of ultrasound in distinguishing between obstructive and nonobstructive jaundice exceeds 90% (33). In the nonjaundiced patient suspected of having bile duct obstruction, the bile duct diameter alone is less accurate in predicting the presence or absence of obstruction, but the ductal size is still a useful test in assessing this group of patients. The accuracy of bile duct size alone in these patients is greater than 80% (34–36).

Earlier ultrasound studies regarding the level and cause of biliary obstruction reported a wide range of accuracies (Table 4.5) (34–37). Koenigsberg et al. (36) in 1979 reported 95% accuracy for the level of obstruction and 81% for the cause. Haubek et al. (35) in 1981 re-

ported 94% accuracy for the level of obstruction and 68% for the cause. In 1982, Baron et al. (34) reported 60% accuracy for the level and 38% for the cause. In 1983, Honickman et al. (37) reported 27% accuracy for the level and 23% for the cause.

More recent studies (2,38) demonstrated quite high accuracies for ultrasound in determining the level and cause of biliary obstruction (see Table 4.5). Laing et al. (2) in 1986 reported 92% accuracy for the level and 71% for the cause. Gibson et al. (38) in 1986 reported 95% accuracy for the level and 88% for the cause. It is clear that the accuracy in a given setting will depend heavily on the quality of the ultrasound machines, the clinical ultrasound expertise, the scanning techniques (2), and the types of patients seen in the clinical practice.

The accuracy is higher when the obstructions are due to tumors in the porta hepatis (38) and lower for choledocholithiasis. The ultrasound technique is extremely important in assessing the level and cause of obstruction. Laing et al. (2) used a technique that optimizes ultrasound accuracy (see above).

TABLE 4.5. *Accuracy of ultrasound in determining the level and cause of bile duct obstruction*

Study	Level of obstruction (%)	Cause of obstruction (%)
Koenigsberg et al., 1979 (36)	95	81
Haubek et al., 1981 (35)	94	68
Baron et al., 1982 (34)	60	38
Honickman et al., 1983 (37)	27	23
Laing et al., 1986 (2)[a]	92	71
Gibson et al., 1986 (38)[b]	95	88

[a] In 91%, the level of obstruction was in the pancreatic head. Causes for obstruction were choledocholithiasis 37.3%, pancreatitis 27.3%, neoplasm 19.1%, stricture 6.4%, undetermined 5.5%, postcholecystectomy 3.6%, and sclerosing cholangitis 0.9%.
[b] The level of obstruction was divided into 2 groups and not 3 as Laing et al. (2) defined. The *hilar group* included obstruction of the proximal 2 cm of the common hepatic duct or the right and left hepatic ducts. The *nonhilar group* included obstructions more than 2 cm distal to the confluence. In 61.5%, the obstruction was hilar and in 38.5% nonhilar. Causes for obstruction were choledocholithiasis 4.6%, pancreatitis 1.5%, neoplasm 86.2%, sclerosing cholangitis 1.5%, choledochal cyst 3%, and Mirizzi syndrome 3%.

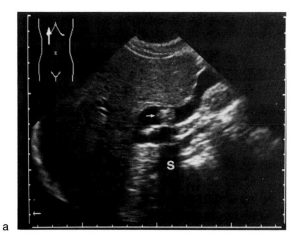

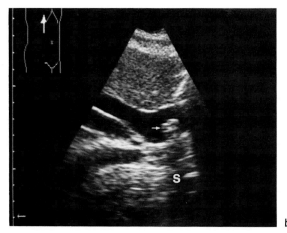

a   b

FIG. 4.10. Nonobstructing calculus in common duct. **a:** Sagittal scan of proximal common duct demonstrates a nonobstructing calculus (*arrow*) with posterior acoustic shadowing (*s*). Notice small amount of fluid between calculus and anterior wall of dilated bile duct. **b:** With patient in left lateral decubitus position, calculus (*arrow*) moved into distal common bile duct, which is larger than proximal duct. Maximum bile duct diameter was 19 mm. *s*, posterior acoustic shadowing.

Choledocholithiasis

In most published series, calculi are the second most common cause of bile duct obstruction after neoplasms (see Table 4.4). Choledocholithiasis may coexist with stones in the gallbladder, or they may be diagnosed after cholecystectomy (retained stone or newly formed stone). The calculus may reside anywhere in the biliary tree, but most calculi cause obstruction at the level of the pancreatic head (2). Therefore complete ultrasound examination of the distal common bile duct with optimal scanning technique is of paramount importance in detecting choledocholithiasis (see above for scanning techniques).

Calculi vary greatly in size, and they may be nonobstructive, intermittently obstructive, or impacted in the distal common bile duct (Figs. 4.10–4.12). When a calculus is free within an enlarged bile duct, the diagnosis is straightforward (Fig. 4.13), whereas an impacted calculus in the pancreatic head is more difficult to perceive because the calculus is surrounded by echogenic solid tissue and the tissue differentiation is reduced. In addition, the pancreatic head is more difficult to visualize than the proximal common duct because of overlying bowel. If one uses optimal scanning techniques (2), this difficulty is minimized. If a small calculus is present in a nondilated duct, the diagnosis is difficult (Fig. 4.14). In a series by Cronan et al. (40), 36% of patients with choledocholithiasis had normal-sized bile ducts; in a series by Laing and Jeffrey (41), 30% had normal-sized ducts.

Early studies indicated that ultrasound had a low sensitivity in detecting choledocholithiasis, ranging from 11% to 25% (40–44). With improved real-time ultrasound technology and optimal scanning techniques of the intrapancreatic portion of the common duct (1,2), the sensitivity has increased to levels between 55% and 80% (1,2,45). The sensitivity is lower for nondilated ducts versus dilated ducts and is lower for stones in the intrapancreatic bile duct versus the proximal duct (1). The CT sensitivity with optimal scanning techniques exceeds 80% (42,46). ERCP remains the most accurate imaging method in the assessment of choledocholithiasis.

Intrahepatic duct calculi are uncommon in the West. However, in Japan, China, Korea, and Southeast Asia, symptomatic intrahepatic duct calculi are quite common (47). These calculi may be a sequela of infestation by *Chlonorchis sinensis* (Chinese liver fluke) and *Ascaris lumbricoides* (roundworm).

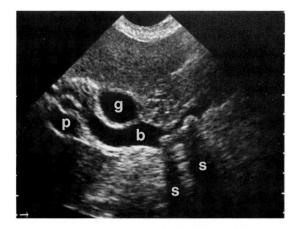

FIG. 4.11. Multiple nonobstructing calculi in bile duct. Scan demonstrates several calculi associated with posterior acoustic shadowing (*s*) in distal common bile duct (*b*). Notice fluid between calculi and anterior wall of distal common bile duct. *p*, right portal vein; *g*, gallbladder neck.

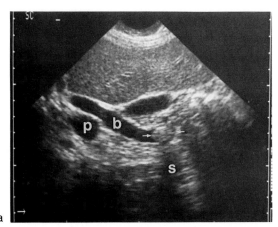
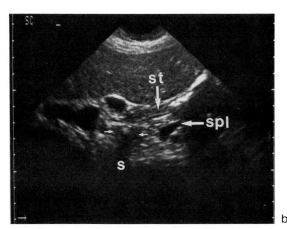

FIG. 4.12. Calculus impacted in distal common bile duct. **a:** Calculus (*arrows*) is impacted in distal common bile duct (*b*). Note that there is no fluid distal to calculus nor between calculus and walls of bile duct. *s*, shadowing posterior to calculus; *p*, pancreas. **b:** Transverse scan [same patient as (*a*)] through distal common bile duct is difficult to interpret in absence of visible fluid in bile duct. However, calculus (*arrows*) was visualized, associated with posterior acoustic shadowing (*s*). *st*, stomach; *spl*, splenic vein.

Biliary Neoplasms

Cholangiocarcinoma is the most common primary biliary neoplasm, but it ranks behind pancreatic neoplasms, choledocholithiasis, and portal lymphadenopathy in causing bile duct obstruction. Cholangiocarcinoma is usually an adenocarcinoma arising from bile duct epithelial cells, and it may arise in any portion of the intrahepatic or extrahepatic biliary tree. About one half of cases arise at the ductal bifurcation (Klatskin tumor) or distal common bile duct, resulting in dilated bile ducts in both hepatic lobes. If the tumor arises in the right or left hepatic ducts, dilated ducts will be present in only one lobe. If the tumor arises in the periphery of the liver, a focal solid liver mass may be the presenting ultrasound finding.

Most tumors are the infiltrating type, causing diffuse annular thickening of the bile duct wall [78% in the series by Choi et al. (48)], whereas a small number are the exophytic and polypoid type. In cases of Klatskin tumors (cholangiocarcinoma arising at the confluence of the left and right hepatic ducts), the most common ultrasound finding is dilated intrahepatic bile ducts, a normal-sized extrahepatic bile duct, and no visible obstructive lesion. Ultrasound may occasionally depict the infiltrating (Fig. 4.15) or exophytic type of primary tumor and perhaps portal lymph node metastases. If the tumor is polypoidal inside the duct, ultrasound is more sensitive in visualizing the tumor (Fig. 4.16) (48,49).

Ultrasound findings similar to cholangiocarcinoma can be seen in other pathologies, and distinction may be difficult: benign stricture, portal lymph node metastases, proximal spread of more distant neoplasm (e.g., pancreatic carcinoma) (Figs. 4.17–4.19).

Biliary cystadenomas and cystadenocarcinomas are rare cystic neoplasms that usually manifest at ultrasound as multiseptated intrahepatic cystic masses.

Pancreatic carcinoma is the most frequent cause of neoplastic obstruction. It is discussed in Chapter 7.

Other Obstructing Lesions

Various other lesions may obstruct the bile ducts: benign stricture, metastases to portal lymph nodes (carci-

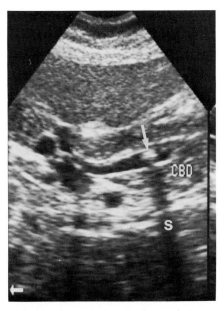

FIG. 4.13. Nonobstructing calculus in normal-sized bile duct. Longitudinal scan of distal common bile duct demonstrates a small calculus (*arrow*) associated with distal acoustic shadowing (*s*). Bile duct was normal in caliber, and calculus was observed to move within bile duct. There was no clinical evidence of obstruction.

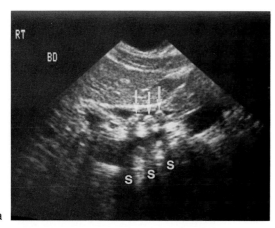 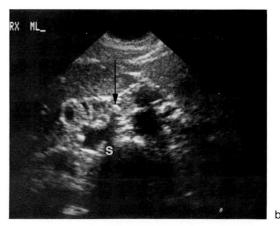

FIG. 4.14. Multiple calculi in nonobstructed bile duct. **a:** Sagittal scan of distal bile duct demonstrates 3 calculi (*arrows*) associated with posterior acoustic shadowing (*s*). Calculi were difficult to visualize because bile duct was small and contained very little fluid. These are nonobstructing calculi. **b:** Transverse scan through distal bile duct demonstrates one of calculi (*arrow*) associated with distal acoustic shadowing (*s*). It was very difficult to appreciate presence of a stone in transverse scan because there was so little fluid within bile duct at this level.

noma, lymphoma), direct spread of tumor (e.g., pancreatic carcinoma, gallbladder carcinoma, hepatocellular carcinoma), pancreatitis, Mirizzi syndrome. Benign strictures are not usually visualized with ultrasound. They present as dilatation of proximal ducts and normal-sized distal ducts and thus can be difficult to distinguish from infiltrating cholangiocarcinoma. Lymph node metastases manifest as multiple discrete hypoechoic masses (Figs. 4.17 and 4.18), but small nodes with reactive fibrosis may be missed by ultrasound. Direct spread of tumor into the porta hepatis may distort the anatomy and make interpretation impossible. Mirizzi syndrome is the extrinsic compression of the common hepatic duct by calculi and inflammation in the gallbladder neck or cystic duct. Ultrasound demonstrates dilated intrahepatic ducts, stones in the cystic duct or gallbladder neck, and a normal-sized distal common bile duct (50).

Cholangitis

Infectious Cholangitis

Intermittent cholangitis consisting of biliary colic, jaundice and fever and chills occurs with intermittent

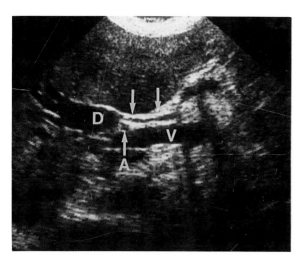

FIG. 4.15. Carcinoma of common bile duct. Walls of common bile duct are thickened (*arrows*), and there is proximal dilatation of bile duct (*D*). *v*, inferior vena cava; *A*, right hepatic artery. (Scan is courtesy of Dr. Peter Cooperberg, Chief of Radiology, St. Paul's Hospital, Vancouver, Canada.)

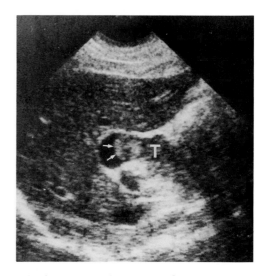

FIG. 4.16. Carcinoma of bile duct. Scan demonstrates an intraluminal solid tumor (*T*) filling common duct. Tumor extends into proximal common hepatic ducts (*arrows*) and causes dilatation of bile ducts proximal to tumor.

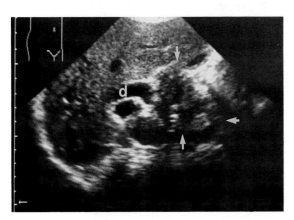

FIG. 4.17. Gastric carcinoma with portal lymph node metastases. Irregular solid masses (*arrows*) are present in porta hepatis, causing obstruction in proximal extrahepatic bile duct (*d*).

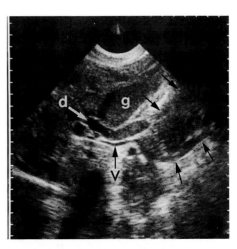

FIG. 4.18. Lymphoma obstructing bile duct. A large solid mass (*arrows*) is present in position of head of pancreas, causing obstruction to distal bile duct (*d*). Note echogenic material in bile duct and in gallbladder (*g*). Echogenic material is sludge secondary to biliary stasis. *v*, inferior vena cava.

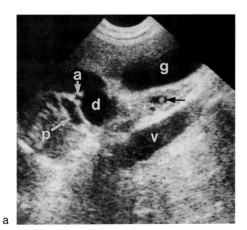

a

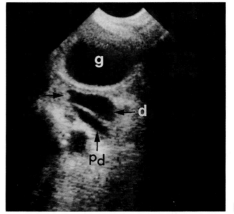

b

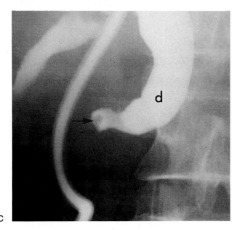

c

FIG. 4.19. Villous adenoma of ampulla of Vater. **a:** Scan through inferior vena cava (*v*) demonstrates a small solid nodule (*arrow*) surrounded by fluid in pancreatic head. There is gross dilatation of extrahepatic bile duct (*d*). *g*, gallbladder; *a*, right hepatic artery; *p*, portal vein. **b:** Transverse scan through pancreatic head demonstrates small solid nodule (*arrow*) causing obstruction and dilatation of pancreatic duct (*pd*) and distal common bile duct (*d*). *g*, gallbladder. **c:** T-tube cholangiogram. Small solid mass (*arrow*) is seen at distal end of common bile duct (*d*), which is grossly dilated.

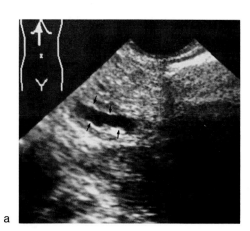
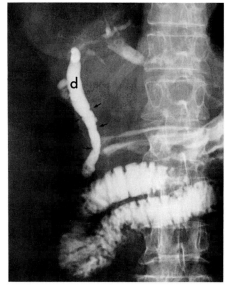

a   b

FIG. 4.20. Sclerosing cholangitis. **a:** Sagittal scan of extrahepatic bile duct demonstrates irregularity of contour of bile duct walls (*arrows*). **b:** Transhepatic cholangiogram demonstrates opacification of common duct (*d*). Note marginal irregularities of contrast column, corresponding to irregularities in ultrasound scan.

bile duct obstruction caused by choledocholithiasis. With complete obstruction, ductal contents may become purulent, and the clinical manifestations of sepsis will overshadow those of cholestasis. Ultrasound demonstrates dilated bile ducts and possibly echogenic bile, gas in the bile ducts, and/or thickened bile duct walls.

Sclerosing Cholangitis

Primary sclerosing cholangitis is a rare condition of unknown etiology consisting of nonbacterial chronic inflammatory narrowing of the bile ducts. The peak incidence is 20 to 40 years of age. It is more common in males (M:F=3:1). About one third of cases are associated with ulcerative colitis or regional enteritis, retroperitoneal fibrosis, or Riedel's thyroiditis. Ultrasound demonstrates widespread segmental and variable bile duct dilation throughout the biliary tree caused by multiple bile duct strictures. Thickening of the bile duct walls may also be visualized (Figs. 4.20 and 4.21). Only the very rare diffuse form of cholangiocarcinoma would give similar appearances to sclerosing cholangitis.

Secondary sclerosing cholangitis results from previous infection, choledocholithiasis, carcinoma, or previous surgery.

Oriental Cholangiohepatitis (Synonym: recurrent pyogenic cholangitis)

Oriental cholangiohepatitis is uncommon in North America but is endemic in areas of China, Japan, Indo-

nesia, and South Africa. It is characterized by biliary infestation with *Chlonorchis sinensis* or *Ascaris lumbricoides* and infection with *Escherichia coli,* resulting in strictures, biliary sludge, and multiple soft pigmented stones. At presentation, ultrasound demonstrates a massively dilated extrahepatic bile duct (up to 4-cm diameter) and dilated intrahepatic ducts together with intraductal calculi and debris (51). The calculi may be difficult to visualize because of their soft friable nature (52).

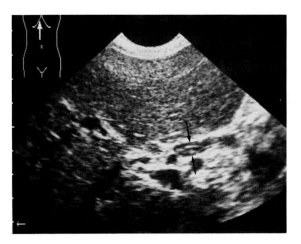

FIG. 4.21. Sclerosing cholangitis. Note diffuse thickening of walls of common duct (*arrows*). There is a very small fluid-filled lumen remaining between endothelial surfaces of bile duct wall.

AIDS-Related Cholangitis

Acalculous inflammation of the bile ducts may occur in patients with acquired immunodeficiency syndrome (AIDS), probably caused by cytomegalovirus or *Cryptosporidium* infection. The bile duct abnormalities are indistinguishable from sclerosing cholangitis and consist of bile duct strictures, multiple focal biliary dilatation, and thickening of bile duct walls (53).

Congenital Abnormalities

Biliary Atresia

Biliary atresia consists of obliteration of some or all the extrahepatic bile duct, and it may be caused by *in utero* infection (54). Biliary atresia (which can be treated surgically with biliary enteric bypass) presents in the neonatal period as cholestatic jaundice, and it can be difficult to distinguish from neonatal hepatitis (which is treated medically). Unfortunately the ultrasound features of both diseases are similar. In biliary atresia, the intrahepatic and extrahepatic bile ducts are normal in size, the liver parenchyma is normal or hyperechoic, and the gallbladder is absent or small (<1.5-cm diameter) in 90% of cases (55). In neonatal hepatitis, the liver parenchyma is normal or hyperechoic, the intrahepatic and extrahepatic bile ducts are normal in size, and the gallbladder is large, normal, small, or nonvisualized. If the gallbladder contracts after a feeding, this suggests a patent bile duct and thus biliary atresia would be unlikely (56).

Biliary isotope scanning may be more useful. In biliary atresia, there is prompt uptake by the liver parenchyma but no excretion into the gut. In neonatal hepatitis, there is poor uptake by the liver parenchyma, but there is some excretion into the bowel.

Caroli's Disease

Caroli's disease is a rare congenital abnormality (autosomal recessive) associated with cystic dilatation of multiple intrahepatic ducts. In one type there is quite marked tubular and saccular dilation of the intrahepatic ducts, which is usually accompanied by intraductal calculi and infection. In the other type, there is less severe ductal dilatation, but there is associated portal hypertension and hepatic fibrosis. The ultrasound examination usually demonstrates multiple dilated intrahepatic bile ducts (tubular and saccular dilatation). Debris and calculi may be visualized within the ducts.

Choledochal Cyst

A choledochal cyst is focal dilatation of the extrahepatic bile duct, which becomes clinically manifest be-

tween 1 and 10 years of age. The classic clinical presentation is jaundice, abdominal pain, and a palpable abdominal mass, although many patients lack one or more of these findings. It occurs more commonly in girls (F:M=4:1) (57). It may be caused by an anomalous pancreatic-biliary junction, which allows reflux of pancreatic enzymes into the bile duct. Three major types of cyst occur: type I, which is concentric dilatation of the common bile duct; type II, which is a diverticulum or asymmetric bulging of the common bile duct; and type III, which is a choledochocele (most uncommon) (58). Ultrasound demonstrates a cyst in the porta hepatis separate from the gallbladder (Figs. 4.22 and 4.23) (59). In some patients the central intrahepatic ducts are dilated. Biliary isotope scanning demonstrates filling of the cyst and subsequent emptying into the gut.

A choledochal cyst may present in the neonatal period, and this may be a separate entity from the choledochal cyst that presents in childhood. The neonate presents with jaundice, a cystic mass, and atresia of the distal common bile duct. Nuclear medicine demonstrates accumulation of bile in the cyst but no excretion into the bowel (60).

Perforation of the Common Duct

Spontaneous perforation of the extrahepatic bile duct presents in the first 3 months of life with jaundice and ascites. The cause is unclear but may be related to an increase in intraductal pressure caused by some obstructive phenomenon associated with a congenital weakness of the wall at the junction of the cystic duct and common hepatic duct. Ultrasound demonstrates generalized ascites and occasionally a loculated fluid collection in the porta hepatis (61,62).

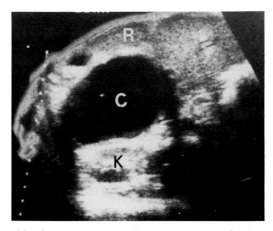

FIG. 4.22. Choledochal cyst. Transverse scan of right upper quadrant in a 5-year-old girl who presented with jaundice. There is a large fluid-filled structure that was a choledochal cyst (*C*) interposed between right hepatic bulb (*R*) and right kidney (*K*). (Scan is courtesy of Dr. David Martin, Department of Radiology, Children's Hospital of Eastern Ontario, Ottawa, Canada.)

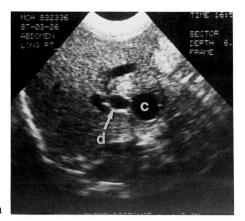
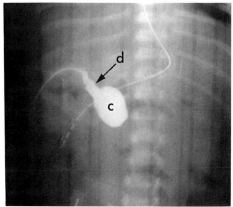

FIG. 4.23. Choledochal cyst. **a:** Longitudinal scan in right upper quadrant demonstrates a small- to moderate-sized choledochal cyst (*c*) at distal end of common bile duct (*d*). **b:** Intraoperative cholangiogram demonstrates choledochal cyst (*c*) presenting as a focal dilatation of distal common bile duct (*d*). (Scan and radiograph are courtesy of Dr. S. Jecquier from Montreal Children's Hospital, Montreal, Canada.)

4.4 POSTOPERATIVE BILIARY TRACT

Biliary Colic Postcholecystectomy

In the presence of biliary colic and jaundice postcholecystectomy, ultrasound is useful to distinguish between obstructive versus nonobstructive jaundice. Ultrasound is also useful but less sensitive in detecting the cause of obstruction. With biliary colic and no jaundice, ultrasound is less useful in detecting the cause of pain. A retained calculus in a nondilated common duct can be visualized in some cases, but in many cases it is missed. ERCP is the imaging test of choice in this situation.

After cholecystectomy 5% to 60% of patients experience persistent upper abdominal pain, and this is called the postcholecystectomy syndrome. Ampullary stenosis with or without choledocholithiasis is a major cause for the syndrome. Zeman et al. (63) showed that hepatobiliary scintigraphy is a good noninvasive technique for differentiating biliary obstruction from other causes of pain in the postcholecystectomy patient.

Biliary-Enteric Anastomosis

A spontaneous fistula may form between the biliary tree and bowel secondary to cholelithiasis and chronic cholecystitis. The gallstone erodes through the walls into the bowel lumen. Gas in the bile ducts is the main ultrasound finding. The gas manifests as linear echogenic foci that may shadow, not shadow, or have a "ring-down" artifact behind them (Fig. 4.24).

With previous surgical anastomosis, nuclear medicine is more useful in assessing patency of the anastomosis, although ultrasound can be useful as well. Gas in the bile ducts implies patency. If the common duct is visible, it should be normal size and often contains debris or gas if the anastomosis is patent. If the common duct contains echo-free fluid or is dilated, obstruction of the anastomosis is suspected (Fig. 4.25).

A common surgical cause for biliary air is a previous sphincterotomy. If the gallbladder is still in place and there is gas within the bile ducts, one must ask about previous sphincterotomy before assuming that the gas is due to a biliary-enteric fistula.

4.5 PITFALLS, ARTIFACTS, AND PRACTICAL TIPS

Pseudo Calculi

The right hepatic artery often indents the proximal common duct, and this may simulate an intraductal calculus. Scanning in the long axis of the artery and using Doppler will confirm the normal anatomy. Surgical clips adjacent to the bile duct from previous cholecystectomy may be mistaken for intraductal calculi or gas (Fig. 4.26). When in doubt, obtain a plain radiograph. Similarly, bowel gas beside the bile duct, especially when the duct is tortuous, can give the appearance of a calculus in the common duct. One avoids this pitfall by following the course of the duct carefully and observing the echogenic focus for evidence of movement or peristalsis. Gas within the bile duct may also simulate a calculus by demonstrating an echogenic focus with distal shadowing. The diagnosis is usually clarified by demonstration of movement of the gas, appearance of "ring-down" artifact behind the echogenic focus, or the presence of multiple foci of gas within the biliary tree (Fig. 4.24).

Pseudo Bile Ducts

Occasionally the common duct becomes massively dilated and the anatomy in the porta hepatis becomes dis-

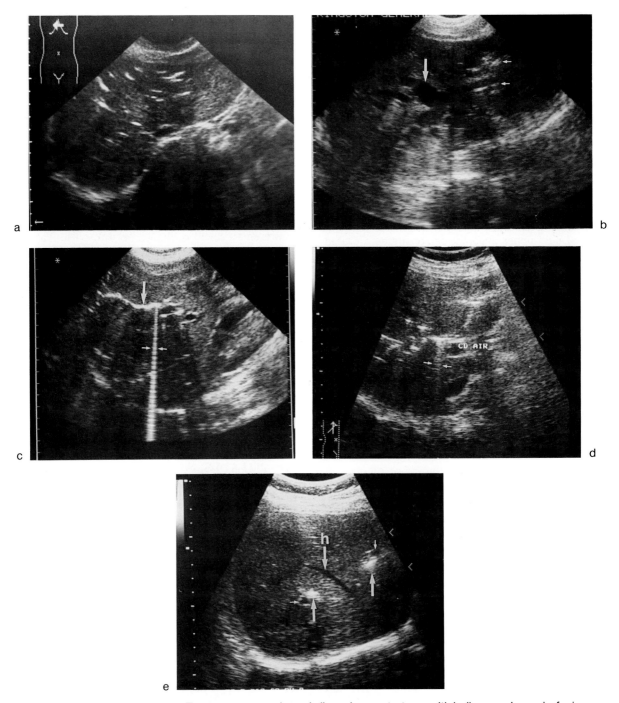

FIG. 4.24. Biliary gas. **a:** Transverse scan through liver demonstrates multiple linear echogenic foci representing gas in intrahepatic bile ducts. No definite posterior shadows nor ring-down artifact is identified. **b:** Transverse scan through liver in another patient demonstrates marked dilatation of right intrahepatic bile duct (*large arrow*). Left intrahepatic bile ducts are nondilated and filled with air (*smaller arrows*). Right hepatic duct is obstructed, and left hepatic duct is anastomosed to bowel. **c:** Strong ring-down artifacts (*smaller arrows*) are posterior to intrahepatic biliary gas, which manifests as hyperechoic linear foci (*larger arrow*). **d:** Air in common duct has a weak posterior ring-down artifact (*arrows*). **e:** Hyperechoic collections of gas (*larger arrows*) are noted within bile ducts, which lie immediately adjacent to portal vein branches (*smaller arrows*). Bile ducts and portal vein branches course together in liver parenchyma. *h*, hepatic vein.

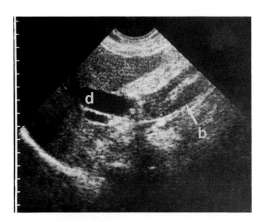

FIG. 4.25. Obstructed biliary-enteric anastomosis. Longitudinal scan of right upper quadrant demonstrates a dilated fluid-filled common duct (*d*). Bile duct is anastomosed to a loop of bowel (*b*) in right upper quadrant. Bile duct should be smaller, and it should contain gas if anastomosis is patent.

torted. The enlarged bile duct may be mistaken for a prominent portal vein and the smaller portal vein for the bile duct. Doppler ultrasound quickly resolves the anatomy. A prominent hepatic artery may be mistaken for the common hepatic duct and prominent intrahepatic hepatic arterial branches for mildly dilated intrahepatic bile ducts. Doppler ultrasound in this case will also resolve the problem.

Pseudo Biliary Gas

Occasionally intrahepatic arterial calcification is extensive enough to simulate biliary gas. Both appear as linear hyperechoic foci that may or may not have weak posterior shadowing (64). Plain radiographs will distinguish between these two possibilities.

Portal venous gas manifests as multiple linear intrahepatic hyperechoic foci and may mimic biliary air (see Chapter 5). Classically portal venous gas resides in the periphery of the liver near the liver capsule and biliary gas more centrally, but the patterns may overlap (65). Portal venous gas usually arises because of bowel ischemia.

Other Intraductal Abnormalities

Echogenic material inside the bile ducts commonly represents a calculus, sludge, or tumor. Blunt abdominal trauma and surgical procedures can traumatize the bile ducts with bleeding into the ducts. Ultrasound will demonstrate echogenic material in the common duct (Fig. 4.27), and this resembles sludge (Fig. 4.18). If blood is suspected, further investigations are required to identify the cause and site of the bleeding (Fig. 4.27).

A drainage tube inside the common duct manifests as two parallel lines inside the common duct (Fig. 4.28).

Practical Tips

To assess the bile ducts optimally with ultrasound, the techniques described by Laing et al. (2) probably give the best results. Begin by scanning the distal common bile duct in the transverse plane with the patient in the semi-upright position turned toward the right. If necessary, 6 to 12 oz of water may be swallowed by the patient to create a scanning window through the gastric antrum.

To visualize the proximal extrahepatic bile duct opti-

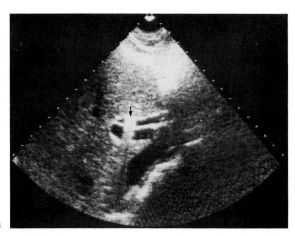
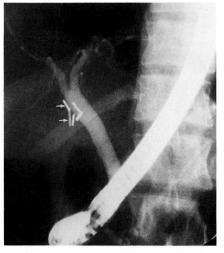

a   b

FIG. 4.26. Metallic clips simulating biliary gas. **a:** Longitudinal scan in right upper quadrant demonstrates an echogenic focus (*arrow*) with posterior ring-down artifact. Appearances suggest gas in bile duct. **b:** Radiograph demonstrates 5 metallic surgical clips (*arrows*) immediately adjacent to contrast-filled bile duct.

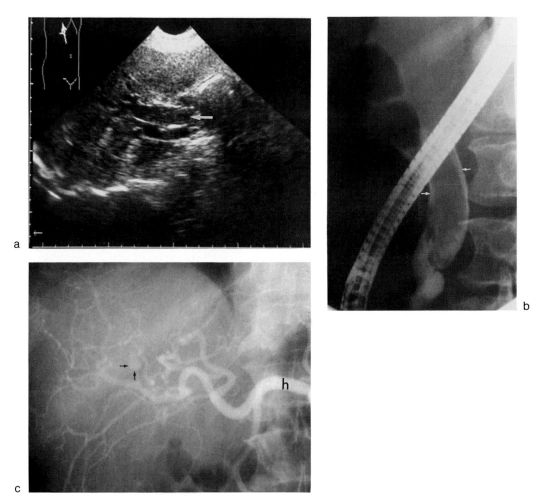

FIG. 4.27. Hemobilia. **a:** Longitudinal scan of proximal common duct demonstrates multiple low-level echoes (*arrow*) within distended bile duct. **b:** ERCP examination demonstrates a filling defect within common bile duct. Note contrast material (*arrows*) between filling defect and walls of the duct. **c:** Celiac angiogram demonstrates opacification of common hepatic artery (*h*). This study demonstrates active extravasation of contrast material (*arrows*) from intrahepatic arteries. This patient had recent blunt abdominal trauma, and angiogram demonstrates source of hemobilia.

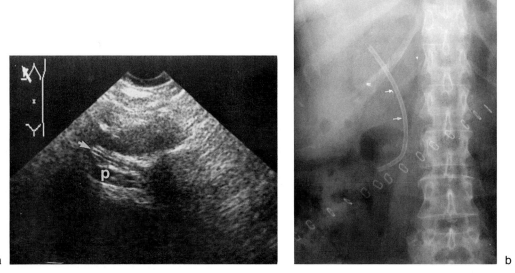

FIG. 4.28. Intrabiliary stent tube. **a:** Longitudinal scan of common duct demonstrates a tube (*arrow*) within nondistended bile duct, which lies anterior to portal vein (*p*). **b:** Radiograph of same patient demonstrates stent tube (*arrows*) extending from porta hepatis down into pancreatic head.

mally, the patient lies flat, turned toward the left side to use the liver as a scanning window. At this position the intrahepatic ducts may be assessed as well.

If the radiologist is not sure of the finding or the diagnosis, he or she must acknowledge this and suggest what further should be performed to assess the biliary tract. For example, if the radiologist demonstrates dilated bile ducts but is not absolutely sure of the cause of obstruction, he or she must pursue this with suggestions as to how the definitive diagnosis can be made.

REFERENCES

Scanning Techniques

1. Laing FC, Jeffrey RB, Wing VW. Improved visualization of choledocholithiasis by sonography. *AJR* 1984;143:949–952.
2. Laing FC, Jeffrey RB, Wing VW, Nyberg DA. Biliary dilatation: defining the level and cause by real-time US. *Radiology* 1986;160:39–42.

Normal Anatomy

3. Brett PN, de Stempel JV, Atri M, Lough JO, Illescas FF. Intrahepatic bile duct and portal vein anatomy revisited. *Radiology* 1988;169:405–407.
4. Lim JH, Ryu KN, Ko YTK, Lee DH. Anatomic relationship of intrahepatic bile ducts to portal veins. *J Ultrasound Med* 1990;9:137–143.
5. Sauerbrei E. Ultrasound of the common bile duct. In: Sanders RC, Hill M, eds. *Ultrasound annual 1983.* New York: Raven Press; 1983:1–46.
6. Lynn JA. Physiology of the extrahepatic biliary tree. In: Wright R, Alberti KGMM, Karran S, Millward-Sadler GH, eds. *Liver and biliary disease: pathophysiology, diagnosis, management.* London, Philadelphia: Saunders; 1979:228–232.
7. Darweesh RMA, Dodds WJ, Hogan WJ, et al. Fatty-meal sonography for evaluating patients with suspected partial common duct obstruction. *AJR* 1988;151:63–68.
8. Fein AB, Rauch RF II, Bowie JD, Halvorson RA Jr, Rosenberg ER. Intravenous cholecystokinin octapeptide: its effect on the sonographic appearance of the bile ducts in normal subjects. *Radiology* 1984;153:499–501.
9. Raptopoulos V, Smith EH, Karellas A, Miranda DK, Tefft CA. Daytime constancy of bile duct diameter. *AJR* 1987;148:557–558.
10. Jacobson JB, Brodey PA. The transverse common duct. *AJR* 1981;136:91–95.
11. Cooperberg PL. High-resolution real-time ultrasound in the evaluation of the normal and obstructed biliary tract. *Radiology* 1978;129:477–480.
12. Dewbury KC. Visualization of normal biliary ducts with ultrasound. *Br J Radiol* 1980;53:774–780.
13. Bruneton JN, Roux P, Fenart D, Caramella E, Occelli JP. Ultrasound evaluation of common bile duct size in normal adult patients and following cholecystectomy. A report of 750 cases. *Eur J Radiol* 1981;1:171–172.
13a. Sample WF, Sarti DA, Goldstein LI, Weiner M, Kadell BM. Gray-scale ultrasonography of the jaundiced patient. *Radiology* 1978;128:719–725.
14. Niederau C, Müller J, Sonnenberg A, et al. Extrahepatic bile ducts in healthy subjects, in patients with cholelithiasis, and in post cholecystectomy patients: a prospective ultrasonic study. *JCU* 1983;11:23–27.
15. Wolson AH. Common bile duct measurements. In: Kurtz A, Goldberg BB, eds. *Atlas of ultrasound measurements.* New York: Raven Press; 1990:102–107.

16. Bressler EL, Rubin JM, McCracken S. Sonographic parallel channel sign: a reappraisal. *Radiology* 1987;164:343–346.
17. Mintz MC, Grumbach K, Arger PH, Coleman BG. Sonographic evaluation of bile duct size during pregnancy. *AJR* 1985;145:575–578.
18. Wu C-C, Ho Y-H, Chen C-Y. Effect of aging on common bile duct diameter: a real-time ultrasonographic study. *JCU* 1984;12:473–478.
19. Siegel MJ. Liver and biliary tract. In: Siegel MJ, ed. *Pediatric sonography.* New York: Raven Press; 1991:115–160.
20. Simeone JF, Butch RJ, Mueller PR, et al. The bile ducts after a fatty meal: further sonographic observations. *Radiology* 1985;154:763–768.
21. Willson SA, Gosink BB, van Sonnenberg E. Unchanged size of a dilated common duct after a fatty meal: results and significance. *Radiology* 1986;160:29–31.
22. Wedmann B, Börsch G, Coenen C, Paassen A. Effect of cholecystectomy on common bile duct diameter: a longitudinal prospective ultrasonographic study. *JCU* 1988;16:619–624.
23. Graham MF, Cooperberg PL, Cohen MM, Burhenne HJ. The size of the normal common hepatic duct following cholecystectomy: an ultrasonographic study. *Radiology* 1980;135:137–139.
24. Mueller PR, Ferrucci JT Jr, Simeone JF, et al. Postcholecystectomy bile duct dilatation: myth or reality? *AJR* 1981;136:355–358.
25. Chang VH, Cunningham JJ, Fromkes JJ. Sonographic measurement of the extrahepatic bile duct before and after retrograde cholangiography. *AJR* 1985;144:753–755.
26. Sauerbrei EE, Cooperberg PL, Gordon P, Li D, Cohen MM, Burhenne HJ. The discrepancy between radiographic and sonographic bile duct measurements. *Radiology* 1980;137:751–755.

Pathology

27. Klingensmith WC III, Johnson ML, Kuni CC, Dunne MG, Fritzberg AR. Complementary role of Tc-99m-diethyl-IDA and ultrasound in large and small duct biliary obstruction. *Radiology* 1981;138:177–184.
28. Zeman RK, Taylor KJW, Rosenfield AT, Schwartz A, Gold JA. Acute experimental biliary obstruction in the dog: sonographic findings and clinical implications. *AJR* 1981;136:965–967.
29. Klingensmith WC III, Whitney WP, Spitzer VM, Klintmalm GB, Koep LM, Kuni CC. Effect of complete biliary-tract obstruction on serial hepatobiliary imaging in an experimental model: concise communication. *J Nucl Med* 1981;22:866–868.
30. Shawker TH, Jones BL, Girton ME. Distal common bile duct obstruction: an experimental study in monkeys. *JCU* 1981;9:77–82.
31. Zeman RK, Taylor KJW, Burrell MI, Gold J. Ultrasound demonstration of anicteric dilatation of the biliary tree. *Radiology* 1980;34:689–692.
32. Graham MF, Cooperberg PL, Cohen MM, Burhenne HJ. Ultrasonographic screening of the common hepatic duct in symptomatic patients after cholecystectomy. *Radiology* 1981;138:137–139.
33. Ferrucci JT, Adson MA, Mueller PR, Stanley RJ, Stewart ET. Advances in the radiology of jaundice: a symposium and review. *AJR* 1983;141:1–20.
34. Baron RL, Stanley RJ, Lee JKT, et al. A prospective comparison of the evaluation of biliary obstruction using computed tomography and ultrasonography. *Radiology* 1982;145:91–98.
35. Haubek A, Pedersen JH, Burcharth E, Gammelgaard J, Hancke S, Willumsen L. Dynamic sonography in the evaluation of jaundice. *AJR* 1981;136:1071–1074.
36. Koenigsberg M, Wiener SN, Walzer A. The accuracy of sonography in the differential diagnosis of obstructive jaundice: a comparison with cholangiography. *Radiology* 1979;133:157–165.
37. Honickman SP, Mueller PR, Wittenberg J, et al. Ultrasound in obstructive jaundice: prospective evaluation of site and cause. *Radiology* 1983;147:511–515.
38. Gibson RN, Yeung E, Thompson JN, et al. Bile duct obstruction: radiologic evaluation of level, cause and tumor resectability. *Radiology* 1986;160:43–47.
39. Salem S, Vas W. Ultrasonography in evaluation of the jaundiced patient. *J Can Assoc Radiol* 1981;31:30–34.

40. Cronan JJ, Mueller PR, Simeone JF, et al. Prospective diagnosis of choledocholithiasis. *Radiology* 1983;146:467–469.
41. Laing FC, Jeffrey RB Jr. Choledocholithiasis and cystic duct obstruction: difficult ultrasonic diagnosis. *Radiology* 1983;146:475–479.
42. Mitchell SE, Clark RA. A comparison of computed tomography and sonography in choledocholithiasis. *AJR* 1984;142:729–733.
43. Einstein DM, Lapin SA, Ralls PW, Halls JM. The insensitivity of sonography in the detection of choledocholithiasis. *AJR* 1984;142:725–728.
44. Gross BH, Harter LP, Gore RM, et al. Ultrasonic evaluation of common bile duct stones: prospective comparison with endoscopic retrograde cholangiography. *Radiology* 1983;146:471–474.
45. Cronan JJ. US diagnosis of choledocholithiasis: a reappraisal. *Radiology* 1986;161:133–134.
46. Jeffrey RB, Federle MP, Laing FC, Wall S, Rego J, Moss AA. Computed tomography of choledocholithiasis. *AJR* 1983;140:1179–1183.
47. Schulman A. Non-western patterns of biliary stones and the role of ascariasis. *Radiology* 1987;162:425–430.
48. Choi BI, Lee JH, Han MC, Kim SH, Yi JG, Kim C-W. Hilar cholangiocarcinoma: comparative study with sonography and CT. *Radiology* 1989;172:689–692.
49. Machan L, Müller NL, Cooperberg PL. Sonographic diagnosis of Klatskin tumors. *AJR* 1986;147:509–512.
50. Becker CD, Hassler H, Terrier F. Preoperative diagnosis of the Mirizzi syndrome: limitations of sonography and computed tomography. *AJR* 1984;143:591–596.
51. Ralls PW, Colletti PM, Quinn MF, Lapin SA, Morris UL, Halls J. Sonography in recurrent oriental pyogenic cholangitis. *AJR* 1981;136:1010–1012.
52. Federle MP, Cello JP, Laing FC, Jeffrey RB. Recurrent pyogenic cholangitis in Asian immigrants: use of ultrasonography, computed tomography and cholangiography. *Radiology* 1982;143:151–156.
53. Dolmatch BL, Laing FC, Federle MP, Jeffrey RB, Cello J. AIDS-related cholangitis: radiographic findings in nine patients. *Radiology* 1987;163:313–316.
54. Morecki R, Glaser JH, Cho S, Balistrero WF, Horwitz MS. Biliary atresia and retrovirus type 3 infection. *N Engl J Med* 1982;307:481–484.
55. Brun P, Gauthier F, Boucher D, Brunelle F. Ultrasound findings in biliary atresia in children. *Ann Radiol* 1985;28:259–263.
56. Weinberger E, Blumhagen JD, Odell JM. Gallbladder contraction in biliary atresia. *AJR* 1987;149:401–402.
57. Reuter K, Raptopoulos VD, Cantelmo N, Fitzpatrick G, Hawes LE. The diagnosis of choledochal cyst by ultrasound. *Radiology* 1980;136:437–438.
58. Alonzo-Lej F, Rever WB Jr, Pessagno DJ. Collective review: congenital choledochal cyst, with a report of 2, and an analysis of 94 cases. *Int Abst Surg* 1959;108:1–30.
59. Kangarloo H, Sarti DA, Sample WF, Amundsen G. Ultrasonographic spectrum of choledochal cysts in children. *Pediatr Radiol* 1980;9:15–18.
60. Torrisi JM, Haller JO, Velcek FT. Choledochal cyst and biliary atresia in the neonate: imaging findings in five cases. *AJR* 1990;155:1273–1276.
61. Bahia JO, Boal DKB, Karl SR, Gross GW. Ultrasonographic detection of spontaneous perforation of the extrahepatic bile ducts in infancy. *Pediatr Radiol* 1986;16:157–159.
62. Haller JO, Condon VR, Berdon WE, et al. Spontaneous perforation of the common bile duct in children. *Radiology* 1989;172:621–624.

Postoperative Biliary Tract

63. Zeman RK, Burrell MI, Dobbins J, Jaffe MH, Choyke PL. Postcholecystectomy syndrome: evaluation using biliary scintigraphy and endoscopic retrograde cholangiopancreatography. *Radiology* 1985;156:787–792.

Pitfalls, Artifacts, and Practical Tips

64. Desai RK, Paushler DM, Armistead J. Intrahepatic arterial calcification mimicking pneumobilia. A potential pitfall in the ultrasound evaluation of biliary tract disease. *J Ultrasound Med* 1989;8:333–335.
65. Pearse BF, Sauerbrei EE, Leddin D. The ultrasound and CT diagnosis of gas in the mesenteric-portal venous system. *J Can Assoc Radiol* 1982;33:269–272.

CHAPTER 5

The Liver

INTRODUCTION

Three major noninvasive imaging techniques are used to assess the liver today: ultrasound, CT, and MRI. Real-time ultrasound is the commonest imaging modality to assess the liver because it is a widespread, inexpensive modality that gives high-resolution images and very good accuracy in assessing many liver diseases. This chapter will describe the normal appearances of the liver and the more common focal and diffuse hepatic disorders.

5.1 SCANNING TECHNIQUES

Scans are performed with a real-time sector probe of the highest frequency possible. A complete study can usually be obtained with the patient supine by placing the probe in various subcostal and intercostal locations to generate long-axis and transverse scans throughout the liver. Care must be taken to include all surfaces of the liver as well as the parenchyma. The American College of Radiology and the American Institute of Ultrasound (1) recommend the following in liver sonography (excerpted from *AIUM Guidelines for Performance of the Abdominal and Retroperitoneal Ultrasound Examination*):

> The liver survey should include both long axis (coronal or sagittal) and transverse views. If possible, views comparing the echogenicity of the liver to the right kidney should be performed. The major vessels (aorta/inferior vena cava) in the region of the liver should be imaged, including the position of the inferior vena cava where it passes through the liver.
> The regions of the ligamentum teres on the left and on the high dome of the right lobe with the right hemidiaphragm and right pleural space should be imaged. The main lobar fissure should be demonstrated.
> Survey of right and left lobes should include visualization of the hepatic veins. The right and left branches of the portal vein should be identified. This analysis can also serve to evaluate for possible intrahepatic bile duct dilatation.

Abbreviations: **CDU,** color Doppler ultrasound; **CT,** computed tomography; **FNH,** focal nodular hyperplasia; **GE junction,** gastroesophageal junction; **GI,** gastrointestinal; **MRI,** magnetic resonance imaging; **PW Doppler,** pulsed wave Doppler.

5.2 NORMAL ANATOMY

The liver is a large solid organ that resides in the right upper quadrant and epigastrium, bounded cranially by the diaphragm, anteriorly by the anterior abdominal wall, posteriorly by the diaphragm and posterior abdominal wall, and laterally (right side) by the diaphragm and right abdominal wall. The diaphragm and lung tissue lie adjacent to a portion of the posterior and right lateral aspect of the liver and thus prevent ultrasound imaging from these areas. Much of the liver is "tucked up" beneath the right ribs, and the ribs themselves are barriers to ultrasound evaluation of the liver. The intercostal spaces are important portals for insonation of the liver for complete hepatic evaluation.

Lobar and Segmental Anatomy

The liver is divided into left and right lobes and the caudate lobe. The right lobe lies entirely to the right of midline and is divided into anterior and posterior segments. The left lobe lies in the epigastrium, with some lying to the left of midline and some to the right of midline. The left lobe is divided into the medial segment (formerly called the quadrate lobe) and the lateral segment (the left-most segment). The caudate lobe is smaller than the right and left lobes, and it lies posterior to the medial segment of the left lobe (Fig. 5.1).

Fissures

The interlobar fissure (or main lobar fissure) forms an incomplete boundary between the right and left lobes. It is oriented in a vertical plane, extending toward the middle hepatic vein from the gallbladder fossa, and it may be visualized in longitudinal and transverse scans as an echogenic line because of the fibrofatty tissue contained in the fissure (Fig. 5.1). In many patients the fissure is not visible because it is small or absent.

The left intersegmental fissure (fissure for the ligamentum teres) lies between the caudal aspects of the medial and lateral segments of the left lobe. This fissure contains the ligamentum teres, which is seen as a round hyperechoic structure in transverse scans because of the fat surrounding the ligamentum teres (Fig. 5.1). The ligamentum teres (remnant of the umbilical vein) courses from the left portal vein through the liver parenchyma to the umbilicus. Outside the liver, the ligamentum teres lies in the free edge of the falciform ligament, which is a peritoneal reflection that courses from the anterior abdominal wall to the anterior surface of the left hepatic lobe.

The fissure for the ligamentum venosum forms the boundary between the caudate lobe posteriorly and the medial segment of the left lobe anteriorly. This fissure is seen as an echogenic line in transverse and sagittal scan planes (Fig. 5.1). The ligamentum venosum is the remnant of the ductus venosus, which conducted blood from the left portal vein to inferior vena cava prenatally. Prenatally, the umbilical vein enters the fetal abdomen at the umbilicus and courses through the left hepatic lobe and carries blood to the left portal vein. Blood flows directly from here to the ductus venosus into the inferior vena cava. (The intrahepatic umbilical vein becomes the ligamentum teres; the intrahepatic ductus venosus becomes the ligamentum venosum.)

Vascular Anatomy

The portal veins, hepatic arteries, and bile ducts course together in the liver parenchyma through the central portions of the lobes and segments. These three vessels form the portal triads, which are surrounded by fibrofatty tissue that causes their walls to be hyperechoic and thus easily visible on ultrasound (Fig. 5.1). The portal veins and hepatic arteries provide the blood supply to the liver.

The main portal vein is formed by the junction of the splenic vein and inferior mesenteric vein, along the posterior aspect of the pancreatic neck. The main portal vein runs obliquely in the porta hepatis and branches into the right and left portal veins, which course into the hepatic parenchyma (Fig. 5.1). The main portal vein has a mean diameter of 10 to 12 mm in the adult with the 95th percentile at 15 mm (2).

In ultrasound scans, the portal vein is usually measured just distal to the junction of the splenic and superior mesenteric veins (2). A scan through the long axis of the portal vein is obtained and the anteroposterior diameter is measured (Fig. 5.1). In most cases, the portal vein tapers slightly as it courses toward the liver. In a small percentage of cases, the portal vein remains the same size or actually enlarges as it approaches the liver. The portal vein diameter should be measured in quiet respiration after 3 to 12 hr of fasting with the patient in supine position. Many variables significantly affect the portal vein diameter (e.g., respiration, previous meals, medications, patient position, patient activity) and sequential measurements on the same people demonstrate quite a lot of variability. In addition, Lafortune et al. (3) have shown that there is no significant difference between the caliber of the portal vein in cirrhotic patients compared with normal patients.

In normal children and adults, inspiration causes an increase in portal vein diameter (as well as splenic vein and superior mesenteric vein diameters), and expiration causes a decrease in the vein diameters (4). Inspiration causes compression of the liver by the descending diaphragm, causing decreased outflow through the hepatic veins. Meanwhile, splanchnic venous flow continues and causes distension of the splenic vein, superior mesenteric vein, and portal vein. The process reverses with expiration.

Three main hepatic veins (right, middle, and left) drain blood from the liver into the inferior vena cava at the level of the diaphragm. Transverse scans often demonstrate all three branches (Fig. 5.1), and sagittal scans or oblique sagittal scans demonstrate the middle or left hepatic vein draining into the inferior vena cava, which courses along the posterior aspect of the liver. The hepatic veins travel between lobes and between segments and thus form part of the visible boundaries between lobes and between segments. The middle hepatic vein lies between the left and right hepatic lobes, the right hepatic vein lies between the anterior and posterior segments of the right lobe, and the left hepatic vein lies between the medial and lateral segments of the left lobe.

The hepatic veins have very little surrounding fibrofatty tissue, and thus the vein walls are much less echogenic than the walls of the portal veins (Fig. 5.1). However, when the sound beam is perpendicular to the hepatic vein wall, a bright specular echo results.

The caudate lobe receives blood supply from branches of the right and left portal veins and right and left hepatic arteries, and blood is drained from the caudate lobe by small hepatic veins that course directly into the inferior vena cava (i.e., venous drainage from the caudate lobe does not flow through the right, middle, nor left hepatic veins).

Liver Size

The right lobe is larger than the left lobe and caudate lobe. The liver is variable in shape and size, and it is difficult to quantify the liver size with ultrasound or other imaging modalities. However, several methods have been postulated to assess liver size (5). In practice, we use the cranio-caudal length of the right hepatic lobe as measured in the right midclavicular line (Fig. 5.2). The upper limit of normal is taken to be 15 cm (5). With diffuse enlargement, the edges of the liver tend to become rounded or bulbous as opposed to wedge-shaped in the normal liver.

Liver Echogenicity

Except for blood vessels and fissures within the liver, the parenchyma has a uniform medium-level echogenicity. In the adult, the liver is slightly more echogenic than normal renal cortex (Fig. 5.2) and slightly less echogenic than the spleen.

Normal Doppler

Portal Vein

Color Doppler ultrasound and PW Doppler are both excellent techniques to assess blood flow in the portal

vein (5a). Color Doppler ultrasound is used for rapid screening for the presence and direction of blood flow in the portal vein and its branches (Fig. 5.3). Note that CDU depicts the *average Doppler shift frequency* and not the maximum flow velocity (6). The main portal vein and left portal vein are usually best evaluated from an anterior approach and the right portal vein from a right intercostal approach (7). Pulsed Wave Doppler demonstrates a characteristic low-velocity continuous flow toward the liver with mild undulations related to cardiac contractions (Fig. 5.3). The velocity of portal venous flow increases during inspiration and after meals.

Hepatic Artery

The hepatic artery flow is evaluated by Color Doppler ultrasound and PW Doppler via an anterior approach (Fig. 5.4). Color Doppler ultrasound is very useful in initial localization for positioning of the PW sample volume. The spectral display demonstrates antegrade flow throughout diastole (Fig. 5.4), indicating a low-resistance system (7). There is more spectral broadening in the hepatic artery compared with the aorta because laminar flow in small arteries is parabolic (i.e., velocities decrease progressively from the center of the lumen to the wall of the vessel) as opposed to "plug" flow in the larger aorta (i.e., velocities are almost the same in the center of the lumen as more peripheral locations in the lumen).

Hepatic Veins

The main hepatic veins are best assessed with transverse scans high in the epigastrium. Color Doppler ultrasound easily demonstrates blood flow toward the inferior vena cava, and PW Doppler yields a characteristic velocity or Doppler frequency profile (Fig. 5.5) (7). In the hepatic veins and inferior vena cava, a triphasic curve is seen, which reflects cardiac activity (Fig. 5.5). The first downward peak represents enhanced flow toward the heart caused by right atrial diastole, and the second downward peak is due to right ventricular diastole. The third component of the curve is an upward peak representing a slight reversal of blood flow (i.e., toward the probe and away from the heart) caused by right atrial contraction.

Normal Variants

The liver shape and specific diameter measurements vary quite a lot with different body types (5). For example, for ectomorphic body types (thin), the average liver depth is 11.4 cm, and for endomorphic body types (heavier), the depth is 14.7 cm. Another variation (Riedel's lobe) can give misleadingly high values for liver size. Riedel's lobe is a bulbous widening of the caudal

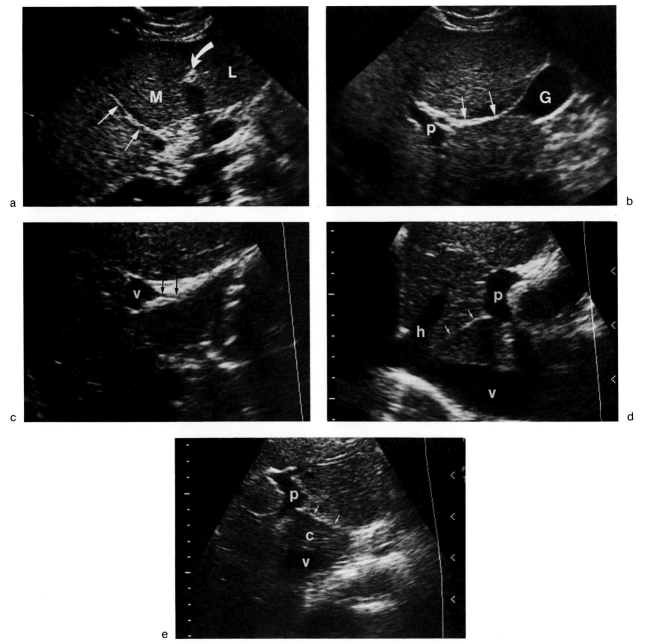

FIG. 5.1. Normal liver anatomy. **a:** main lobar fissure and ligamentum teres—transverse. Transverse scan demonstrates main lobar fissure (*straight arrows*), which separates right and left hepatic lobes. Ligamentum teres (*curved arrow*) divides left lobe into medial (*M*) and lateral (*L*) segments. **b:** main lobar fissure—longitudinal. Longitudinal scan demonstrates main lobar fissure (*straight arrows*) coursing from gallbladder (*G*) to portal vein bifurcation (*P*). **c:** ligamentum teres—longitudinal. Sagittal scan of left hepatic lobe demonstrates a very small umbilical vein (*arrows*) arising from left portal vein (*v*) and coursing toward umbilicus. Broad band of hyperechoic material is fibrofatty tissue surrounding ligamentum teres. Note that a small umbilical vein occasionally can be seen in normal people such as this. **d:** fissure for ligamentum venosum—sagittal. Sagittal scan through left hepatic lobe demonstrates a thin echogenic line (*arrows*) that is the fissure for ligamentum venosum. It courses from left portal vein (*p*) to anterior aspect of inferior vena cava (*v*). *In utero,* the ductus venosus is a patent vein carrying blood from left portal vein into inferior vena cava. *h,* middle hepatic vein. **e:** fissure for ligamentum venosum—transverse. Transverse scan through liver demonstrates fissure for ligamentum venosum (*arrows*) separating caudate lobe (*c*) from left hepatic lobe. *v,* inferior vena cava; *p,* left portal vein.

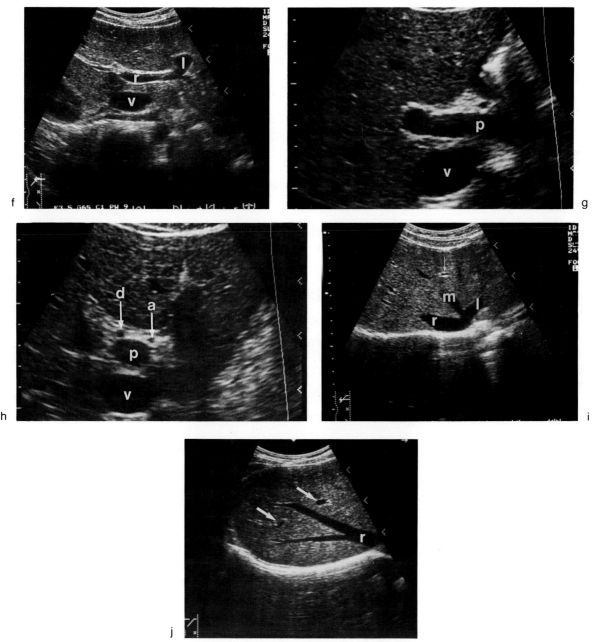

FIG. 5.1. *continued.* **f:** normal portal vein branches. Transverse scan through liver demonstrates normal left (*l*) and right (*r*) portal vein branches within the liver. *v*, inferior vena cava. **g:** normal portal vein. Oblique scan in right upper quadrant demonstrates long axis of main portal vein (*p*). Internal diameter of portal vein measures 11 mm. Note low-level echoes within lumen in this individual. In real-time scan, this represented visible blood flow within the portal vein. *v*, inferior vena cava. **h:** normal portal vein—transverse. Transverse scan of porta hepatis demonstrates normal main portal vein (*p*) immediately anterior to inferior vena cava (*v*). Extrahepatic bile duct (*d*) lies along anterior-right aspect of main portal vein, and proper hepatic artery (*a*) lies along anterior-medial aspect of main portal vein. **i:** main hepatic veins. Transverse scan through liver demonstrates right (*r*), middle (*m*), and left (*l*) hepatic veins joining together to form the inferior vena cava. *Arrow,* portal vein branch. **j:** normal hepatic veins and portal veins. Transverse scan through right hepatic lobe demonstrates right hepatic vein (*r*), which forms the boundary between anterior and posterior segments of right hepatic lobe. Portal vein branches (*arrows*) course within hepatic segments. Walls of portal vein branches are hyperechoic, whereas walls of hepatic veins are less echogenic. (Scans (c), (d), (e), (g), and (h) are courtesy of Dr. Steve Valentine, Resident, Department of Radiology, Queen's University, Kingston, Canada.)

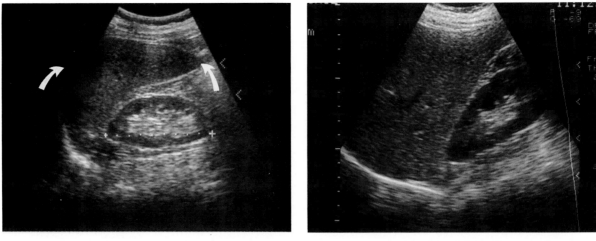

FIG. 5.2. Normal liver size and echogenicity. **a:** Sagittal scan through right hepatic lobe demonstrates length of right lobe (*arrows*). Normal length is ≤15 cm. **b:** Sagittal scan of right hepatic lobe in another person, demonstrating that liver parenchyma is slightly more echogenic than the renal cortex at the same level. This is the expected normal appearance.

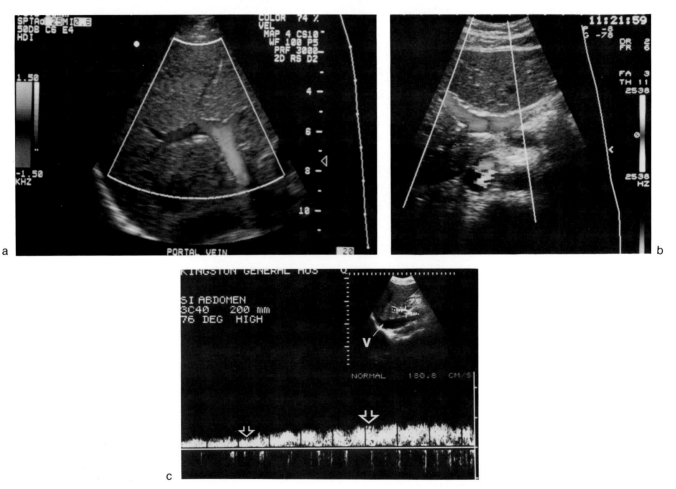

FIG. 5.3. Doppler ultrasound of portal veins. (*See color images of parts a and b in the color plate section, which follows page 50.*) **a:** Blood flow in main portal vein is toward liver (hepatopedal). It is coded red because flow is toward the ultrasound probe. Flow in right portal vein is away from the probe and thus coded blue. [Scan is courtesy of Advanced Technology Laboratories (ATL).] **b:** Color Doppler of portal vein bifurcation. Blood flow in right portal vein is coded red because its net flow is toward the ultrasound probe. Flow in left portal vein is coded red because net flow is slightly away from the probe. **c:** Pulsed wave spectrum. Sagittal scan of right upper quadrant demonstrates pulsed wave Doppler cursor in main portal vein. *v*, inferior vena cava. Doppler spectrum (*arrows*) demonstrates blood flow toward the liver. Blood flow is low velocity and continuous, with mild temporal fluctuations in peak velocity caused by cardiac pulsations. Note increase in the velocity toward right of the graph with patient inspiration.

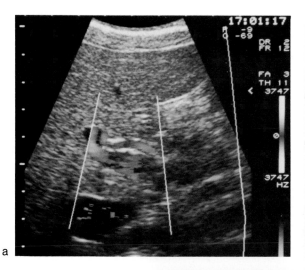

a

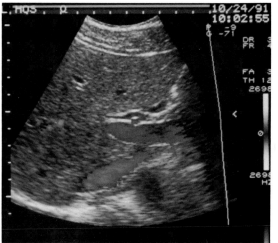

b

c

FIG. 5.4. Doppler ultrasound of hepatic artery. (*See color images of parts a and b in the color plate section, which follows page 50.*) **a:** Color Doppler of hepatic artery. Oblique scan of right upper quadrant demonstrates proper hepatic artery anterior to portal vein. Flow in proximal portion of the artery is red (toward probe) and in distal portion blue (away from probe). This represents blood flow toward the liver. (Scan is courtesy of Mr. Tyler Sauerbrei.) **b:** Color Doppler of right hepatic artery. Right hepatic artery is a small circle with red in it (flow toward probe). It lies posterior to common duct (no color flow) and anterior to portal vein (red). Note blue color in the inferior vena cava (flow away from probe). **c:** Pulsed wave spectrum of hepatic artery. Note forward flow in diastole (*arrows*). This indicates relatively low resistance to hepatic artery flow.

aspect of the right hepatic lobe (Fig. 5.6). (The right lobe normally tapers to a wedge shape in sagittal scans.) A Riedel's lobe is usually seen in women.

In some patients the normal left hepatic lobe extends to the anterior aspect of the spleen. In these cases the rim of liver tissue adjacent to the spleen can be mistaken for a perisplenic fluid collection adjacent to the more echogenic splenic parenchyma. However, with the optimal gain settings and the appropriate probe, there should be no confusion (see Chapter 6).

Occasionally the left hepatic lobe is quite small, and very little liver tissue is seen in the epigastrium. Careful inspection usually allows visualization of the ligamentum teres, which divides the small left lobe into medial

and lateral segments. A small left hepatic lobe may cause suboptimal epigastric scans because bowel replaces the liver here.

5.3 PATHOLOGY

Neoplasms

Metastases

Metastases are the commonest hepatic neoplasms in ultrasound and CT practice. Ultrasound is commonly used for the initial assessment of possible liver metas-

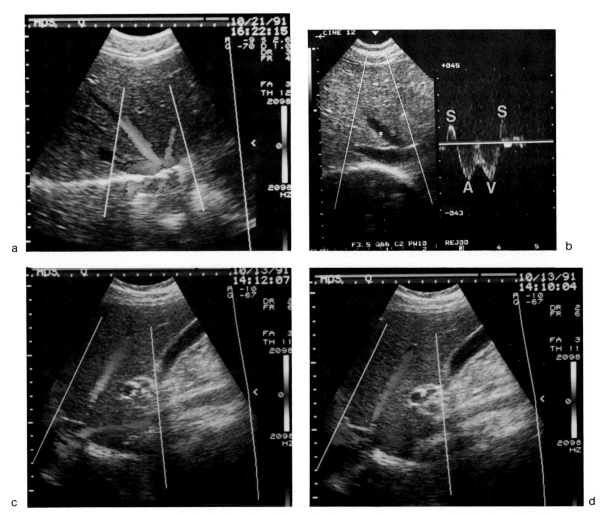

FIG. 5.5. Doppler ultrasound of hepatic veins. (*See color images of parts **a, c,** and **d** in the color plate section, which follows page 50.*) **a:** Color Doppler ultrasound—transverse. Blood flow in right, middle, and left hepatic veins is toward inferior vena cava. Flow in middle and left hepatic veins is coded blue (flow away from probe). (Scan is courtesy of Mr. Peter Sauerbrei.) **b:** Pulsed wave ultrasound spectrum. Transverse scan demonstrates PW spectrum of blood flow in middle hepatic vein. Most of the time, flow is toward the inferior vena cava and thus away from the probe: the spectrum demonstrates flow below baseline (A,V). For short time intervals, flow is away from inferior vena cava and thus toward the probe: the spectrum demonstrates flow above baseline (s). A, atrial diastole; V, ventricular diastole; S, atrial systole. **c:** Color Doppler ultrasound—sagittal. Blood flow throughout middle hepatic vein is toward the inferior vena cava at this time. Flow in hepatic vein is coded blue (flow away from probe). Flow in inferior vena cava is toward right atrium. **d:** Color Doppler—sagittal. Same patient as (c), slightly later in same cardiac cycle. Cine loop function allows color depiction of flow a fraction of a second later when there is momentary reversal of flow in hepatic vein. This corresponds to "S" component of spectrum in (b).

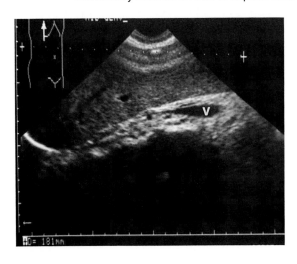

FIG. 5.6. Riedel's lobe. Sagittal scan demonstrates a long right hepatic lobe (about 18 cm in length). There is slight widening of distal aspect of right hepatic lobe. This is a normal variant. *v,* inferior vena cava.

tases and for follow-up during therapy. Although ultrasound provides an accurate imaging method for assessing the liver in neoplastic disease, well-performed CT scans are more accurate for detecting hepatic neoplasms (8). In addition, it is easier to monitor the progression of multiple hepatic tumors on sequential CT scans than sequential ultrasound scans because CT scans provide a complete set of slices through the liver in a reproducible, annotated way, whereas real-time ultrasound cannot provide this as easily. Wernecke et al. (8a) demonstrated that for liver metastases more than 2 cm in diameter, ultrasound, CT, and MRI were 100% sensitive in their detection. However, the detection rate of sonography for lesions of 1 to 2 cm was 61% compared with 74% for CT and 77% for MRI. The detection rate of sonography for lesions less than 1 cm was 20% compared with 49% for CT and 31% for MRI. Despite these shortcomings, ultrasound is used very widely to provide reasonably accurate information in the initial and follow-up assessments for liver metastases.

The ultrasound pattern of liver metastases is quite varied, and there is no consistent relation between ultrasound patterns and type of tumor that allows one to specify the primary malignancy (9). The various ultrasound patterns include multiple hypoechoic, hyperechoic, and isoechoic foci (Fig. 5.7). The echo pattern may be mixed, there may be anechoic foci especially with necrotic or hemorrhagic components, and some metastases may calcify (Fig. 5.7). Occasionally metastatic disease may be solitary or confined to one segment or lobe, in which case surgical resection of part of the liver is possible (Fig. 5.7). Uncommonly, liver metastases may present as a diffuse process throughout the liver, and differentiation from normal or other diffuse liver diseases may be difficult.

Although one cannot predict the primary neoplasm from the ultrasound pattern of the liver metastases, there are some patterns that are more common in certain diseases and thus may alter or influence the differential diagnosis. Calcified metastases (Fig. 5.7) most commonly are associated with carcinoma of the colon, although other tumors may do this (e.g., neuroblastoma in children, breast carcinoma, osteosarcoma, ovarian carcinoma, malignant melanoma, gastric carcinoma) (10). Metastatic sarcomas tend to become necrotic and fluid-filled more frequently than carcinomas. If multiple tumors with central fluid collections and fluid–debris levels are present, metastatic sarcomas would be a primary consideration (11).

The presence of liver metastases may be confirmed by ultrasound-guided fine needle aspiration for cytology, but in many cases, the imaging results taken together with the clinical and laboratory data give strong enough evidence to "make" the diagnosis. In follow-up assessment during and after therapy, one often sees a change in the ultrasound texture of the metastases, but the size and number of metastases provide a more reliable indicator of response to therapy. For sequential ultrasound scans in metastatic disease, one must scan the liver in a thorough and consistent way in transverse and sagittal/coronal planes to make comparisons with previous exams.

Carcinoma

Hepatocellular carcinoma (hepatoma) is more common in Asia and Africa than North America or Europe (12). Many hepatomas arise in patients with cirrhosis. In North America, up to 5% of patients with cirrhosis may develop hepatocellular carcinoma.

The patients may present with a deterioration of liver function, pain, weight loss, and an abdominal mass. At presentation many patients have disease extension beyond the liver, either by direct extension outside the liver capsule or by invasion and extension through the portal or hepatic veins (12).

Ultrasound, CT, or MRI may demonstrate a large solitary tumor, a dominant tumor with "satellite" tumors, or a diffuse infiltrative pattern. The ultrasound pattern may be hypoechoic, hyperechoic, isoechoic, or mixed (Fig. 5.8). It is not uncommon to visualize tumor extension into the portal or hepatic veins. Smaller tumors containing mainly tumor cells tend to be hypoechoic, whereas large tumors containing hemorrhage, necrosis, and fibrosis tend to be hyperechoic (13). A definitive diagnosis usually requires needle aspiration or biopsy. On imaging, the differential diagnosis includes metastases, large benign tumors such as adenomas and focal nodular hyperplasia, and abscesses.

Hemangioma

Cavernous hemangiomas are benign liver tumors of vascular origin, and they constitute the most common hepatic neoplasm (14). They range in size from very small to very large. Although hemangiomas are usually solitary, multiple hemangiomas are not uncommon. Most hemangiomas are asymptomatic and not clinically significant, although large hemangiomas may cause abdominal discomfort and may bleed. Benign hemangiomas may be mistaken for other liver tumors, and the main role of ultrasound and other imaging techniques is to distinguish hemangiomas from malignant tumors.

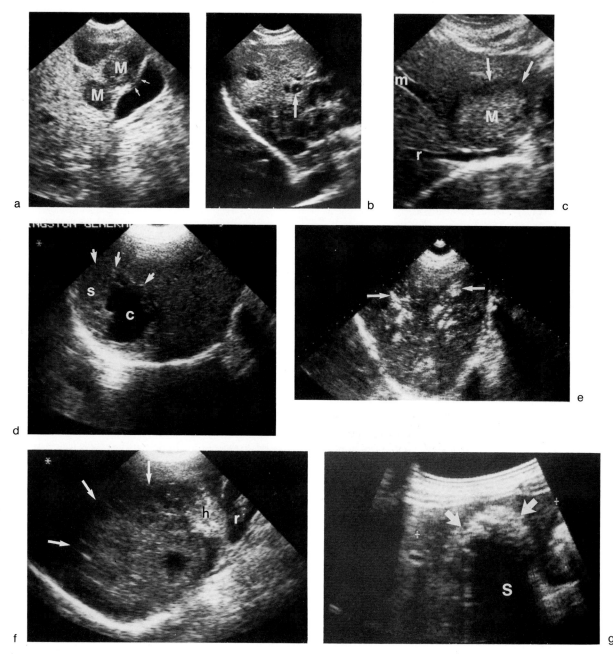

FIG. 5.7. Liver metastases. **a:** Hypoechoic metastases. Sagittal scan of right hepatic lobe demonstrates multiple discrete hypoechoic solid masses (*M*). These are metastatic foci from ureteric transitional cell carcinoma. One of the masses invades through gallbladder wall (*arrows*). **b:** Hypoechoic metastases with target appearance. Some of metastatic foci (*arrow*) have a central echogenic focus, simulating a target appearance. This is an uncommon manifestation of liver metastases. This ultrasound appearance can also be seen in fungal abscesses and lymphoma. Needle aspiration biopsy would be required for differentiation. In this patient, foci were due to metastases from malignant melanoma. **c:** Isoechoic liver metastases. Transverse scan of left hepatic lobe demonstrates a large isoechoic mass (*M*) in left hepatic lobe. Note hypoechoic halo (*arrows*) around mass. *m*, middle hepatic vein; *r*, right hepatic vein. **d:** Cystic metastases. Metastatic foci may be partly cystic. In this example, in right hepatic lobe, some of the tumor (*arrows*) is cystic (*c*), but much of it is solid (*s*) and more difficult to appreciate. **e:** Hyperechoic metastases. Sagittal scan through right hepatic lobe demonstrates multiple nonshadowing hyperechoic metastases (*arrows*). These arose from a mucinous adenocarcinoma of the bowel. **f:** Metastases of mixed echogenicity. Sagittal scan through right hepatic lobe demonstrates large tumor masses (*arrows*) in posterior aspect of right hepatic lobe. Some of the metastatic tumor mass is isoechoic, some is hypoechoic, and a component is hyperechoic (*h*). *r*, right kidney. These are metastases from carcinoid tumor of the small bowel. **g:** Calcified liver metastases. Sagittal scan through superficial aspect of right hepatic lobe demonstrates a solid tumor (*cursors*). Part of solid tumor is calcified (*arrows*), associated with distal acoustic shadowing (*s*). This is a calcified metastatic focus from mucinous adenocarcinoma from the colon.

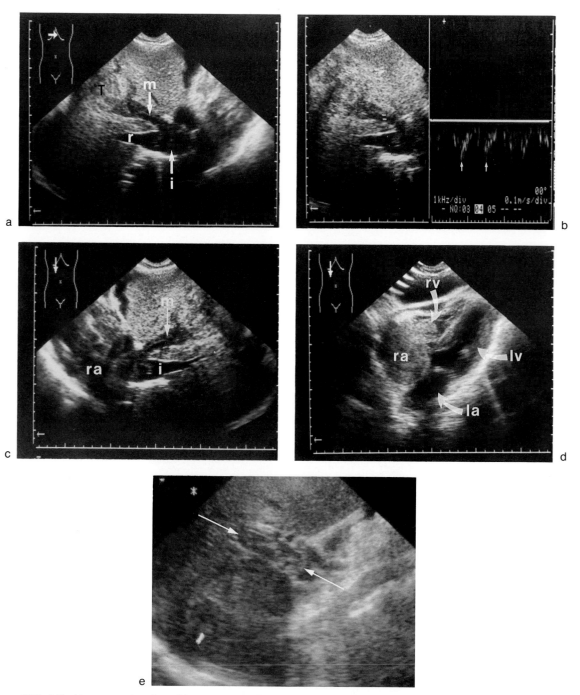

FIG. 5.8. Venous extension of hepatoma. **a:** Transverse scan of liver demonstrates a solid tumor (*T*) in liver parenchyma with extension into middle hepatic vein (*m*) and into inferior vena cava (*i*). *r*, right hepatic vein. Part of tumor is hyperechoic and part is hypoechoic. **b:** Duplex Doppler of the intravascular tumor. Cursor is placed within middle hepatic vein. Doppler spectrum demonstrates arterial blood flow (*arrows*) within intravascular material. This differentiates intravascular tumor from bland thrombus. Bland thrombus would not have arterial blood flow within it. **c:** Sagittal scan of middle hepatic vein (*m*) demonstrates extension of tumor into inferior vena cava (*i*) and from there into right atrium (*ra*). **d:** Oblique scan through heart demonstrates tumor filling and distending right atrium (*ra*) and extending through tricuspid valve apparatus into the right ventricle (*rv*). *la*, left atrium; *lv*, left ventricle. **e:** Extension into portal vein. Scan of a different patient demonstrates tumor (*arrows*) filling portal vein. This was tumor extension from a hepatoma in right hepatic lobe.

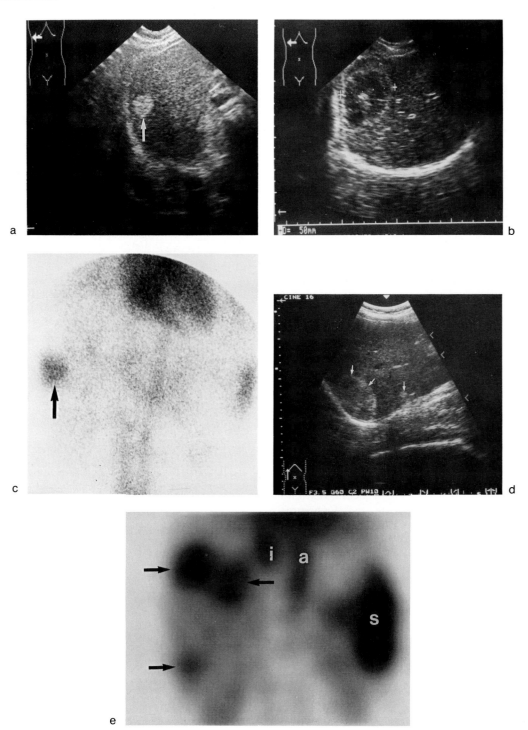

FIG. 5.9. Liver hemangioma. **a:** Characteristic hemangioma. Transverse scan of right hepatic lobe demonstrates a well-defined hyperechoic focus (*arrow*) measuring 2.4 cm in diameter. This is the most common appearance for a liver hemangioma. In absence of other liver lesions and absence of a primary malignancy, this is almost certainly a benign hemangioma. **b:** Hemangioma, atypical appearance. Transverse ultrasound scan demonstrates a 5-cm diameter hypoechoic solitary mass in periphery of the liver. There is a small central hyperechoic focus within the mass. **c:** Red cell–labeled isotope scan in same patient as (b) is characteristic of a liver hemangioma. It demonstrates increased uptake (*arrow*) at site of tumor noted in (b). **d:** Multiple liver hemangiomas. Sagittal scan of right hepatic lobe demonstrates multiple masses within the liver (*arrows*). Smaller ones were uniformly hyperechoic, and the large one was of mixed echogenicity. **e:** Red cell–labeled isotope scan in a coronal tomographic plane demonstrates three hemangiomas (*arrows*) in this plane. *i*, inferior vena cava; *a*, abdominal aorta; *s*, spleen.

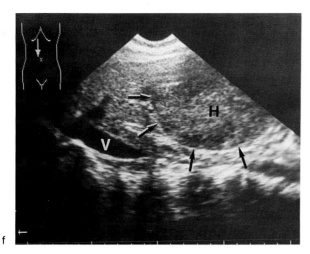
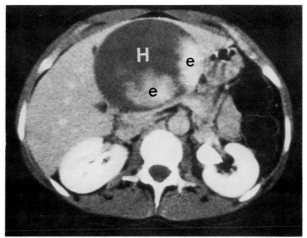

f

g

FIG. 9. *continued.* **f:** Large atypical hemangioma. Sagittal ultrasound scan of right hepatic lobe demonstrates a very large solid mass (*arrow*) arising in caudal aspect of right hepatic lobe. The mass is partly hypoechoic and partly isoechoic compared with normal liver tissue. *v*, inferior vena cava. **g:** Dynamic CT scan in same patient as (f). This demonstrates preferential enhancement (*e*) in periphery of the mass. Later CT scans demonstrated filling-in of central portion of the mass, and this is characteristic for hemangioma (*H*).

On ultrasound, most hemangiomas are well-defined, uniformly hyperechoic, rounded foci less than 3 cm in diameter (Fig. 5.9) (15,16). Acoustic enhancement may be visualized posterior to hemangiomas, especially with large lesions. Some hemangiomas have a complex echo pattern caused by hypoechoic areas that may be hemorrhage, thrombosis, or fibrosis (Fig. 5.9) (16). Occasionally, hemangiomas are predominantly hypoechoic (Fig. 5.9).

In a patient without evidence of a primary malignancy, the finding of a small round hyperechoic focus in the liver is strongly suggestive of a hemangioma (17). Although the differential diagnosis theoretically includes hepatocellular carcinoma, liver cell adenoma, focal nodular hyperplasia, and solitary metastasis, this common characteristic finding (in the above patient) does not warrant further investigation with dynamic CT, angiography, red cell–labeled isotope scan, or biopsy.

For hemangiomas less than 1.5 cm in diameter, dynamic CT scans and red cell–labeled isotope scans are often unsuccessful. However, for larger lesions these techniques are quite successful and quite specific in their findings to indicate a hemangioma. The latter techniques are useful when the lesions are greater than 1.5 cm in diameter, when the echo pattern is mixed, and when there is a history of a primary malignancy (18). Needle biopsy is usually reserved for patients in whom the imaging modalities are not sufficiently characteristic to allow a reasonably confident diagnosis.

Adenoma

The vast majority of liver adenomas occur in young women, often with a history of taking oral contraceptives (19). The tumor is usually solitary and well-defined, and the echo pattern is quite variable, ranging from hypoechoic to isoechoic to hyperechoic to mixed cystic and solid, depending on the presence and age of internal hemorrhage. Adenomas vary in size from small to very large (>10-cm diameter). On ultrasound one cannot distinguish between adenoma and focal nodular hyperplasia if there is no internal hemorrhage (20). Because patients may present with spontaneous hemorrhage into an adenoma, an adenoma should be removed (21).

Focal Nodular Hyperplasia

Focal nodular hyperplasia is an uncommon benign tumor that also occurs in young women and is associated with oral contraceptives. It is usually solitary and asymptomatic, and hemorrhage is rare. It may contain a central scar, and it may range up to 20 cm in diameter. On ultrasound the mass may be slightly hypoechoic, isoechoic, or slightly hyperechoic (20). Internal hemorrhage or cystic degeneration is rare. A central scar will manifest as a nonshadowing hyperechoic focus within the mass (Fig 5.10) (22).

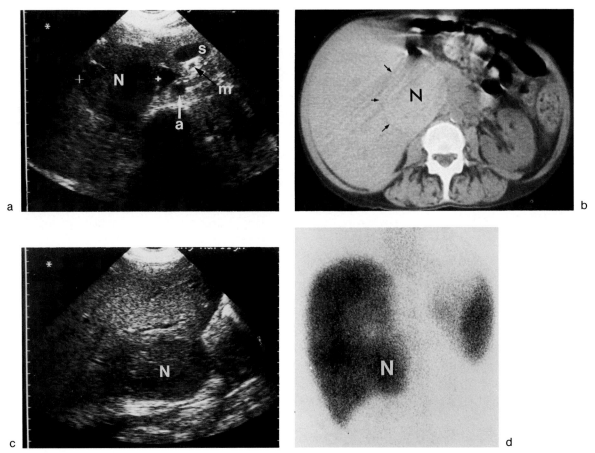

FIG. 5.10. Focal nodular hyperplasia. **a:** Transverse ultrasound scan demonstrates a large solid mass (*N*) arising in caudate lobe of the liver. *a*, abdominal aorta; *m*, superior mesenteric artery; *s*, splenic vein. **b:** CT scan in same scan plane as (a) demonstrates large isodense mass (*N, arrows*) arising in caudate lobe. **c:** Sagittal scan through liver demonstrates hypoechoic mass (*N*) in caudate lobe. **d:** Isotope scan demonstrates that the mass (*N*) takes up isotope the same as the rest of liver parenchyma.

Distinction between adenoma and FNH on ultrasound may be impossible. A hemorrhagic focus (hyperechoic if acute; cystic if old) inside the tumor would favor an adenoma. A central hyperechoic scar would favor FNH. A homogeneous solid solitary mass in a young woman usually will require further evaluation with liver radionuclide scintigraphy, which can help distinguish between adenoma and FNH. Adenomas usually do not take up radionuclide, whereas FNH does take up radionuclide (there are exceptions).

Lymphoma

After the spleen, the liver is the most commonly affected extralymphatic organ in Hodgkin's and non-Hodgkin's lymphoma (23). Lymphoma commonly involves the liver at the time of autopsy (50% or more of patients with Hodgkin's and non-Hodgkin's lymphoma)

(24) but is much less common in clinical imaging practice. Discrete hypoechoic foci are the most common finding in both types of lymphoma, although diffuse textural abnormality may also be seen (Fig. 5.11). Occasionally foci are anechoic and may simulate cysts (Fig. 5.11). Hyperechoic foci (Fig. 5.12) and target lesions can be seen in non-Hodgkin's lymphoma (24). Calcifications may occur in hepatic lymphoma deposits, most commonly after therapy.

Leukemia

Leukemia involves the liver uncommonly. With diffuse microscopic deposits in acute lymphocytic and acute myelogenous leukemia, ultrasound will be normal. Larger discrete foci are often hypoechoic or even anechoic. Small areas of central necrosis may give rise

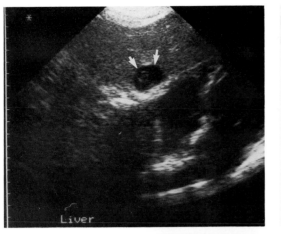

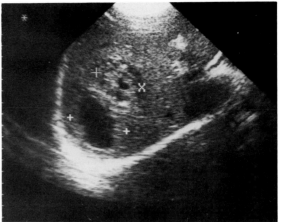

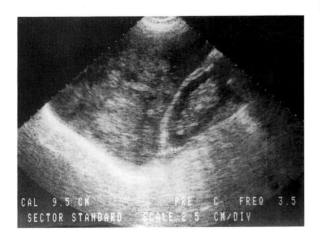

FIG. 5.11. Lymphoma of the liver. **a:** Transverse scan through left hepatic lobe demonstrates an ovoid, hypoechoic mass (*arrows*) in posterior aspect of left hepatic lobe. This was a focal solid deposit of lymphoma. **b:** Transverse scan through right hepatic lobe in same patient demonstrates a large mass of mixed echogenicity in posterior aspect. Portions of the mass are hypoechoic and others are hyperechoic. This was another deposit of lymphoma. **c:** Sagittal scan in right hepatic lobe of another patient demonstrates an anechoic mass in the liver associated with posterior acoustic enhancement. Although these findings are suggestive of a simple cyst, this was a solid deposit of lymphoma. When the gain was increased, low-level echoes became apparent inside the tumor.

FIG. 5.12. Sagittal scan demonstrates multiple hyperechoic foci throughout the right hepatic lobe, representing infiltration with lymphoma.

to hyperechoic central foci within the hypoechoic tumors (25).

Portal Lymphadenopathy

Enlarged lymph nodes in the porta hepatis may be due to neoplastic or inflammatory diseases. In ultrasound practice most cases are due to metastatic deposits or lymphoma. Sagittal scans through the inferior vena cava and portal vein demonstrate solid masses between these two veins, and transverse scans may demonstrate extension from the portal vein toward the celiac axis (Fig. 5.13).

Cysts

Simple Cyst

Simple hepatic cysts are quite common incidental findings in people older than 50 years of age (26). Most commonly they are small and few in number and usually do not present a diagnostic problem, even when there is a history of primary malignancy or fever of unknown origin. Simple cysts have the following ultrasound characteristics: anechoic interior, sharply defined posterior

wall, and posterior acoustic enhancement (Fig. 5.14). A liver cyst may have an irregular border because of its interface with surrounding liver parenchyma. This type of irregularity of the contour, in practice, does not create confusion between a simple cyst and a lesion with cystic and solid components. Occasionally other lesions can mimic simple cysts (e.g., lymphoma). If there is clinical suspicion of a lesion other than a simple cyst, a fine needle aspiration can be performed.

A simple cyst may rarely become very large and thereby symptomatic because of local pressure effects. Drainage will relieve the symptoms, but reaccumulation of the fluid is the rule (27). If there is hemorrhage into a simple cyst (spontaneous, blunt trauma, or after needle or drainage procedure), the walls may become thickened and irregular and there may be multiple internal echoes (Fig. 5.15). In these cases sequential scans and comparison with previous scans would resolve any diagnostic uncertainty.

Polycystic Disease

Simple liver cysts (often ten or more) are present in up to 50% of patients with diagnosed polycystic renal dis-

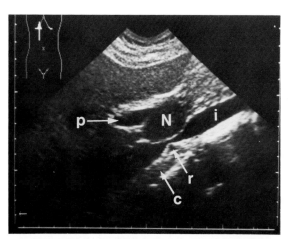

a

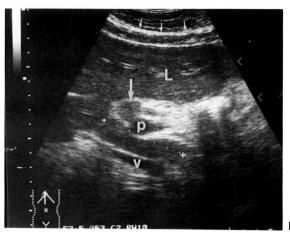

b

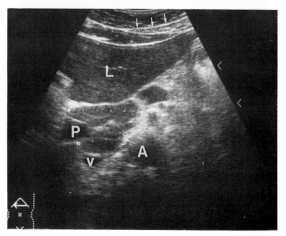

c

FIG. 5.13. a: Portal lymphadenopathy. Sagittal scan through inferior vena cava (*i*) demonstrates an enlarged lymph node (*N*) indenting anterior aspect of inferior vena cava and posterior aspect of portal vein (*p*). *r*, right renal artery; *c*, crus of the diaphragm. **b:** Portal lymphadenopathy. Sagittal scan through porta hepatis demonstrates several hypoechoic masses (*cursors*) between portal vein (*p*) and inferior vena cava (*v*), and (*arrow*) between portal vein and liver parenchyma (*L*). *Small arrows,* linea alba. **c:** Portal lymphadenopathy. Transverse scan of same patient as (b) demonstrates multiple enlarged lymph nodes extending from aorta (*A*) into porta hepatis adjacent to portal vein (*p*) and inferior vena cava (*v*). *L,* left hepatic lobe; *small arrows,* left rectus abdominis muscle.

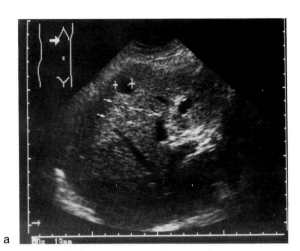
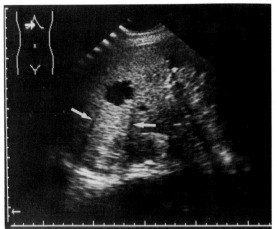

a

b

FIG. 5.14. Liver cysts. **a:** Transverse scan of right hepatic lobe demonstrates typical appearance of a small simple liver cyst. The liver cyst (*cursors*) is anechoic and has a sharply defined posterior wall associated with posterior acoustic enhancement (*arrows*). **b:** Transverse scan of another patient demonstrates a simple cyst (*arrow*) in right hepatic lobe. Note slightly irregular wall. This is a common finding and does not detract from diagnosis of a simple cyst. Note thin refractive shadows posterior to edges of the cyst and posterior acoustic enhancement.

ease (Fig. 5.16) (28). Whenever multiple hepatic cysts are present, one should examine the kidneys to assess for polycystic renal disease. Usually, the cystic disease of the kidneys is more widespread and obvious, but occasionally the cystic liver disease is more severe than the renal component.

Infection

Granuloma

Healed granulomas often present as small punctate calcifications in the spleen but also in the liver (Fig. 5.17). These may have posterior acoustic shadowing. Previous histoplasmosis infection is the most common cause, but tuberculosis can also cause calcified granulomas. Histoplasmosis is especially common in North America in the Great Lakes Basin and in the midwestern United States.

Metallic clips or gas in the intrahepatic bile ducts or portal veins can mimic calcified granulomas, but the strong reverberation artifacts posterior to metal clips and the linearity of intrabiliary/intravascular gas allows differentiation (see Chapter 4).

Pyogenic Abscess

The vast majority of liver abscesses in North American ultrasound practice are pyogenic abscesses (29). There is a male predominance, most are solitary, and most occur in the right lobe. Liver abscesses are commonly caused by anaerobic organisms from the gut.

These organisms reach the liver via the bile ducts, portal veins, hepatic arteries, lymphatic channels, or direct spread. Abscesses may also be secondary to trauma (surgical and nonsurgical), and infection may complicate simple cysts or necrotic tumors. In some cases, no causes can be found (29).

On ultrasound examination, there is quite a variable presentation, although most pyogenic abscesses are hypoechoic, rounded, fluid-filled masses with variable degrees of internal echoes or debris (Fig. 5.18). There may be diffuse low-level echoes, clumps of irregular echogenicity, fluid–debris levels, or septations. A few abscesses will have hyperechoic gas collections within them, signifying a gas-producing organism or a fistula to bowel. The borders of the abscess are usually distinct, and ultrasound may demonstrate a thick wall.

Most solitary abscesses can be drained percutaneously even when septations are present because septations are usually incomplete. Ultrasound or CT may be used for guidance of needle and catheter placements. When multiple abscesses are present, it is still useful to percutaneously drain the dominant abscess because smaller abscesses (<2 cm) often respond to antibiotic therapy after drainage of the dominant cavity.

Echinococcus Granulosus (Hydatid Disease) and Echinococcus Multilocularis

Infestation with echinococcus granulosus is quite common in sheep-raising and cattle-raising areas of the world. The definitive host is the dog, which passes the eggs in its stool. These eggs are swallowed by interme-

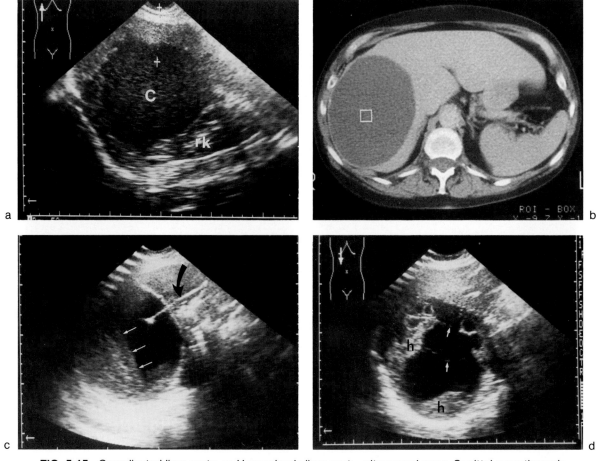

FIG. 5.15. Complicated liver cysts. **a:** Hemorrhagic liver cyst—ultrasound scan. Sagittal scan through right hepatic lobe demonstrates a large mass (c) in right hepatic lobe adjacent to right kidney (rk). Note multiple low-level echoes throughout the mass. **b:** Hemorrhagic liver cyst—CT scan. CT scan through same mass as (a) demonstrates a well-defined low-density lesion within right hepatic lobe. Needle aspiration revealed old blood. Follow-up scans demonstrated no evidence of a neoplasm. **c:** Sagittal scan in right hepatic lobe of another patient demonstrates a large cystic mass with a fluid–debris level (arrows) within it. Needle aspiration (curved arrow) demonstrated crystalline material within a simple liver cyst. **d:** A complex cystic mass is demonstrated in this sagittal scan through right hepatic lobe in another patient. A scan several years ago demonstrated a large simple cyst. The patient had an episode of hemorrhage into this cyst, which was confirmed by needle aspiration. Follow-up scan several months later demonstrated several hyperechoic areas (h) in periphery of the cyst and thin septations (arrows) within the cyst. This is an old, organizing hemorrhagic cyst. This is an uncommon finding. Without previous history, this would be suspicious for a neoplasm.

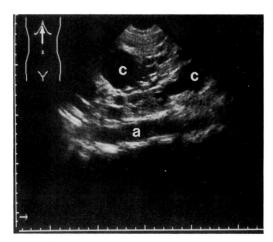

FIG. 5.16. Polycystic disease of the liver. Sagittal scan through left hepatic lobe demonstrates multiple, various size cysts (c) in an enlarged left hepatic lobe, which lies anterior to abdominal aorta (a).

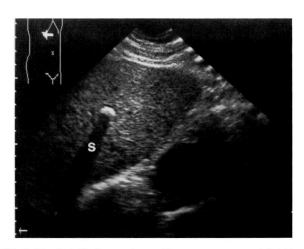

FIG. 5.17. Calcified granuloma. Transverse scan of right hepatic lobe demonstrates a solitary hyperechoic focus with posterior acoustic shadowing (s).

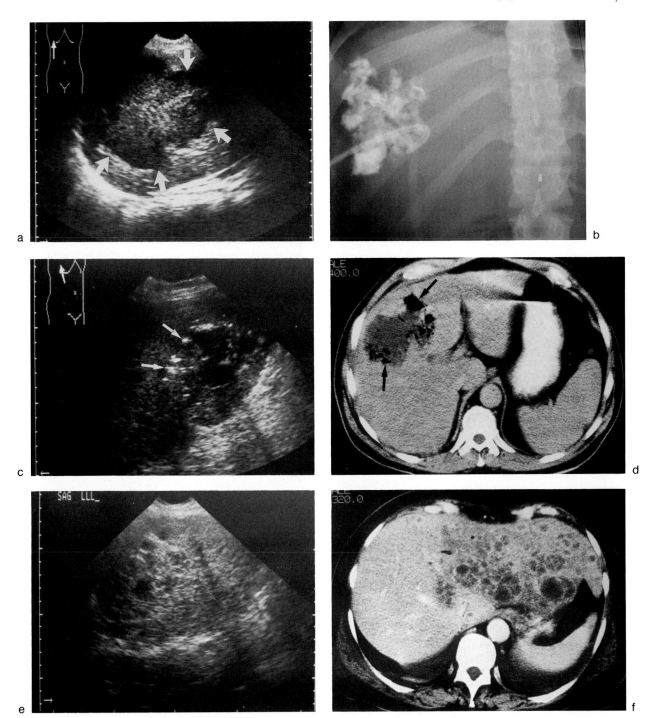

FIG. 5.18. Liver abscesses. **a:** Sagittal scan of right hepatic lobe demonstrates an irregularly marginated mass (*arrows*) filling much of right hepatic lobe. This mass contains multiple medium-level echoes. Needle aspiration demonstrated pus within this mass. **b:** Plain radiograph of same patient as (a) demonstrates placement of a drainage catheter within this abscess. After aspiration of pus, some contrast material was injected, which demonstrates very irregular margins of the collapsed abscess cavity. **c:** Oblique scan through right hepatic lobe of another patient demonstrates multiple hypoechoic areas in liver parenchyma associated with small hyperechoic foci (*arrows*), which represent gas in the abscess. **d:** CT scan through same area as (c) demonstrates low-density gas bubbles (*arrows*) within periphery of this liver abscess. **e:** Multiple small abscesses. Sagittal scan through left hepatic lobe of another patient demonstrates diffuse heterogeneity in liver parenchyma associated with some small, poorly defined hypoechoic areas. **f:** CT scan of same patient as (e) demonstrates enlargement of left hepatic lobe caused by numerous hypodense areas that represent locules of pus.

diate hosts such as sheep or cattle and occasionally humans. The eggs travel to the liver via the portal vein and become embedded in hepatic capillaries.

The gross morphology of the stages of hepatic infestation are

1. *Unilocular fertile cysts.* This is composed of an endocyst lining, which produces fluid and embryonic larvae (scolices), and a pericyst, which is a surrounding fibrotic rind of tissue. Ultrasound will often reveal a double line comprising the wall of the cyst. The inner line is the endocyst and the outer line is the pericyst (30). Fine internal echoes arise from multiple tiny scolices (hydatid sand) (31).

2. *Daughter cysts.* Daughter cysts are separate endocyst formations within the large cyst. Sonography demonstrates cysts and septations within the large cyst.

3. *Cysts with detached endocyst.* Ultrasound demonstrates an undulating membrane within the cyst fluid.

4. *Organizing cysts.* The cyst fills with an echogenic gelatinous material that may mimic a solid mass (Fig. 5.19).

5. *Degenerated, heavily calcified cyst.* Cysts are collapsed and contain internal and wall calcifications. These are now innocuous. Sonography demonstrates a hyperechoic, shadowing focus (Fig. 5.19).

Needle aspiration of an echinococcal cyst may cause an anaphylactic reaction. Surgical removal is the treatment of choice.

Echinococcus multilocularis (hepatic alveolar echinococcus) is another parasite that may also cause human liver disease, but the ultrasound appearances are quite different from echinococcus granulosus (32). The main

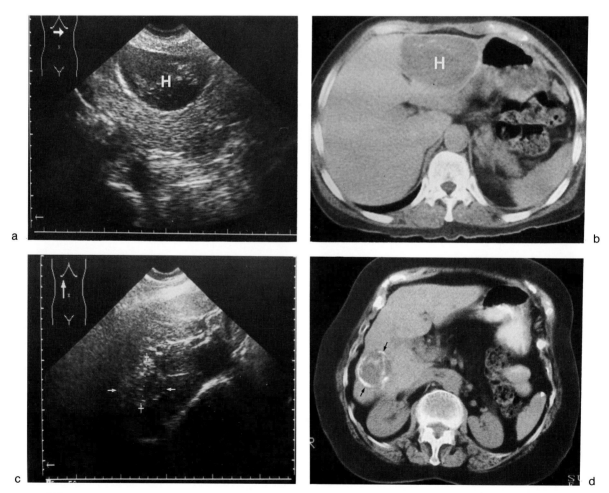

FIG. 5.19. Hydatid disease of the liver. **a:** Transverse ultrasound scan through left hepatic lobe demonstrates a hypoechoic mass (*H*) in anterior aspect of left hepatic lobe. This mass contains some low-level echoes. Note thick echogenic rind of tissue surrounding the mass. This corresponds to fibrotic pericyst. **b:** CT scan through same area as (a) demonstrates a hypodense mass in same place. This was a hydatid cyst without any observable calcification in the walls. **c:** Organizing hydatid cyst. Ultrasound scan through right hepatic lobe demonstrates a rounded mass (*arrows*) with multiple hyperechoic foci in periphery. **d:** CT scan of same patient as (c) demonstrates calcifications (*arrows*) in wall of the organized hydatid cyst in liver parenchyma.

host is often the fox, and the intermediate hosts are usually wild rodents such as field mice. Humans become infested by ingesting the eggs from fox-contaminated wild berries or by direct contact with foxes. Endemic areas include central Europe, Commonwealth of Independent States, Japan, and certain areas of North America (Alaska, northern Canada, and central North America).

Liver lesions are infiltrative, and they extend into large areas of the liver. There is a tendency to stenose bile ducts, hepatic veins, and portal veins; to necrose; to become infected; and to calcify with microcalcifications. Sonography demonstrates hyperechoic poorly marginated masses that may simulate liver tumors. If the lesion is necrotic, a large central fluid collection may be present. Microcalcifications are seen in up to 50% of cases. Early diagnosis is important because only surgical therapy is effective.

Fungal Abscess

Liver fungal infection occurs in immunocompromised people. The most common organism is *Candida albicans*. Candidiasis and other fungal infections (e.g., aspergillosis) may cause small abscesses in the liver, giving rise to several different appearances on ultrasound (33–35).

The earliest manifestation is a wheel-within-a-wheel appearance (34). An outer hypoechoic rim corresponds to fibrosis, an inner hyperechoic rim corresponds to inflammatory tissue, and the central small hypoechoic focus represents necrosis (Fig. 5.20). This evolves into a bull's-eye appearance that is missing the small central hypoechoic focus (Fig. 5.20) (33). The most common pattern is a small, uniformly hypoechoic focus, and the last type is a tiny (2–5-mm diameter) hyperechoic focus, which is seen late in the disease process.

Amebic Abscess

Amebic abscesses occur most commonly in warm climates (caused by infestation with *Entamoeba histolytica* from food or water). Most abscesses are solitary, and most arise in the right lobe. Sonographic features are similar to pyogenic abscesses, and imaging findings do not allow distinction (Fig. 5.21) (36).

Trauma

Traumatic liver injury may occur with blunt abdominal trauma, during abdominal surgery, or during percutaneous biopsy. In blunt abdominal trauma, multiorgan injury is possible, and CT scanning is usually the best initial imaging test (37,38). Ultrasound is useful in monitoring known hepatic injuries and in initial assessment if CT is not available or if the patient cannot be moved.

The right lobe is more commonly affected than the left lobe. Traumatic lesions include liver contusion, intrahepatic hematoma, and laceration. If the parenchymal damage extends to the periphery, a subcapsular hematoma may form, and if the capsule tears, perihepatic hematomas and intraperitoneal blood may be present (Fig. 5.22).

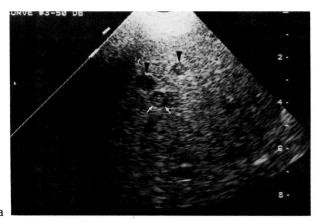
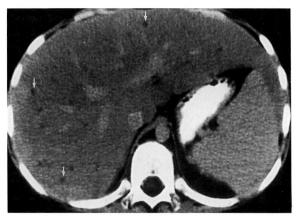

a

b

FIG. 5.20. Liver candidiasis. **a:** Transverse scan through right hepatic lobe demonstrates a small focal lesion (*arrows*) with an outer hypoechoic ring, an inner hyperechoic ring, and a small central hypoechoic focus. This appearance is called "wheel-within-a-wheel" appearance. Outer hypoechoic ring corresponds to fibrosis, inner hyperechoic ring corresponds to inflammatory tissue, and small central hypoechoic focus corresponds to necrosis. Two other similar foci (*arrowheads*) have less well-defined interior structures. **b:** CT scan of same patient demonstrates several tiny hypodense foci (*arrows*) within liver parenchyma. This particular scan plane fails to demonstrate wheel-within-a-wheel appearance of small foci. (Scans are courtesy of Dr. Howard Greenberg, Department of Radiology, Health Sciences Center, Winnipeg, Canada.)

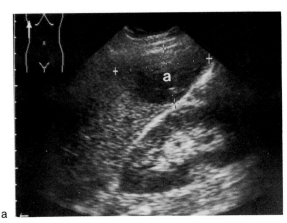
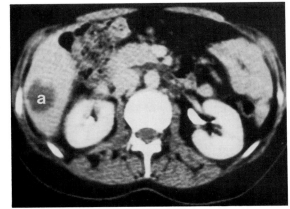

a

b

FIG. 5.21. Amebic liver abscess. **a:** Sagittal scan of right hepatic lobe demonstrates an ill-defined hypoechoic mass (a) in caudal aspect of right hepatic lobe. A few ill-defined low-level echoes are within this collection. **b:** CT scan through tip of right hepatic lobe demonstrates same amebic abscess (a). The lesion is hypodense, and its borders are ill-defined.

In the acute phase or first few days after injury, a liver contusion will present as an ill-defined hyperechoic area on ultrasound (Fig. 5.22). A recent hematoma will be iso- or hyperechoic compared with liver parenchyma. After several days, the hematoma becomes hypoechoic as red cells break down and hemoglobin is resorbed (Fig. 5.22). A laceration will appear as a linear fluid collection, often extending to the liver surface.

Contusions may resolve in a few weeks, whereas larger intrahepatic hematomas may take months to resorb. On occasion, a bile pseudocyst or pseudoaneurysm may develop (39). Fibrous scar tissue (linear echogenic foci) or calcification may be later sequelae of liver trauma.

Diffuse Diseases

Fatty Changes

Fat content in the liver increases quickly in a number of conditions by the accumulation of triglycerides within hepatocytes. Fat accumulation commonly occurs in obesity, chemotherapy, and alcoholic liver disease. Less common causes include diabetes mellitus, hyperalimentation, and Cushing syndrome/disease. Fat may accumulate diffusely throughout the liver or in a number of nonuniform ways: lobar distribution, focal mass-like accumulation, diffuse infiltration with focal areas of sparing, and patchy ill-defined zones. A number of authors have recognized pitfalls associated with focal fatty deposits that could be mistaken for tumors or abscesses (40–43) or pitfalls associated with focal areas of sparing in generalized fatty infiltration, which also can be mistaken for focal pathology (44–46). It is recognized that the fat content may change quickly (in weeks) if the underlying stimulus to fatty deposition changes. This is re-flected in dramatic changes in ultrasound and CT scan appearances.

Sonography of diffuse fatty infiltration demonstrates hepatomegaly, hyperechoic liver parenchyma, and increased sound attenuation (Fig. 5.23). Focal fatty deposits manifest as discrete hyperechoic segments, ill-defined hyperechoic masses, or discrete hyperechoic masses (Fig. 5.23). In a patient with a known primary malignancy, a CT scan may be necessary to establish the fatty nature of focal collections. With diffuse fatty infiltration and zonal or focal sparing, sonography demonstrates mass-like hypoechoic areas or geographic-like zones of relatively hypoechoic tissue (Fig. 5.23). The characteristic locations of sparing are in the quadrate lobe adjacent to the portal vein (46) and adjacent to the gallbladder.

To distinguish between tumors and fatty changes, note that fatty depositions do not cause a mass effect on hepatic vessels, whereas tumors do cause a distortion of vessels. Computed tomography may be required in some cases (Fig. 5.23), and occasionally a needle biopsy is required.

Cirrhosis

Cirrhosis is a diffuse liver process that is a response to various insults to the liver tissue (e.g., alcohol abuse, hepatitis). Fibrous tissue forms around the central veins and surrounding venous sinusoids, and this causes altered blood flow and pressures in the portal venous system. In the liver, blood flows from portal vein radicles through venous sinusoids (which course among hepatocytes) to central veins, which empty into the hepatic veins. When the disease process becomes advanced, imaging techniques will demonstrate abnormalities.

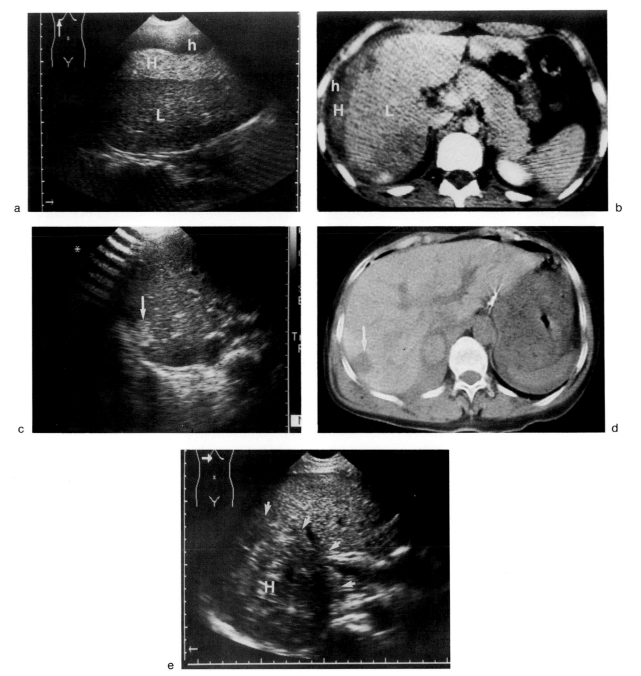

FIG. 5.22. Liver trauma. **a:** Ultrasound scan after recent blunt abdominal trauma demonstrates two collections along anterolateral aspect of right hepatic lobe (*L*). The most superficial collection is hypoechoic (*h*), and the collection immediately adjacent to the liver is hyperechoic (*H*). **b:** CT scan demonstrates two collections of fluid adjacent to liver (*L*). The most peripheral (*h*) is least dense, and the inner collection (*H*) is slightly denser. These represent two collections of blood of different density adjacent to liver after blunt abdominal trauma. **c:** Ultrasound scan of another patient with a focal intraparenchymal contusion and hematoma. Ultrasound scan demonstrates a fairly well-defined hyperechoic focus (*arrow*) in peripheral parenchyma of right hepatic lobe. **d:** CT scan of same patient as (c) demonstrates a hypodense focal collection (*arrow*) in periphery of right hepatic lobe posteriorly. After several weeks, this lesion gradually resorbed. **e:** Transverse scan of right hepatic lobe in another patient after blunt abdominal trauma demonstrates a large area (*arrows, H*) of inhomogeneous texture in right hepatic lobe. This represents lacerations and hematoma in liver parenchyma.

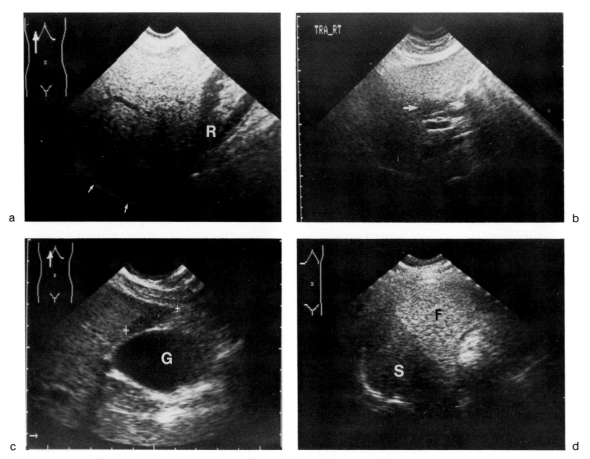

FIG. 5.23. Fatty changes in the liver. **a:** Generalized fatty infiltration in liver. Liver parenchyma is hyper-echoic compared with cortex of right kidney (*R*). In this case, sound attenuation is increased: Posterior half of liver is poorly identified. *Arrows*, right hemidiaphragm. **b:** Fatty infiltration with sparing in left hepatic lobe. This is a sagittal scan through a liver with generalized fatty infiltration and a focal area of sparing (*arrows*) anterior to portal vein and bile duct. This is a common area for focal sparing and should not be mistaken for a tumor. **c:** Sagittal scan through gallbladder (*G*) demonstrates another common area for focal sparing (*cursors*) adjacent to gallbladder and at periphery of the liver. **d:** Transverse scan through right hepatic lobe demonstrates a segmental area of fatty infiltration (*F*) and a segmental area of sparing (*S*).

With advanced cirrhosis, ultrasound demonstrates decreased size of the right lobe and medial segment of the left lobe, and enlargement of the caudate lobe and lateral segment of the left lobe (47). The caudate–right lobe ratio may be useful in assessing for cirrhosis. The width of the right lobe is measured from the lateral margin of the right lobe to the lateral edge of the main portal vein. The caudate width is taken from this point to the medial margin of the caudate lobe. A ratio of greater than 0.65 is very suggestive of cirrhosis. The average ratio in normal adults is 0.37 (48). The liver surface becomes finely lobulated (Fig. 5.24), and the intrahepatic veins are compressed. There is increased sound attenuation by the liver, the parenchyma is hyperechoic and the parenchyma may be finely inhomogeneous. Secondary signs of advanced cirrhosis include ascites, splenomegaly and formation of portosystemic collaterals veins (see below).

Viral Hepatitis

Viral hepatitis may be caused by type A, type B, or non-A non-B virus. In acute hepatitis, ultrasound demonstrates hypoechoic liver parenchyma, mild liver enlargement, and hyperechoic portal vein walls (compared with normal) (Fig. 5.25) (49). The hypoechoic parenchyma may be caused by swelling of hepatocytes and the hyperechoic portal vein walls by inflammatory and fibrous changes in and around the walls of the portal vein radicles. In chronic hepatitis, fibrous tissue and inflammatory cells may be distributed more widely in the liver tissue and thus give rise to hyperechoic liver parenchyma and a decrease in echogenicity of the walls of the portal vein radicles. Although ultrasound abnormalities are commonly seen in cases of viral hepatitis, the ultrasound findings are usually not diagnostic. The definitive diagnosis depends on clinical assessment and other tests.

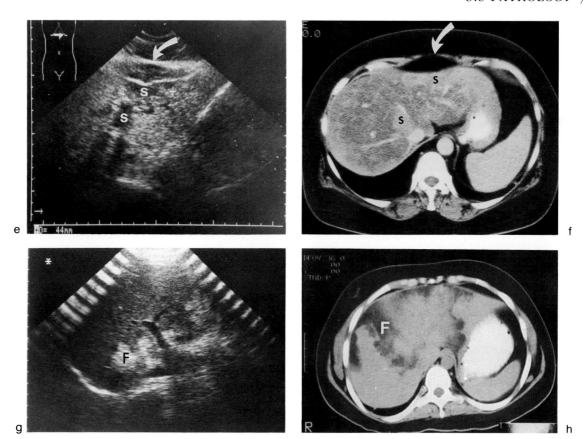

FIG. 23. *continued.* **e:** Transverse scan through left hepatic lobe of another patient demonstrates areas of increased echogenicity interspersed with areas of focal sparing (*s*). This is a more unusual distribution of focal sparing in generalized fatty infiltration. *Curved arrow*, linea alba. **f:** CT scan of same patient as (e) demonstrates a fatty liver with peripheral islands of sparing (*s*). *Curved arrow*, linea alba. **g:** Ultrasound scan of another patient with regional and focal areas of fatty infiltration in an otherwise normal liver. On ultrasound, regions of focal fatty infiltration (*F*) present as hyperechoic foci. **h:** CT scan of same patient as (g) demonstrates areas of decreased CT density (*F*) caused by focal fatty infiltration. (Scans (g) and (h) are courtesy of Dr. Linda Hutton, Department of Radiology, University Hospital, University of Western Ontario, London, Canada.)

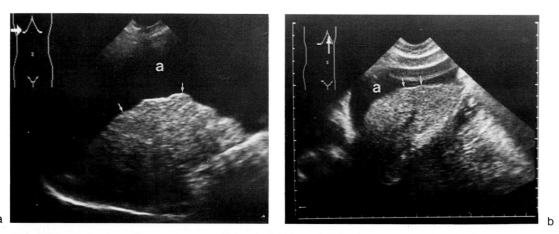

FIG. 5.24. Cirrhosis. **a:** Transverse scan through right hepatic lobe demonstrates that right hepatic lobe is shrunken and that it has a grossly lobulated contour (*arrows*). Note large amount of ascites (*a*) adjacent to liver. Without presence of ascites, lobulated contour of liver in cirrhosis is more difficult to perceive. **b:** Sagittal scan through left hepatic lobe in another patient with cirrhosis demonstrates finely lobulated contour of liver surface (*arrows*). This degree of lobulation is very difficult to perceive without ascites. *a*, ascites.

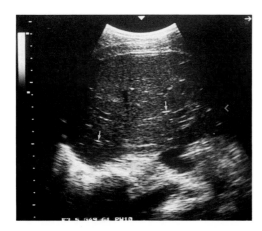

FIG. 5.25. Viral hepatitis. In this transverse scan through right hepatic lobe, walls of portal veins appear relatively more echogenic than usual (*arrows*). Hepatic parenchyma is hypoechoic because of swelling of hepatocytes, and portal vein walls are more echogenic than usual because of inflammatory and fibrous changes in and around walls of portal veins.

Right Heart Failure

Right heart failure implies increased pressure and volume of blood in the hepatic venous system and thus increased fluid content in the liver. Ultrasound will demonstrate enlargement of the hepatic veins and inferior vena cava, some generalized liver enlargement (depending on the severity of cardiac compromise), and decreased echogenicity of the liver ("superscan" of liver) (Fig. 5.26). The Doppler pattern of blood flow in the hepatic veins may also be altered depending on the severity of right heart failure and the cause. Doppler evaluation of the portal vein may demonstrate inferior vena cava–like pulsatility in the portal vein blood flow (50).

AIDS

Patients with AIDS commonly have intra-abdominal abnormalities detectable by ultrasound. The ultrasound findings are nonspecific and multisystem (51). In a series of 155 patients with AIDS (51), 46% had hyperechoic liver parenchyma, 45% splenomegaly, 37% lymphadenopathy, and 29% hyperechoic renal cortex. Less common findings in the liver included liver abscess and metastatic Kaposi sarcoma. The lymphadenopathy was commonly in the porta hepatis and peripancreatic tissue and thought to represent reactive hyperplasia.

In a series of 22 patients with AIDS, Grumbach et al. (52) demonstrated that the hyperechoic liver parenchyma could be due to granulomatous hepatitis (secondary to mycobacterium infection or talc granulomas) or hepatic steatosis (fatty liver). The liver was enlarged in 41% of cases in this study. A normal liver ultrasound did not rule out hepatitis.

Portal Vein Hypertension

Portal hypertension is increased blood pressure within the portal vein, and the cause of portal hypertension is increased resistance to blood flow. The location of the increased resistance may be at various sites (e.g., the portal vein itself, the small intrahepatic portal vein radicles, the hepatic parenchyma, the hepatic veins), and the causes are varied. The most common cause of portal hypertension in North America is cirrhosis, which represents an abnormality of the hepatic parenchyma. If the ultrasound examination demonstrates normal hepatic veins and normal main portal vein and major branches, the cause of the portal hypertension is probably intrahepatic.

Diameter of the Portal Vein

It is unlikely that portal vein diameter is a clinically useful measurement to distinguish between normals and portal hypertension (50). In an angiographic study, Lafortune et al. (3) demonstrated no significant difference in venous size between normals and those with portal hypertension.

Respiratory Variation in Diameter of the Portal Vein

In normal individuals, respiration causes significant variations in portal blood flow and in the size of the portal vein (53–55). In portal hypertension, Doppler and imaging ultrasound demonstrate less or no respiratory variation in blood flow and in venous diameter. In fact this is quite a good sign in assessing for portal hypertension. When respiratory variations are reduced (<20%),

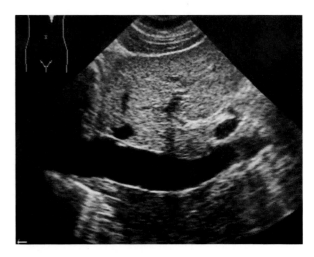

FIG. 5.26. Right heart failure. Sagittal scan demonstrates enlargement of inferior vena cava and excellent sound propagation through liver caused by increased water content.

the sensitivity for portal hypertension being present is greater than 80% and the specificity greater than 95% (53–55).

Doppler Evaluation of the Portal Vein

With chronic liver disease, the resistance to blood flow in the portal vein increases and the portal vein pressure increases. In response, increased blood flow develops in the splenic circulation, and the reasons for this are unknown (56,57). In addition, portosystemic veins develop to drain blood away from the high pressure portal system to the systemic veins. Increased splenic blood flow will maintain normal volume flow into the portal vein in the face of increased resistance and the portosystemic shunts. However, this compensatory mechanism of increased splenic blood flow will eventually fail to maintain normal portal vein flow as liver resistance increases further and portosystemic collaterals enlarge.

In portal hypertension, if normal volume flow is maintained, the Doppler examination will demonstrate a normal pattern of flow toward the liver. As the compensatory mechanism fails, volume flow will gradually decrease, and this may be detected with careful scanning techniques, although the time taken and the built-in errors in the volume flow calculations make this an impractical test in most ultrasound departments. However, in practices with many portal hypertension patients, volume flow determinations may be a useful tool to sequentially evaluate patients.

If portal vein flow decreases close to zero, Doppler

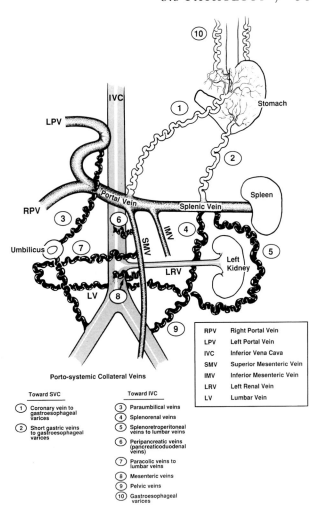

FIG. 5.28. Portosystemic collateral veins—schematic diagram.

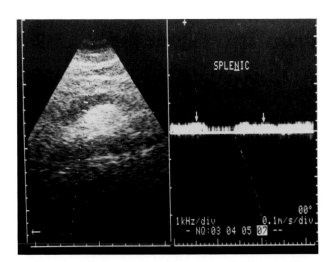

FIG. 5.27. Retrograde flow in splenic vein in portal hypertension. Transverse scan of epigastrium demonstrates PW Doppler cursor in splenic vein. Doppler spectrum (*arrows*) demonstrates blood flow toward the probe and thus away from the liver. In portal hypertension, blood flow is usually toward the liver (hepatopedal), but in a small percentage of cases the flow may be hepatofugal (i.e., away from the liver).

examination will demonstrate a to-and-fro motion inside the portal vein. Hepatofugal flow (blood flow away from the liver) is uncommon without a surgical shunt (Fig. 5.27). Occasionally, however, intrahepatic arterioportal shunts form, and this may cause reversal of blood flow in the portal vein.

As portal vein flow gradually decreases in more advanced cirrhosis, blood flow in the hepatic artery increases, and this leads to enlargement of the hepatic artery (58).

Portosystemic Collateral Veins

As a response to increased pressure in the portal vein, tiny existing veins enlarge to shunt blood away from the portal vein to the systemic veins, thus bypassing the liver parenchyma (59–62). Portosystemic collaterals may drain toward the superior vena cava or toward the inferior vena cava (Fig. 5.28). Drainage toward the superior vena cava occurs through gastroesophageal varices which often cause GI bleeding. Drainage toward the inferior vena cava occurs through multiple pathways (Fig. 5.28) that usually do not cause bleeding because they are remote from mucosal surfaces. These pathways, however, form large-caliber vessels that shunt a lot of blood away from bowel directly into the systemic circulation. Ammonia and other products in this blood may give rise to encephalopathy.

The following are the common portosystemic collateral veins that may be seen with ultrasound.

Toward Superior Vena Cava

Coronary Vein. (Shunt: Portal vein to superior vena cava.) The coronary vein receives blood from the stomach, the paraesophageal veins, and the venous plexus in the wall of the distal esophagus. A portion of the coronary vein (right gastric vein) runs in the lesser omentum (i.e., gastrohepatic ligament) *toward* the GE junction, and another portion (the left gastric vein) returns *from* the GE junction in the retroperitoneum to empty into the splenic vein or portal vein. In portal hypertension, the retroperitoneal coronary vein is often enlarged (i.e., >5-mm diameter), and this can be seen best with sagittal ultrasound scans (Fig. 5.29) (59). Sagittal scans will also demonstrate tortuous veins in the lesser omentum deep to the left hepatic lobe, corresponding to the coronary vein within the lesser omentum. Doppler examination often (but not always) demonstrates reversed venous flow toward the GE junction in the retroperitoneal coronary vein (left gastric vein). A coronary vein that measures greater than 7 mm in diameter is seen in severe portal hypertension where the probability of esophageal bleeding is high (63).

Short Gastric Veins. (Shunt: Splenic vein to superior vena cava.) Short gastric veins normally drain blood away from the stomach through the gastrosplenic ligament to the splenic vein. In portal hypertension, blood flow may be reversed, carrying blood from the splenic vein to gastroesophageal varices. Coronal and transverse scans through the spleen will demonstrate enlarged short gastric veins along the medial aspect of the spleen adjacent to the stomach (Fig. 5.29).

Toward Inferior Vena Cava

Paraumbilical Veins. (Shunt: Left portal vein to external iliac vein.) Paraumbilical veins enlarge and drain blood away from the left portal vein to the anterior abdominal wall near the umbilicus and thence into epigastric veins of the anterior abdominal wall and into the external iliac veins. Right parasagittal scans demonstrate a patent vein with a diameter greater than 3 mm (62) arising from the left portal vein and coursing through the liver in the ligamentum teres toward the umbilicus (Fig. 5.30). Doppler (CDU or PW) will usually demonstrate blood flow toward the umbilicus (Fig. 5.30).

Splenorenal Veins. (Shunt: Splenic vein to left renal vein.) Splenorenal veins run in the splenorenal ligament. Coronal and transverse scans demonstrate tortuous vessels between the splenic hilum and left renal hilum (Fig. 5.31).

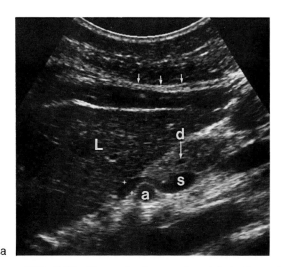 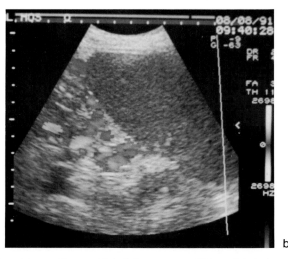

a   b

FIG. 5.29. (*See color image of part* ***b*** *in the color plate section, which follows page 50.*) **a:** Dilated coronary vein. Sagittal scan demonstrates a slightly dilated coronary vein (i.e., left gastric vein) arising from splenic vein (*s*) and passing over splenic artery (*a*). Note pancreatic duct (*d*) in body of pancreas. *L,* left hepatic lobe; *arrows,* linea alba; ++, inner diameter of left gastric vein is slightly dilated (7 mm). **b:** Short gastric veins—color Doppler ultrasound. Transverse scan through spleen in another patient demonstrates multiple tortuous enlarged veins medial to spleen. Blood flow is coded red and blue in these veins because some loops have flow toward the probe (*red*) and some away from the probe (*blue*).

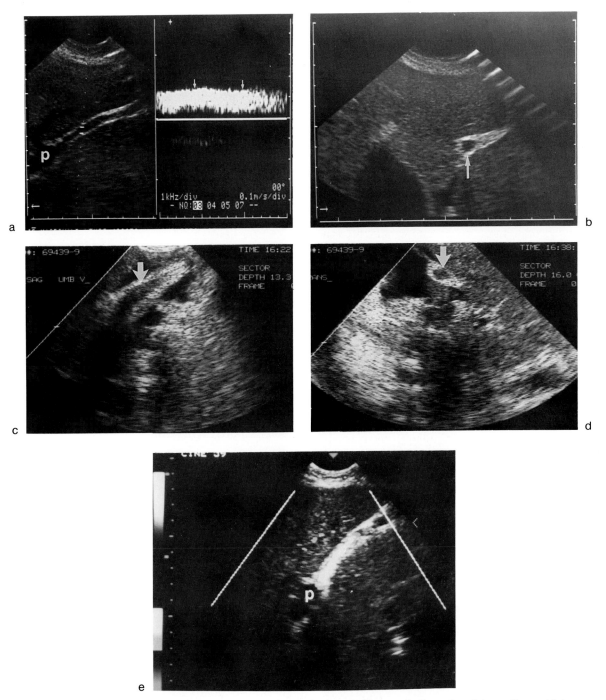

FIG. 5.30. Recanalized paraumbilical veins. (*See color image of part* **e** *in the color plate section, which follows page 50.*) **a,b:** Sagittal and transverse scans through left hepatic lobe demonstrate a recanalized paraumbilical vein (PW Doppler *cursor*). Doppler spectrum analysis (*small arrows*) demonstrates blood flow from left portal vein (*p*) toward the umbilicus. *Large arrow*, paraumbilical vein. **c,d:** Sagittal and transverse scans of another patient with an enlarged paraumbilical vein (*arrow*). Note echogenic material filling paraumbilical vein in this patient. Doppler examination demonstrated no blood flow within the vein. This represented thrombosis within a previously patent recanalized paraumbilical vein. **e:** Color Doppler flow study in another patient demonstrates blood flow (*yellow* and *red*) in recanalized paraumbilical vein from left portal vein (*p*) toward umbilicus.

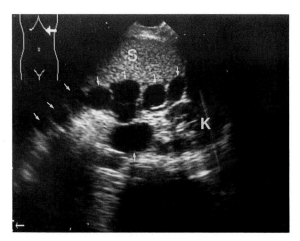

FIG. 5.31. Splenorenal veins—portosystemic collaterals. Transverse scan through spleen (*S*) demonstrates large tortuous veins (*arrows*) between spleen and left kidney (*K*). These veins could be traced to the left renal vein, which was enlarged.

Splenoretroperitoneal Veins. (Shunt: splenic vein to lumbar veins.) The retroperitoneal veins connect the splenic vein to the lumbar veins, and these drain blood from the splenic vein into the inferior vena cava in portal hypertension. Transverse ultrasound scans will demonstrate tortuous veins passing from the renal hilus lateral to the left kidney.

Peripancreatic Veins or Pancreaticoduodenal Veins. (Shunt: superior mesenteric vein to inferior vena cava.) These are retroperitoneal collaterals that shunt blood from the superior mesenteric vein directly into the inferior vena cava (Fig. 5.32).

Paracolic Veins. (Shunt: superior mesenteric vein to lumbar veins.) These are retroperitoneal paracolic veins that shunt blood into the lumbar veins and thence into the inferior vena cava.

Mesenteric Veins. (Shunt: superior mesenteric vein to inferior vena cava.) These collaterals lie in the small bowel mesentery. They shunt blood directly from the superior mesenteric vein into the inferior vena cava.

Pelvic Veins. (Shunt: inferior mesenteric vein to iliac veins.) Multiple collaterals may form in the pelvic walls, including hemorrhoidal veins.

Less common portosystemic collaterals include intrahepatic collaterals, which course between the portal vein or its main branches through the posterior segment of the right hepatic lobe toward the bare area and into the inferior vena cava (64).

Other Sequelae (Splenomegaly, Ascites)

Splenomegaly is often present in portal hypertension. Using the method of measurement outlined in Chapter 6, one can calculate splenic weight. Two hundred grams is taken to be the upper limit of normal in average size adults.

In advanced cirrhosis, some ascites is often present (Fig. 5.24). This may be related to the primary liver disease, the portal hypertension, or some complication such as portal vein thrombosis or hepatic vein occlusion.

Surgical Portosystemic Shunts

Surgical shunts are classified as selective or nonselective (50). Nonselective shunts decompress the entire portal venous system and the most common are the following:

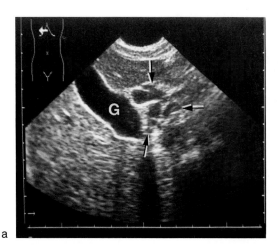

a

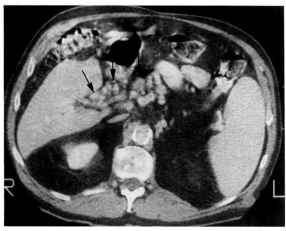

b

FIG. 5.32. Duodenal varices—portosystemic collaterals. **a:** Transverse scan through gallbladder (*G*) demonstrates multiple tortuous blood vessels (*arrows*) medial to gallbladder and adjacent to duodenum. **b:** CT scan through same area demonstrates multiple tortuous enhancing veins (*arrows*) adjacent to gallbladder fossa and duodenum. These represent paraduodenal enlarged veins that are shunting blood from portal system to systemic system.

1. *Portocaval (side-to-side).* The side of the portal vein is joined to the side of the inferior vena cava.
2. *Portocaval (end-to-side).* The portal vein is severed. The splenic end of the portal vein is joined to the side of the inferior vena cava.
3. *Proximal splenorenal shunt.* Splenectomy is performed. The hepatic end of the splenic vein is anastomosed to the side of the left renal vein.
4. *Mesocaval interposition.* Graft material is used to join the side of the superior mesenteric vein to the side of the inferior vena cava.

A reliable and simple test to assess for shunt patency in a nonselective shunt is Doppler assessment of the main portal vein or the main portal vein branches. If hepatofugal flow is present (i.e., flow away from the liver), this indicates shunt patency (65,66). The high-pressure portal venous blood is now shunted to the lower-pressure systemic veins, and thus flow should be away from the liver if the shunt is patent. If sequential scans demonstrate a switch from hepatofugal to hepatopetal flow, this is very suspicious for shunt occlusion, usually by thrombosis.

Direct imaging and Doppler assessment of the portosystemic anastomoses can be performed in many instances (especially for portocaval shunts and proximal splenorenal shunts), but bowel gas may prevent this in some.

A Warren shunt (distal splenorenal shunt) is a common *selective* portosystemic shunt. The splenic vein is severed, but the spleen is left in place. The splenic end of the splenic vein is attached to the side of the left renal vein. This decompresses gastroesophageal varices into the left renal vein. However, blood flow in the superior mesenteric vein maintains blood flow in the portal vein toward the liver. Therefore, in a patent Warren shunt, Doppler will normally demonstrate portal vein flow toward the liver. Hepatofugal flow suggests that blood is shunting away from the superior mesenteric vein to the splenic vein and left renal vein.

Other Portal Vein Abnormalities

Portal Vein Thrombosis

Nonneoplastic thrombus may form in the main portal vein and its branches for several reasons: hypercoagulation states (e.g., polycythemia, systemic infections), cirrhosis, regional inflammatory conditions (e.g., pancreatitis), trauma, extrinsic compression (e.g., portal lymphadenopathy). In infants, the main causes are dehydration, sepsis, and catheterization of the umbilical vein (67). The clinical findings are often nonspecific or absent, and the diagnosis is usually made at ultrasound or CT. In patients with chronic liver disease, a sudden exacerbation of the illness with decreased liver function and onset of ascites may be due to acute thrombosis of the portal vein.

Ultrasound often demonstrates an echogenic thrombus within the portal vein (Fig. 5.33). The echogenicity is usually less than or equal to normal liver parenchyma, and the clot may fill or partially fill the vein. Recently formed thrombus may be almost anechoic and thus difficult to visualize. The vein may be normal diameter or mildly enlarged. Rarely, a long-standing thrombus may

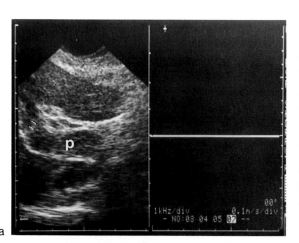
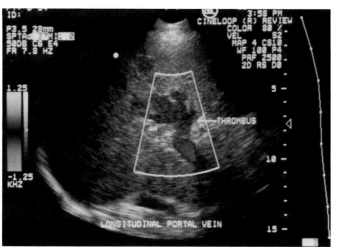

FIG. 5.33. *(See color image of part **b** in the color plate section, which follows page 50.)* Portal vein thrombosis. **a:** Scan through long axis of portal vein (*p*) demonstrates echogenic material filling lumen of portal vein. Note PW Doppler cursor within proximal portion of portal vein. Corresponding Doppler study on right side of the picture demonstrates no evidence of blood flow within the portal vein. **b:** Color Doppler ultrasound. Oblique scan demonstrates some slow flow in main portal vein toward the probe and thus toward the liver (*dark red color*). Intrahepatic portal vein branches are filled with echogenic thrombus. There is no flow detected in these branches. (Scan is courtesy of Advanced Technology Laboratories [ATL].)

become calcified. If the thrombus fills the main portal vein, Doppler (CDU or PW) fails to demonstrate blood flow within it (Fig. 5.33) (68). If color Doppler ultrasound demonstrates a patent portal vein, no further evaluation is necessary, but a lack of color flow does not always indicate occlusion (very slow flow may not register on the Doppler examination) and other tests are needed for confirmation (68). If the clot has retracted away from the vein walls or if there is recanalization within the clot or if periportal collateral veins have developed, Doppler will demonstrate blood flow within these channels. If portal vein obstruction persists for 1 month or more, periportal collateral veins may enlarge and carry all the portal blood flow past the occluded main portal vein into the liver (69). These collateral veins are portoportal collaterals, which are called cavernous transformation of the portal vein, and they form in 30% of patients with portal vein occlusion (70). In place of a single portal vein, several serpiginous veins are present (Fig. 5.34) in the porta hepatis. Doppler evaluation demonstrates blood flow toward the liver.

Portal Vein Tumor

Extension of neoplasm into the portal vein is occasionally seen in ultrasound practice. The most common cause is extension of hepatocellular carcinoma into portal vein branches. Approximately one-third of patients with hepatocellular carcinoma will have demonstrable portal vein tumor on ultrasound, whereas 1% or less of liver metastases will have venous extension (71).

Ultrasound imaging may demonstrate continuity between the liver tumor and the portal vein extension. In other cases, it may be impossible to distinguish between tumor and bland thrombus with imaging. Pulsed Doppler may demonstrate arterial tumor blood flow within the intravenous tumor, and this will make the definitive diagnosis of tumor versus bland thrombus.

Portal Vein Gas

Ultrasound can demonstrate portal venous gas in adults (72), usually secondary to ischemic bowel disease: gas enters the splanchnic veins from the bowel lumen (usually colon) and flows through the portal vein into the peripheral portal vein branches and into the peripheral liver parenchyma. Ultrasound demonstrates peripheral linear echogenic collections, which usually do not shadow (Fig. 5.35). One may visualize echogenic material (microbubbles of gas) flowing inside the splanchnic veins (Fig. 5.35) (73). Biliary gas is usually more centrally and ventrally located, but it may also be located peripherally. Bile flows from the periphery toward the porta hepatis and carries biliary gas toward the porta hepatis. Thus, biliary gas is usually more centrally located than portal venous gas.

In infants, the cause of portal venous gas is necrotizing enterocolitis. The ultrasound findings of portal venous gas may precede the plain film findings and thus alert the pediatricians to the probable diagnosis, which must be treated promptly.

Hepatic Vein Occlusion (Budd-Chiari Syndrome)

Budd-Chiari syndrome implies obstruction of one or more of the major hepatic veins (right, middle, left) and possibly the intrahepatic inferior vena cava. This is a rare condition that may be caused by membranous obstruction of the intrahepatic inferior vena cava (primary Budd-Chiari syndrome), hypercoagulation states leading to hepatic vein thrombosis, and liver diseases that cause mechanical compression of the hepatic veins and inferior vena cava (e.g., liver tumors and cirrhosis). The cause is often not found. The clinical symptoms depend on the extent and duration of the obstruction. In acute cases, findings include abdominal pain, ascites, and an enlarged tender liver.

Ultrasound demonstrates hepatomegaly and ascites (74–76) in the acute phase. The liver parenchyma is usually homogeneous but occasionally may be diffusely patchy and inhomogeneous (Fig 5.36). In long-standing cases, the caudate lobe enlarges and is relatively hypoechoic. This is thought to be related to the separate venous drainage from the caudate lobe via multiple small veins directly into the inferior vena cava. If the main hepatic veins are significantly obstructed, these caudate veins remain as the only effective venous drainage sys-

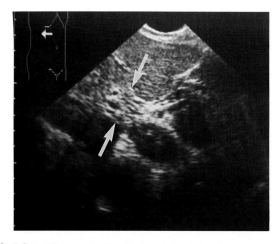

FIG. 5.34. ''Recanalization'' of portal vein (porto-portal collateral veins). Oblique scan through porta hepatis demonstrates multiple, various size serpiginous vessels (*arrows*) in place of normal portal vein. These represent periportal venous collaterals, which carry blood from gut to liver, bypassing thrombosed portal vein.

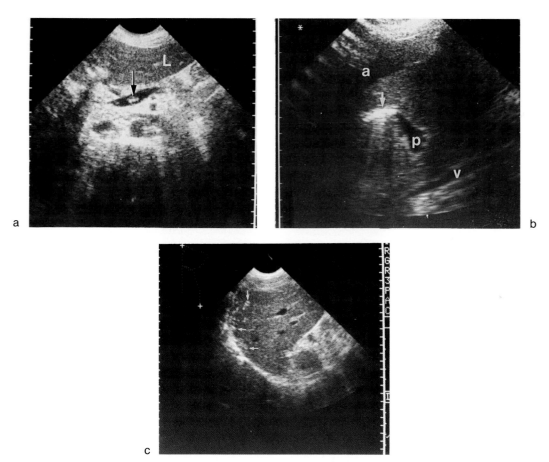

FIG. 5.35. Portal venous gas. **a:** Transverse scan through left hepatic lobe (*L*) demonstrates echogenic material (*arrow*) flowing in splenic vein toward the liver. These represented bubbles of gas as documented on a CT scan of the same day. The patient had ischemic colitis. **b:** Sagittal scan through right hepatic lobe of another patient demonstrates echogenic material (*arrows*) within an intrahepatic portal vein branch. This represents gas within one of main branches of intrahepatic portal vein. *a*, ascites; *p*, portal vein; *v*, inferior vena cava. **c:** Sagittal scan through right hepatic lobe of another patient with portal venous gas demonstrates multiple linear echogenic foci in periphery of the liver (*arrows*), representing gas within peripheral portal venous branches and gas within liver parenchyma.

tem of the liver. In some chronic cases, multiple collateral veins may be visible in the porta hepatis.

Color Doppler ultrasound is the best ultrasound technique to assess for patency of the three main hepatic veins (77), although PW duplex ultrasound is useful in many circumstances (Fig. 5.36). Sensitive color Doppler units will detect flow in narrow vessels that may be quite difficult to visualize with real-time imaging and therefore also difficult to assess with PW Doppler. This is frequently the case in advanced cirrhosis, where the liver is small and the hepatic veins are difficult to visualize, and in hepatomegaly, where the hepatic veins may be compressed.

Patients with hepatic vein occlusion are treated with a decompressive shunt. A mesoatrial shunt is a synthetic graft that joins the superior mesenteric vein and right atrium and thus bypasses the liver. A cavoatrial shunt joins together the inferior vena cava and right atrium. The graft lies deep to the anterior abdominal wall and is easily assessed for patency with color Doppler ultrasound or PW duplex ultrasound (77).

Liver Transplantation

Imaging ultrasound and Doppler ultrasound are useful in assessing the liver before and after transplantation. If the portal vein is occluded or small in the recipient, surgical anastomosis will be impossible. If Doppler ultrasound demonstrates normal flow in a normal-sized portal vein in the recipient, surgery can be performed. If ultrasound demonstrates no flow in the portal vein or

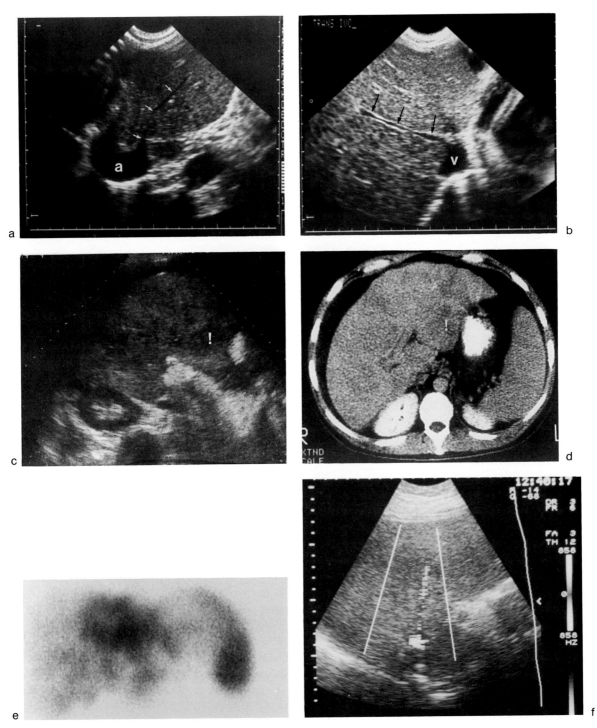

FIG. 5.36. Budd-Chiari syndrome. (*See color image of part f in the color plate section, which follows page 50.*) **a,b:** Sagittal and transverse scans through left hepatic lobe demonstrate marked narrowing of left and middle hepatic veins (*arrows*). *a*, right atrium; *v*, inferior vena cava. This patient had myelofibrosis. **c:** Transverse scan through right hepatic lobe of another patient demonstrates multiple ill-defined hypoechoic areas (*!*) within liver parenchyma in a patient with Budd-Chiari syndrome. These changes may occur secondary to hepatic vein occlusion. **d:** CT scan through same area as (c) demonstrating multiple ill-defined hypodense areas(*!*). **e:** Isotope liver scan of same patient as (c) and (d) demonstrates multiple ill-defined areas of decreased photon emission corresponding to hypoechoic areas on ultrasound and hypodense areas on CT. Liver parenchyma will return to normal appearances after successful treatment of Budd-Chiari syndrome. **f:** Color Doppler ultrasound. Sagittal scan demonstrates slow blood flow (*dark blue*) in a very small hepatic vein. This vessel was not visible on 2-D real-time imaging. Blood flow is coded *blue* (away from the probe) and thus toward inferior vena cava.

only a small amount of flow in periportal collaterals, angiography is required to outline precisely the vascular anatomy in the recipient. In children with biliary atresia (a common reason for pediatric liver transplantation), up to 25% may have associated anomalies including anomalies of the inferior vena cava and hepatic arteries, which may be detected with sonography (78).

After liver transplantation, the most feared complication is acute thrombosis of the hepatic artery, which will lead to hepatic infarction (79). The hepatic artery provides most of the blood supply to the transplanted liver, whereas it delivers a relatively small proportion of the blood supply to the native liver. Color Doppler ultrasound is the preferred method of finding the hepatic artery and diagnosing an occluded or severely stenotic vessel. If Doppler fails to show hepatic arterial blood flow, angiography is needed, because a delay in treating acute thrombosis will worsen the prognosis.

Sonography is also well suited to identify other vascular complications such as inferior vena cava thrombosis, portal vein thrombosis, and portal vein stenosis (79). However, Doppler evaluation of hepatic artery impedance patterns has not been useful in assessing for rejection (80,81).

Ultrasound is also the best method to diagnose other postoperative complications such intrahepatic and extrahepatic fluid collections, parenchymal alterations in rejection, and bile duct obstruction (82).

5.4 PITFALLS, ARTIFACTS, AND PRACTICAL TIPS

Hyperechoic Liver

The liver echogenicity is compared with the echogenicity of the right renal cortex in a parasagittal scan. For this comparison, the right kidney must be normal. Liver parenchyma is slightly more echogenic than normal renal cortex. In a hyperechoic liver, the difference is accentuated. If in doubt, one scans a known normal for comparison. If the liver parenchyma is quite hyperechoic and it attenuates sound more than usual, it will be difficult to rule out small focal lesions. In these cases a CT scan is helpful to rule out focal lesions.

In clinical practice, the most common cause of a hyperechoic liver is fatty infiltration, which can be caused by many factors. However, other pathologies can certainly cause hyperechoic liver parenchyma, and a biopsy may be required to make the definitive diagnosis depending on the clinical circumstances.

Pseudo Tumors Associated with a Hyperechoic Liver

In a fatty liver, it is quite common to have zones of normal echogenicity in the liver as well. These can be small or large, and they may be fairly well defined or quite poorly defined. Commonly they lie adjacent to the gallbladder fossa and porta hepatis, but they may occur anywhere in the liver. These can be mistaken for tumors, but the presence of hyperechoic liver parenchyma and the characteristic locations of the areas usually are sufficient to make the diagnosis (Fig. 5.23). If the borders are ill-defined and the shape is geographic, this is also very suggestive. In larger lesions, if there is no distortion of the liver vasculature, this also favors focal sparing. A CT scan or biopsy is usually not required.

Hemangiomas Versus Other Hyperechoic Neoplasms

Other hyperechoic neoplasms such as metastases may simulate hemangiomas, but this is quite uncommon in clinical practice. Hemangiomas, however, are very common, and in the clinical setting of a healthy person with no primary malignancy, the findings of a uniformly hyperechoic well-defined mass in the liver are sufficient to make the diagnosis of liver hemangioma. Even in the presence of known primary malignancy, characteristic findings on ultrasound are strongly suggestive of a hemangioma (Fig. 5.9). However, hemangiomas may be mixed in echogenicity or hypoechoic, and in these circumstances further investigation is required to make the diagnosis (Fig. 5.9).

Cysts Versus Homogeneous Solid Masses

Various neoplasms in the liver are hypoechoic on ultrasound, and some may simulate a simple cyst. It is usually possible to alter the gain settings or scan planes to demonstrate that these contain low-level echoes. Most solid masses will not have sharply defined posterior walls, and most will not have posterior acoustic enhancement. Rarely, a hypoechoic solid mass may simulate a simple cyst in all respects despite the sonographer's best efforts (Fig. 5.11). In these cases, other findings in the abdomen often suggest the correct diagnosis.

Diaphragmatic Muscle Slips

The surface of the liver along the right lateral abdominal wall may be indented by intercostal muscles, which can become quite prominent (Fig. 5.37). In cross section these may simulate tumors in the periphery of the liver, but scans performed parallel to the muscles demonstrate these to be muscles.

Diaphragm Artifacts

Mirror image artifacts of liver parenchyma and structures within the liver are quite common in clinical prac-

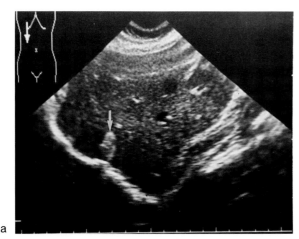
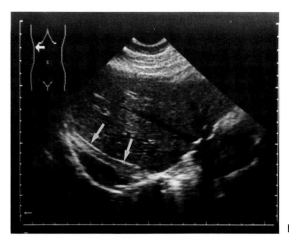

a   b

FIG. 5.37. Diaphragmatic muscle slips. **a:** Sagittal scan through right hepatic lobe demonstrates a hyperechoic focus (*arrow*) in posterior aspect of right hepatic lobe. This could be mistaken for a tumor. **b:** Transverse scan through right hepatic lobe of same patient demonstrates that hyperechoic focus represents a linear structure (*arrows*) indenting the liver. This is a prominent diaphragmatic muscle slip impinging into liver parenchyma.

tice. Real intrahepatic structures are projected cranial to the diaphragm, and these are usually recognized as artifacts. Occasionally a pleural effusion may be simulated, but close inspection of the structures above the diaphragm indicates that they represent duplication of echoes from structures within the liver (see Chapter 2).

Portal Venous Gas Versus Biliary Gas

Biliary gas in the liver is much more common than portal venous gas. The clinical history of biliary surgery or recent biliary manipulation will often clarify the situation if there is a problem in distinguishing these two entities on the ultrasound scan. Although portal venous gas is usually in the periphery of the liver and biliary gas is more centrally located, the positions can be reversed and the ultrasound findings can be confusing.

Hepatic Vein Occlusion Versus Stenosis

On real-time imaging alone it may be impossible to distinguish between complete occlusion of the hepatic veins and marked narrowing. Sensitive color flow Doppler, however, will improve the ability to distinguish between these. Transverse scans high in the epigastrium give optimal Doppler evaluation of the middle and left hepatic veins, because blood flow is almost parallel to the insonating beam. However, if blood flow is very slow in the hepatic veins, color Doppler ultrasound may not detect it. Angiography may be required to differentiate in these cases.

Doppler Assessment of Portal Vein Thrombosis

In some circumstances (e.g., portal hypertension) portal vein flow may be very slow and not detected by color Doppler or pulsed Doppler assessment. If no flow is demonstrated in the Doppler examination, it may be necessary to confirm occlusion by angiography (83). It is useful to change the patient's position and examine the portal vein in inspiration and expiration in an attempt to stimulate portal vein flow. Scanning the portal vein after a meal may also help augment the portal vein flow. The main portal vein can be difficult to assess because the Doppler angle is close to 90°. A better approach is a transverse scan in the epigastrium to assess the left portal vein where the Doppler angle approaches zero. A scan obtained from the right midaxillary line of the right portal vein will also allow optimal assessment of portal venous flow.

REFERENCES

Scanning Techniques

1. Guidelines for performance of the abdominal and retroperitoneal ultrasound examination. *J Ultrasound Med* 1991;10:576–577.
2. Perlmutter GS. Ultrasound measurements of the pancreas. In: Goldberg BB, Kurtz AB, eds. *Atlas of ultrasound measurements.* New York: Raven Press; 1990:124.
3. Lafortune M, Marleau D, Breton G, Viallet A, Lavoie P, Huet PM. Portal venous measurements in portal hypertension. *Radiology* 1984;151:27–30.
4. Kurol M, Forsberg L. Ultrasonographic investigation of respiratory influence on diameters of portal vessels in normal subjects. *Acta Radiol Diagn* 1986;27:675–680.

Normal Anatomy

5. Wolson AH. Liver. In: Goldberg BB, Kurtz AB, eds. *Atlas of ultrasound measurements*. New York: Raven Press; 1990:99–100.
5a. Becker CD, Cooperberg PL. Sonography of the hepatic vascular system. *AJR* 1988;150:999–1005.
6. Middleton WD. Color Doppler ultrasonography: image interpretation and optimization. In: *Syllabus. Color Doppler ultrasonography course*. AIUM Annual Meeting February 23–24, 1991;15–18.
7. Taylor KJW, Burns PN, Woodcock JP, Wells PNT. Blood flow in deep abdominal and pelvic vessels: ultrasonic pulsed Doppler analysis. *Radiology* 1985;154:487–493.

Pathology

8. Berland LL. Screening for diffuse and focal liver disease: the case for hepatic computed tomography. *JCU* 1984;12:83–89.
8a. Wernecke K, Rummeny E, Bongartz G, et al. Detection of hepatic masses in patients with carcinoma: comparative sensitivities of sonography, CT, and MR imaging. *AJR* 1991;157:731–739.
9. Hillman BJ, Smith EH, Gammelgaard J, Holm HH. Ultrasonographic—pathologic correlation of malignant hepatic masses. *Gastrointest Radiol* 1979;4:361–365.
10. Bruneton JN, Ladree D, Caramella E, Mathieu D, Roux P. Ultrasonographic study of calcified hepatic metastases: a report of 13 cases. *Gastrointest Radiol* 1982;7:61–63.
11. Wooten WB, Green B, Goldstein HM. Ultrasonography of necrotic hepatic metastases. *Radiology* 1978;128:447–450.
12. LaBerge JM, Laing FC, Federle MP, Jeffrey RB Jr, Lim RC Jr. Hepatocellular carcinoma: assessment of resectability by computed tomography and ultrasound. *Radiology* 1984;152:485–490.
13. Sheu J-C, Sung J-L, Chen D-S, et al. Ultrasonography of small hepatic tumors using high resolution linear-array real-time instruments. *Radiology* 1984;150:797–802.
14. Sherlock S, Dick D. The impact of radiology on hepatology. *AJR* 1986;147:1116–1122.
15. Bruneton JN, Drouillard J, Fenart D, Roux P, Nicolau A. Ultrasonography of hepatic cavernous hemangiomas. *Br J Radiol* 1983;56:791–795.
16. Mirk P, Rubaltelli L, Bazzocchi M, et al. Ultrasonographic patterns in hepatic hemangiomas. *JCU* 1982;10:373–378.
17. Bree RL, Schwab RE, Neiman HL. Solitary echogenic spot in the liver: is it diagnostic of a hemangioma? *AJR* 1983;140:41–45.
18. Freeny PC, Marks WM. Patterns of contrast enhancement of benign and malignant neoplasms during bolus dynamic and delayed CT. *Radiology* 1986;160:613–618.
19. Mathieu D, Bruneton JN, Drouillard J, Pointreau CC, Vasile N. Hepatic adenomas and focal nodular hyperplasia: dynamic CT study. *Radiology* 1986;160:53–58.
20. Majaewski A, Gratz KF, Brölsch C, Gebel M. Sonographic pattern of focal nodular hyperplasia of the liver. *Eur J Radiol* 1984;4:52–57.
21. Welch TJ, Sheedy PF II, Johnson CM, et al. Focal nodular hyperplasia and hepatic adenoma: comparison of angiography, CT, ultrasound, and scintigraphy. *Radiology* 1985;156:593–595.
22. Scatarige JC, Fishman EK, Sanders RC. The sonographic "scar sign" in focal nodular hyperplasia of the liver. *J Ultrasound Med* 1982;1:275–278.
23. Sekiya T, Meller ST, Cosgrove DO, McCready VR. Ultrasonography of Hodgkin's disease in the liver and spleen. *Clin Radiol* 1982;33:635–639.
24. Ginaldi S, Bernadino ME, Jing BS, Green B. Ultrasonographic patterns of hepatic lymphoma. *Radiology* 1980;136:427–431.
25. Lepke R, Pagani JJ. Sonography of hepatic chloromas. *AJR* 1982;138:1176–1177.
26. Taylor KJW, Viscomi GN. Ultrasound diagnosis of cystic disease of the liver. *J Clin Gastroenterol* 1980;2:197–204.
27. Saini S, Mueller PR, Ferrucci JT Jr, et al. Percutaneous aspiration of hepatic cysts does not provide definitive therapy. *AJR* 1983;141:559–560.
28. *Deleted in proof.*
29. Wilson SR, Arenson AM. Sonographic evaluation of hepatic abscesses. *J Can Assoc Radiol* 1984;35:174–177.
30. Esfahani F, Rooholamini SA, Vessal K. Ultrasonography of hepatic hydatid cysts: new diagnostic signs. *J Ultrasound Med* 1988;7:443–450.
31. Lewall DB, McCorkell SJ. Hepatic echinococcal cysts: sonographic appearance and classification. *Radiology* 1985;155:773–775.
32. Didier D, Weiler S, Rohmer P, et al. Hepatic alveolar echinococcosis: correlative ultrasound and CT study. *Radiology* 1985;154:179–186.
33. Ho B, Cooperberg PL, Li DKB, et al. Ultrasonography and computed tomography of hepatic candidiasis in the immunosuppressed patient. *J Ultrasound Med* 1982;1:157–159.
34. Pastakia B, Shawker TH, Thaler M, O'Leary T, Pizzo PA. Hepatosplenic candidiasis: wheels within wheels. *Radiology* 1988;166:417–421.
35. Fletcher BD, Magill HL. Wheel-within-a-wheel pattern in hepatosplenic infections (Letter to the editor). *Radiology* 1988;169:578–579.
36. Ralls PW, Barnes PF, Radin DR, Colletti P, Halls J. Sonographic features of amebic and pyogenic liver abscesses: a blinded comparison. *AJR* 1987;149:499–501.
37. Stalker HP, Kaufman RA, Towbin R. Patterns of liver injury in childhood. CT analysis. *AJR* 1986;147:1199–1205.
38. Savolaine ER, Grecos GP, Howard J, White P. Evolution of CT findings in hepatic hematoma. *J Comput Assist Tomogr* 1985;9:1090–1096.
39. Esensten M, Ralls PW, Colletti P, Halls J. Posttraumatic intrahepatic biloma: sonographic diagnosis. *AJR* 1983;140:303–305.
40. Wang S-S, Chiang J-H, Tsai Y-T, et al. Focal fatty infiltration as a cause of pseudotumors: ultrasonographic patterns and clinical differentiation. *JCU* 1990;18:401–409.
41. Baker MK, Wenker JC, Cockerill EM, Ellis JH. Focal fatty infiltration of the liver: diagnostic imaging. *Radiographics* 1985;5:923–939.
42. Yoshikawa J, Matsui O, Takashima T, et al. Focal fatty change of the liver adjacent to the falciform ligament: CT and sonographic findings in five surgically confirmed cases. *AJR* 1987;149:491–494.
43. Scatarige JC, Scott WW, Donovan PJ, Siegelman SS, Sanders RC. Fatty infiltration of the liver: ultrasonographic and computed tomographic correlation. *J Ultrasound Med* 1984;3:9–14.
44. White EM, Simeone JF, Mueller PR, et al. Focal periportal sparing in hepatic fatty infiltration: cause of hepatic pseudomass on ultrasound. *Radiology* 1987;162:57–59.
45. Berland LL. Focal areas of decreased echogenicity in the liver at the porta hepatis. *J Ultrasound Med* 1986;5:157–159.
46. Sauerbrei EE, Lopez M. Pseudotumor of the quadrate lobe in hepatic sonography: a sign of fatty infiltration in the liver. *AJR* 1986;147:923–927.
47. Torres WE, Whitmire LF, Gedgaudas-McClees K, Bernadino ME. Computed tomography of hepatic morphological changes in cirrhosis of the liver. *J Comput Assist Tomogr* 1986;10:47–50.
48. Harbin WP, Robert NJ, Ferrucci JT Jr. Diagnosis of cirrhosis based on regional changes in hepatic morphology: a radiological and pathological analysis. *Radiology* 1980;135:273–283.
49. Kurtz AB, Rubin CS, Cooper HS, et al. Ultrasound findings in hepatitis. *Radiology* 1980;136:717–723.
50. van Leeuwen MS. Doppler ultrasound in the evaluation of portal hypertension. In: Taylor KJW, Strandness DE, eds. *Clinics in diagnostic ultrasound. Duplex Doppler Ultrasound*. New York: Churchill Livingstone; 1990:53–76.
51. Yee JM, Raghavendra BN, Horii SC, Ambrosino M. Abdominal sonography in AIDS: a review. *J Ultrasound Med* 1989;8:705–714.
52. Grumbach K, Coleman BG, Gal AA, et al. Hepatic and biliary tract abnormalities in patients with AIDS. Sonographic–pathologic correlation. *J Ultrasound Med* 1989;8:247–254.
53. Bolondi L, Gandolfi L, Arienti V, et al. Ultrasonography in the diagnosis of portal hypertension: diminished response of portal vessels to respiration. *Radiology* 1982;142:167–172.

54. Bolondi L, Mazziotti A, Arienti V, et al. Ultrasonographic study of portal venous system in portal hypertension and after portosystemic shunt operations. *Surgery* 1984;95:261–264.

55. Zoli M, Dondi C, Marchesini G, et al. Splanchnic vein measurements in patients with liver cirrhosis: a case control study. *J Ultrasound Med* 1985;4:641–646.

56. Witte CL, Witte MH, Renert W, Corrigan JJ Jr. Splenic circulatory dynamics in congestive splenomegaly. *Gastroenterology* 1974;67:498–505.

57. Vorobioff J, Bredfeldt JE, Groszmann RJ. Hyperdynamic circulation in portal-hypertensive rat model: a primary factor for maintenance of chronic portal hypertension. *Am J Physiol* 1983;244:G52–G57.

58. Toni R, Bolondi L, Gaiani S, et al. Accessory ultrasonographic findings in chronic liver disease: diameter of splenic and hepatic arteries, fasting gallbladder volume and course of left portal vein. *JCU* 1985;13:611–618.

59. Subramanyan BR, Balthazar EJ, Madamba MR, Raghavendra BN, Horii SC, Lefleur RS. Sonography of portosystemic venous collaterals in portal hypertension. *Radiology* 1983;146:161–166.

60. Jultner H-V, Jeeney JM, Ralls PW, Goldstein LI, Reynolds TB. Ultrasound demonstration of porto systemic collaterals in cirrhosis and portal hypertension. *Radiology* 1982;142:459–463.

61. Glazer GM, Laing FC, Brown TW, Gooding GAW. Sonographic demonstration of portal hypertension: the patent umbilical vein. *Radiology* 1980;136:161–163.

62. Saddekni S, Hutchinson DE, Cooperberg PL. The sonographically patent umbilical vein in portal hypertension. *Radiology* 1982;145:441–443.

63. Lafortune M, Marleau D, Breton G, et al. Portal venous system measurements in portal hypertension. *Radiology* 1984;151:27–30.

64. Mori H, Hayashi K, Fukuda T, et al. Intrahepatic portosystemic venous shunt: occurrence in patients with and without liver cirrhosis. *AJR* 1987;149:711–714.

65. Lafortune M, Patriquin H, Pomier G, et al. Hemodynamic changes in portal circulation after portosystemic shunts: use of duplex sonography in 43 patients. *AJR* 1987;149:701–706.

66. Patriquin H, Lafortune M, Weber A, Blanchard H, Garel L, Roy C. Surgical portosystemic shunts in children: assessment with duplex Doppler US. Work in Progress. *Radiology* 1987;165:25–28.

67. Slovis TL, Haller JO, Cohen HL, Berdon WE, Watts FB. Complicated appendiceal inflammatory disease in children: pyelophlebitis and liver abscess. *Radiology* 1989;171:823–825.

68. Tessler FN, Gehring BJ, Gomes AS, et al. Diagnosis of portal vein thrombosis: value of color Doppler imaging. *AJR* 1991;157:293–296.

69. Kauzlaric D, Petrovic M, Barmeir E. Sonography of cavernous transformation of the portal vein. *AJR* 1984;142:383–384.

70. Weltin G, Taylor KJ, Carter AR, Taylor CR. Duplex Doppler: identification of cavernous transformation of the portal vein. *AJR* 1985;144:999–1001.

71. Subramanyam BR, Balthazar EJ, Hilton S, Lefleur RS, Horii SC, Raghavendra BN. Hepatocellular carcinoma with venous invasion: sonographic–angiographic correlation. *Radiology* 1984;150:793–796.

72. Pearse BF, Sauerbrei EE, Leddin D. The ultrasound and CT diagnosis of gas in the mesenteric–portal venous system. *J Can Assoc Radiol* 1982;33:269–272.

73. Merritt CR, Goldsmith JP, Sharp MJ. Sonographic detection of portal venous gas in infants with necrotizing enterocolitis. *AJR* 1984;143:1059–1062.

74. Harter LP, Gross BH, St Hilaire J, Filly RA, Goldberg HI. CT and sonographic appearance of hepatic vein obstruction. *AJR* 1982;139:176–178.

75. Makuuchi M, Hasegawa H, Yamazaki S, Moriyama N, Takayasu K, Okazaki M. Primary Budd-Chiari syndrome: ultrasonic demonstration. *Radiology* 1984;152:775–779.

76. Menu Y, Alison D, Lorphelin JM, Valla D, Belghiti J, Nahum H. Budd-Chiari syndrome: ultrasound evaluation. *Radiology* 1985;157:761–764.

77. Grant EG, Perrella R, Tessler FN, Lois J, Busuttil R. Budd-Chiari syndrome: the results of duplex and Doppler imaging. *AJR* 1989;152:377–381.

78. Abramson SJ, Berdon WE, Altman RP, Amodio JB, Levy J. Biliary atresia and noncardiac polysplenic syndrome: US and surgical considerations. *Radiology* 1987;163:377–379.

79. Wozney P, Zajko AB, Bron KM, Point S, Starzl TE. Vascular complications after liver transplantation: a 5 year experience. *AJR* 1986;147:657–663.

80. Taylor KJW, Morse SS, Weltin CG, Riely CA, Flye MW. Liver transplant recipients: portable duplex ultrasound with correlative angiography. *Radiology* 1986;159:357–363.

81. Marder DM, De Marino GB, Sumkin JH, Sheahan DG. Liver transplant rejection: value of the resistive index in Doppler ultrasound of hepatic arteries. *Radiology* 1989;173:127–129.

82. Letourneau JG, Day DL, Ascher NL, et al. Abdominal sonography after hepatic transplantation; results in 36 patients. *AJR* 1987;149:299–303.

83. Tessler FN, Gehring BJ, Gomes AS, et al. Diagnosis of portal vein thrombosis: value of color Doppler imaging. *AJR* 1991;157:293–296.

CHAPTER 6

The Spleen

INTRODUCTION

The spleen is the single largest ductless lymphoid gland of the human body. The mean weight is estimated at 180 g for men and 150 g for women (1). Its functions are to filter the bloodstream of unwanted elements and to participate in the immune response.

Sonography is the screening modality of choice in the evaluation of the spleen because it is faster, less expensive, safer, and more readily available than CT or isotope scanning. In fact, it can detect subtle textural changes that may be missed by CT scanning. It is also the modality of choice for monitoring splenic hematoma or cyst and for guiding percutaneous procedures such as aspiration biopsy or drainage.

6.1 SCANNING TECHNIQUE

Scanning the spleen constitutes an integral part of the routine ultrasound examination of the upper abdomen. No special patient preparation is required. Routinely, a 3.5- or 5-MHz real-time transducer is used, depending on patient's size.

The spleen is usually scanned by having the patient lying on the right side and then gradually turning toward the supine position. The ultrasound probe is placed at or near the left midaxillary line, either caudal to the ribs or between ribs. From these locations, coronal and transverse scans of the spleen are obtained during various phases of inspiration.

6.2 NORMAL ANATOMY

Usual Normal Anatomy

The spleen is a relatively superficial structure, lying in the left upper quadrant of the abdomen, usually between the ninth and eleventh ribs.

Superiorly, it is covered by the diaphragm; inferiorly, it is related to the splenic flexure of the colon and the left kidney; posterolaterally, it is bounded by the lower chest and upper abdominal wall; and medially, it is adjacent to the gastric fundus and the tail of the pancreas. Two important features should be remembered when performing percutaneous procedures: the left lung may extend as far as the lower border of the spleen and the spleen may occasionally be posterior to the left kidney.

There is a wide range of normal configuration. The shape varies according to the size of the colic impression, from that of a curved wedge to a tetrahedron (Figs. 6.1 and 6.2). The contour is usually smooth, but clefts and lobulations may be seen (2), caused by variations of fusion during development (Figs. 6.3 and 6.4). Variations of normal size are wide and appear to be related to race, age, and sex. As a general observation, Caucasians

---

Abbreviations: **AIDS,** acquired immune deficiency syndrome; **CDU,** color Doppler ultrasound; **CT,** computed tomography; **EBV,** Ebstein-Barr virus; **g,** gram; **IM,** infectious mononucleosis; **MRI,** magnetic resonance imaging; **PWD,** pulsed wave Doppler; **SI,** splenic index; **SW,** splenic weight; **T$_h$,** thickness at hilum.

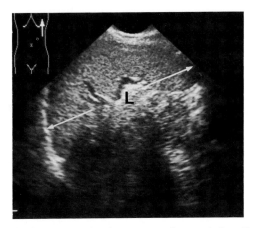

FIG. 6.1. Normal spleen: coronal scan. *L*, length.

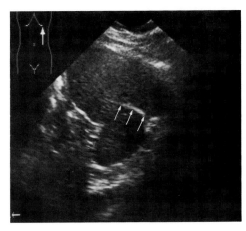

FIG. 6.3. Splenic cleft: coronal scan. Echogenic line (*arrows*) represents a cleft.

usually have larger spleens than blacks and Orientals (1). The organ tends also to be larger in males, in adults, and in tall people (1). Its size has been extensively estimated by different modalities including radiography, isotope, CT, and ultrasound scanning. For a detailed discussion on the matter, the reader is referred to the excellent review by Perlmutter (1).

In our department, for adults, we use the Downey technique to estimate the splenic weight (SW). The technique is based on a retrospective study of 81 autopsy patients (3).

$$SW \text{ (grams)} = 0.43 \times L \times W \times T_h$$

L = length W = width T_h = thickness at hilum.

Length (L) is measured as the longest dimension in a sagittal, parasagittal, or coronal plane, independent of spatial orientation of the spleen. The other diameters are obtained in the transverse plane. Thickness (T_h) is mea-

sured from the hilum perpendicular to the medial concave–lateral convex surfaces. Width (W) is measured as the greatest dimension perpendicular to the thickness (Figs. 6.1 and 6.2).

In children, Dittrich et al. (4) established a sonographic nomogram for the splenic volume in relation to the body length. However, Rosenberg et al. (5) proposed a much simpler method. Splenic size in children was estimated by measuring, in a coronal view that included the hilum, the greatest longitudinal distance between the dome and the tip of the spleen (splenic length) (Fig. 6.5). The upper limits of normal splenic length, correlated with age, are summarized in Table 6.1.

The normal texture of the spleen is uniform, consisting of multiple low-amplitude echoes. The echogenicity is usually slightly greater than that of the normal liver and higher than that of the normal renal cortex.

The blood flow in the splenic vessels at the splenic hilus and adjacent to the pancreatic body is easily demon-

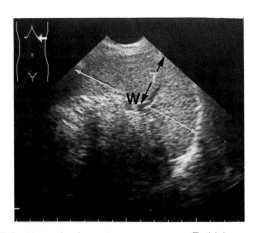

FIG. 6.2. Normal spleen: transverse scan. *T*, thickness at hilum; *W*, width.

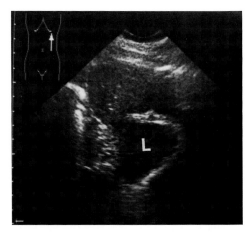

FIG. 6.4. Splenic lobulation: coronal scan. Lobulation (*L*) may be mistaken for an abnormal mass.

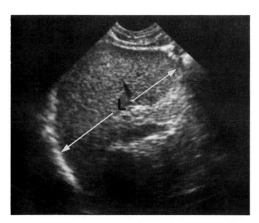

FIG. 6.5. Normal spleen in a child. This is coronal plane in which length (*L*) is measured after Rosenberg technique to estimate splenic size in children. This child is 10 years old. Actual length of spleen at hilus measures 11 cm.

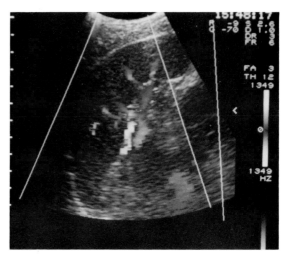

FIG. 6.6 Normal splenic vessels: CDU—coronal scan. *(See color image in color plate section B, which follows page 242.)*

strated by pulsed wave Doppler (PW) and color Doppler ultrasound (CDU). PW Doppler and CDU will also demonstrate flow within the intrasplenic vessels even when these are not apparent on real-time scanning (Figs. 6.6 and 6.7). *Both figures also appear in the color plate section, which follows page 50.* Color Doppler ultrasound allows accurate placement of the cursor for pulsed Doppler analysis. The flow in the splenic vein is similar to the portal vein flow, demonstrating continuous flow and low velocity (6). The flow in the splenic artery demonstrates a systolic peak and low-velocity flow toward the spleen in diastole.

The upper limit for normal splenic vein diameter is 10 mm (7). The vein usually dilates in normal people during inspiration. In portal hypertension, this respiratory response is decreased or lost (8). The vein leaves the spleen at the hilus and runs posterior to the body and tail of the pancreas, anterior to the left adrenal gland.

Normal Variants

Accessory Spleens

Accessory spleens are present in about 10% of the general population (9). In nearly 90% of cases, there is only one. In the remainder, there are two or more. They appear as small spherical nodules of homogeneous texture, usually at the splenic hilus. They measure, in most cases, between 1 to 3 cm in diameter, but sometimes they may be larger (9). Diagnosis is normally suggested by their location and texture (Fig. 6.8). This can be confirmed by a sulfur colloid scan, but this is usually not required.

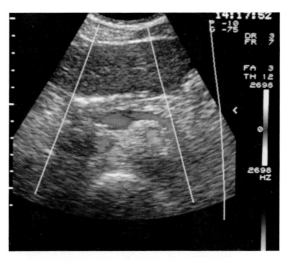

FIG. 6.7 Normal splenic vessels: CDU—transverse scan. Flow toward transducer is colored in blue. Red color indicates flow away from transducer. Intrasplenic vessels are well depicted in color Doppler scan, which allows accurate placement of cursor for PWD analysis. *(See color image in color plate section B, which follows page 242.)*

TABLE 6.1. *Age and splenic length in 230 infants and children—Suggested upper limit*

Age	Splenic length, upper limit (cm)
3 months	6.0
6 months	6.5
12 months	7.0
24 months	8.0
48 months	9.0
60 months	9.5
8 years	10.0
10 years	11.0
12 years	11.5
15 years (girls)	12.0
15 years (boys)	13.0

From Rosenberg et al., ref. 5, with permission.

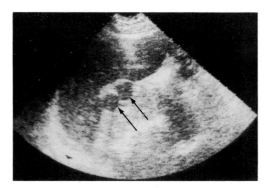

FIG. 6.8. Accessory spleen: coronal scan. Two accessory spleens (*arrows*) appear as round masses in splenic hilus.

Wandering Spleen

This rare developmental anomaly is due to a long mesentery, which results from failure of fusion of the dorsal gastric mesentery with the dorsal peritoneum. The spleen moves around within the abdominal cavity and may undergo torsion on its long mesentery. The ectopic spleen can be identified by ultrasound, CT, and isotope scanning (10).

6.3 PATHOLOGY

Congenital Anomalies

Developmental splenic anomalies are associated with abnormal viscero-atrial situs and complex cardiovascular malformations. Two types are described: polysplenia and asplenia.

Polysplenia (11,12)

Polysplenia occurs more commonly in males. Sonography may detect the multiple retrogastric splenuli and associated anomalies such as

1. biliary atresia
2. interruption of the inferior vena cava with azygous/ hemi-azygous continuation (Fig. 6.9a,b)

Asplenia (11,12)

Asplenia is more common in females. Sonography may detect the following features (Fig. 6.10a,b):

1. absence of splenic tissue
2. horizontal midline liver
3. inferior vena cava and aorta on same side of the spine
4. subdiaphragmatic anomalous pulmonary venous return
5. congenital heart defects

The presence of Howell-Jolly bodies in the peripheral blood is an additional diagnostic clue.

Both of these anomalies are infrequent. Prognosis is usually poor, with 80% to 90% of affected infants dying in the early postnatal period (13).

Splenomegaly

Despite the large number of publications proposing methods to estimate splenic size (1), many departments do not yet apply strict criteria to define enlargement of the spleen. They still follow the "eyeballing" technique: "If it looks big, it's big." One reason for this is that many formulae are too complex and cumbersome for a busy practice. Another reason is the wide variation of normal limits.

A spleen is considered enlarged when the estimated SW exceeds 200 g (3). The formula to calculate SW has been presented in the section on normal anatomy. The acquired data base applies only to the adult population. Alternatively, one may use the modified *Splenic Index* (SI) proposed by Strijk et al. (14), using the formula:

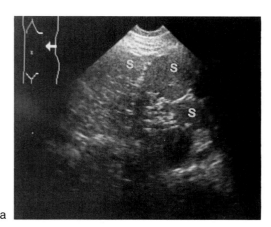

a

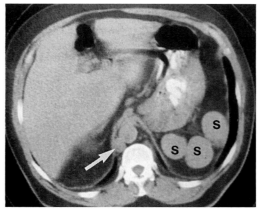

b

FIG. 6.9. Polysplenia. Ultrasound (**a**) and CT (**b**) scans demonstrate multiple splenuli (*s*) and dilated azygous vein (*arrow*).

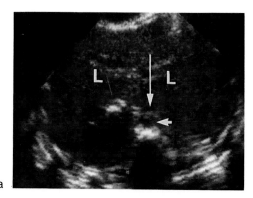 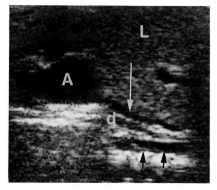

FIG. 6.10. Asplenia. **a:** transverse scan; **b:** parasagittal scan. No spleen could be identified in this infant. Note horizontal midline liver (L) and inferior vena cava (*long arrow*) lying on top of aorta (*short arrows*). A, atrium; d, crus of diaphragm.

$$SI = \frac{L}{(cm)} \times \frac{W}{(cm)} \times \frac{T_h}{(cm)}$$

where L is the longest *cranio-caudad* dimension. The upper limit of normal SI is estimated at 480. In children, the technique proposed by Rosenberg et al. (5) is used.

Splenomegaly is associated with many different systemic and metabolic disorders, caused by either reactive proliferation of lymphocytes or phagocytes, or to infiltration by neoplastic cells or lipid-laden macrophages or to vascular congestion. Focal splenic lesions may cause enlargement, although not necessarily so.

Infections (histoplasmosis, IM) usually produce minimal to moderate splenomegaly (SW < 500 g). Moderate splenomegaly (SW < 2,000 g) (Fig. 6.11a,b) is seen in vascular congestion (portal hypertension) and in collagen diseases or autoimmune disorders (e.g., rheumatoid arthritis, systemic lupus) (15). However, massive splenomegaly (SW > 2,000 g) (Fig. 6.11c) can be seen in patients with chronic malaria, hematologic disorders (e.g., chronic granulocytic leukemia, myelofibrosis, polycythemia vera), and malignant lymphoma (15).

Sonography provides an objective method to evaluate splenic size and to follow up splenomegaly. It is free of radiation risks and therefore particularly useful in the young and in pregnant patients.

Splenic Trauma

The spleen is the most commonly injured organ in blunt abdominal trauma. Rib fractures and left hemothorax are frequent associated findings (16).

No study is available that compares the accuracy of ultrasound, CT, and isotope scanning in the evaluation of splenic trauma. However, in contrast to isotope scanning, ultrasound detects abdominal fluid collections and alterations in splenic texture. High-resolution CT scanning certainly provides excellent anatomical detail. Unfortunately, it is occasionally restricted by the patient's size and frequently by artifacts caused by the presence of monitoring leads, various catheters, and tubes. It is also less readily available and more time-consuming than ultrasound.

Splenic injury may consist of (a) laceration or contusion of the parenchyma without capsular tear; (b) parenchymal and capsular laceration or fragmentation; and (c) disruption of hilar vessels.

Contusions cause only inhomogeneities in the splenic parenchyma. In mild cases, the textural abnormalities on ultrasound may be subtle and thus overlooked (Fig. 6.12). Pulp laceration is associated with intraparenchymal hematoma, which, when fresh (within 24 hr), appears hyperechoic (Fig. 6.13). During resorption, it becomes hypoechoic or echo-free (Fig. 6.14). In the healing phase, the splenic texture may return to normal, or there may be an echogenic linear scar or a residual pseudocyst. At times, lacerations may be seen as irregular echo-free gaps separating the fractured splenic fragments (Fig. 6.15). If the capsule is intact, bleeding from a parenchymal injury is contained within the capsule, resulting in a subcapsular hematoma that manifests as a fluid collection compressing the spleen (Fig. 6.16). Although MRI is not commonly used in splenic trauma, this modality may give a tissue-specific diagnosis of subcapsular hematoma (17).

Intraperitoneal blood (hemoperitoneum) is associated with capsular disruption. Sonography is highly sensitive in detecting intraperitoneal fluid, which should always alert to the possibility of injury to the solid organs, particularly the spleen. Free blood accumulates around the spleen, in the lesser sac, or in the recesses of the greater peritoneal cavity. Large hemoperitoneum usually occurs with extensive injuries (18,19). Lupien and Sauerbrei (20) have shown that, on follow-up sonograms, intraperitoneal fluid usually disappears within 4 weeks, whereas intrasplenic contusions and hematomas take months to resolve.

Some authors tried to predict the outcome of nonsurgical management of splenic injuries based on CT or

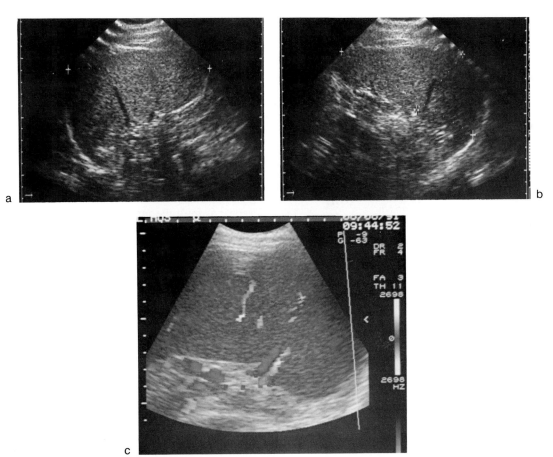

FIG. 6.11 Splenomegaly. *(See color image of part **c** in color plate section B, which follows page 242.)* **a:** parasagittal scan; **b:** transverse scan. This example illustrates moderate splenomegaly (SI = 1,274) in a patient with IM. **c:** Massive splenomegaly: scan with CDU. SI measures >2,000 in this patient with cirrhosis. The varices at the splenic hilus are well demonstrated by CDU.

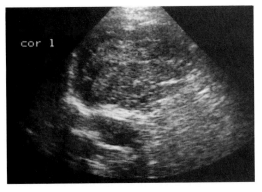

FIG. 6.12. Splenic contusion: coronal scan. Texture of spleen is disorganized, but no focal mass or fluid collection is seen.

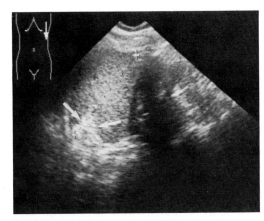

FIG. 6.13. Echogenic splenic hematoma. Fresh hematoma like this one *(arrows)* often appears strongly echogenic.

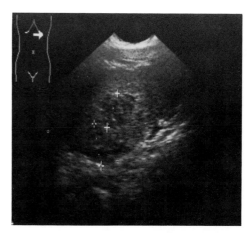

FIG. 6.14. Hypoechoic splenic hematoma. This transverse scan shows two echo-poor hematomas that are 1 week old.

clude infection of a hematoma, rupture of a pseudocyst, and splenosis, which is autotransplantation of splenic tissue in the thorax or peritoneal cavity after severe splenic trauma (24).

Inflammatory and Infectious Diseases

Calcified Granuloma

Calcified granuloma are relatively common incidental findings. They are thought to be caused by previous granulomatous infection such as histoplasmosis. They appear as multiple small bright echoes, often with posterior acoustic shadowing (Fig. 6.17). They are of no clinical significance.

Splenic Abscess

Rare in the past, splenic abscess is seen more frequently in present-day clinical practice. Patients with decreased immune response (e.g., AIDS) and patients with bacterial endocarditis are particularly at risk. High mortality results from delayed diagnosis.

Four categories are recognized: (a) pyogenic embolic infections (usually from infective endocarditis); (b) posttraumatic infection; (c) sickle cell anemia; and (d) spread from infections in adjacent organs (25).

ultrasound findings (21,22). It is felt that, although CT and ultrasound are reliable in quantifying the extent of splenic injury, therapeutic choices should be based on hemodynamic variables and clinical assessment. Imaging modalities should be used primarily to detect the injury and monitor its evolution. Since the use of CT and ultrasound, there has been a marked decrease in splenectomies and in peritoneal lavage (23).

Complications of splenic injuries are rare. They in-

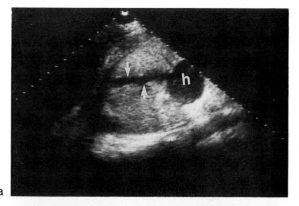

a

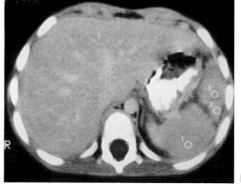

b

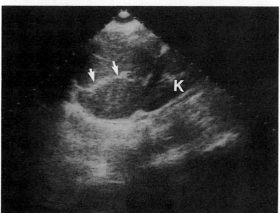

c

FIG. 6.15. Splenic laceration. **a:** parasagittal sonogram; **b:** corresponding CT scan. Laceration appears as an irregular sonolucent line (*arrows*) separating fractured splenic fragments. Note hypoechoic hematoma (*h*). (Sonogram from Lupien and Sauerbrei, ref. 20, with permission.) **c:** Splenic laceration. This parasagittal scan shows an echogenic line (*arrows*) representing scarring from splenic laceration. *K*, kidney.

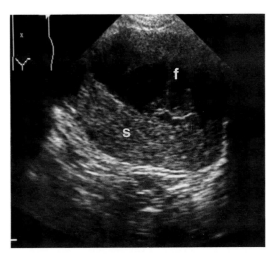

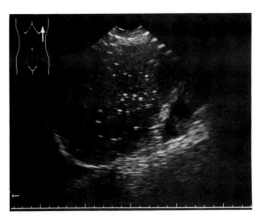

FIG. 6.17. Splenic granuloma. Note multiple small bright echoes with faint posterior shadowing.

FIG. 6.16. Subcapsular hematoma. Septated fluid collection (f) compresses on splenic contour (s).

Splenic abscesses show a wide spectrum of sonographic appearances. Many appear as echo-free or hypoechoic collections that resemble a liquefying hematoma or cyst (Fig. 6.18a). Some may have septations or internal debris, simulating hydatid disease. Only a few show bubbles of gas, which appear as highly reflective echoes (26). Occasionally, tiny "target" lesions are seen representing microabscesses (Fig. 6.18b). Diagnosis can be confirmed by percutaneous aspiration under ultrasound guidance.

Infectious Mononucleosis

Infectious mononucleosis is a worldwide self-limited infection caused by EBV. Transmission is usually through the oropharyngeal route during close personal contact but may also occur after transfusion of infected blood.

The disease most commonly affects young adults in the 15- to 25-year age group. Clinical manifestations include fever, sore throat, palatine petechiae, erythematous macopapular eruption, bilateral supraorbital edema, lymphadenopathy, and splenomegaly. Splenomegaly is seen in about 50% of the patients, with the greatest enlargement occurring during the second and third weeks of illness (27). Laboratory findings consist of abnormal liver function tests, an absolute increase in lymphocytes and monocytes, and the development of persistent antibody against EBV.

The role of ultrasound in IM is to exclude biliary obstruction, to look for abdominal lymphadenopathy, and to document and monitor splenomegaly. Ishibashi et al. (28) found that enlargement of the spleen is usually mod-

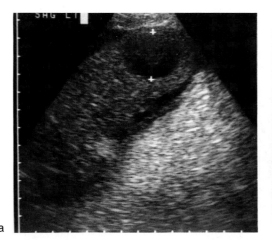

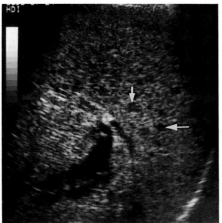

FIG. 6.18. Splenic abscess. a: Pus was aspirated percutaneously from this hypoechoic collection. Patient had subacute bacterial endocarditis. b: Multiple tiny "target" lesions (arrows) are seen in this young patient who was human immunodeficiency virus–positive. They are probably microabscesses but may also be lymphomatous deposits.

erate (SW < 2,000 g) but greater with IM than with acute viral hepatitis. Occasionally, splenomegaly may be massive (SW > 2,000 g), with potential risk of rupture (29). The patients should be advised to refrain from arduous activities (e.g., sports) until massive splenomegaly subsides.

Cystic Disease of the Spleen

Nonparasitic Cysts

Nonparasitic cysts are uncommon and are classified as true or false cysts with a ratio of 1:4 true–false (30). True cysts, containing an epithelial lining, are thought to be developmental and are divided into mesothelial or epidermoid subtypes. False cysts, occurring more commonly in older age groups, have no cellular wall. They are presumed to be related to previous trauma or infarction. Clinical manifestations are usually benign, consisting in many instances of a "heavy sensation" or pain in the left upper quadrant.

Most cysts are small, but some may be quite large. Huge cysts may compress splenic tissue around it. Benign uncomplicated cysts appear as well-defined echo-free lesions with enhanced through transmission (Fig. 6.19). It is not possible to distinguish by sonography a true cyst from a false cyst.

When low-amplitude echoes or septations are seen within the cyst, this may indicate that the cyst has been complicated by hemorrhage or infection. A few cases of very echogenic cysts simulating solid masses have been reported (31). Internal echoes represent cholesterol crystals or breakdown products of hematoma after hemorrhage (Fig. 6.20a,b). Sonography performs better than CT in demonstrating the complex architecture of a cyst containing an organizing hematoma (30). Symptomatic cysts may be aspirated or decompressed percutaneously under CT or ultrasound guidance (32). Splenic cyst has

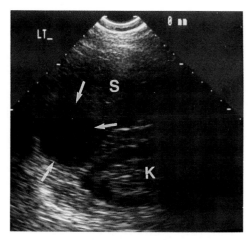

FIG. 6.19. Benign splenic cyst: sagittal scan. This well-defined round fluid collection (*arrows*) is typical of a benign cyst. *S*, spleen; *K*, kidney.

been diagnosed antenatally in the fetus (33). Spontaneous rupture of splenic cysts has also been reported (34).

Hydatid Cysts

Hydatid cysts in the spleen are rare, seen only in 2% of patients with echinococcal disease, which is caused most commonly by *Echinococcus granulosis* in North America.

Clinical symptomatology associated with splenic hydatidosis is usually vague and not helpful. Sonographically, the cyst appears most commonly as a calcified mass containing fluid (35). Membranes and fine particles representing debris and hydatid sand may be seen within the cystic cavity. Small daughter cysts are sometimes identified. Sonography is superior to CT in demonstrating the internal characteristics of the lesion (Fig. 6.21), particularly when the wall is not heavily calcified.

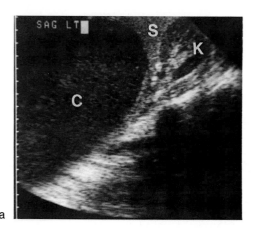
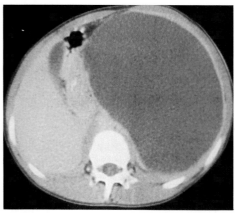

FIG. 6.20. Echogenic cyst. **a:** parasagittal sonogram; **b:** corresponding CT scan. This large splenic cyst is filled with low-amplitude echoes caused by cholesterol crystals. *C*, cyst; *S*, normal spleen; *K*, kidney.

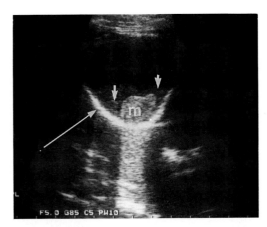

FIG. 6.21. Hydatid cyst. Thickened echogenic wall (*long arrows*) is due to calcification. Low-amplitude echoes (*short arrows*) represent hydatid sand. Large solid mass (*m*) represents calcified daughter cyst.

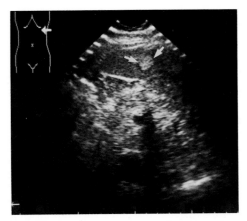

FIG. 6.22. Splenic hemangioma. Small splenic hemangioma is usually hyperechoic (*arrows*), with an appearance similar to liver hemangioma.

Diagnosis should be suspected in endemic areas and should be confirmed by appropriate serologic tests. Hydatid cysts have been safely aspirated percutaneously under CT or ultrasound guidance (36).

Splenic Neoplasms

Splenic Hemangioma

Primary neoplasms of the spleen are rare. These include fibroma, lymphangioma, chondroma, plasmocytoma, and sarcoma. Hemangioma is the most common benign primary neoplasm of the spleen (37).

Most splenic hemangiomas are small single lesions of about 1 to 2 cm in diameter found incidentally on routine screening. Some, however, may be large, measuring up to 17 cm, presenting usually as a nontender palpable mass or splenomegaly. A few may be pedunculated, projecting outside the normal confines of the spleen. Rupture of a large hemangioma has been reported in the past. When multiple, they may be part of generalized angiomatosis (37).

Sonographically, small lesions are echogenic round masses resembling hemangiomas in the liver (Fig. 6.22). Large hemangiomas may be entirely echogenic or may contain small cystic spaces. Some masses may contain calcification (38).

Splenic Lymphoma

Primary lymphoma of the spleen is extremely rare, with non-Hodgkin lymphoma being the most common (39). It manifests either as splenomegaly, or multiple small intrasplenic masses or as a single large mass that may contain calcification, without evidence of other lesions elsewhere (40).

The spleen is more commonly involved in systemic lymphoma, which ranks as the eighth most common malignancy (41). Evaluation of the spleen in lymphoma patients constitutes an important part of staging, because splenic involvement affects prognosis and treatment. Close to 35% of patients have splenic involvement at presentation. This rises to nearly 70% at autopsy (15).

Lymphomatous infiltration results frequently in splenomegaly, which is usually moderate to massive. However, at least 33% of splenic enlargement in lymphoma patients is due to benign causes. Furthermore, to make the issue more complex, the spleen may be normal in size although it is affected by lymphoma. This is seen in about one third of lymphoma patients with splenic involvement (42). Because of this, surgical staging is often necessary.

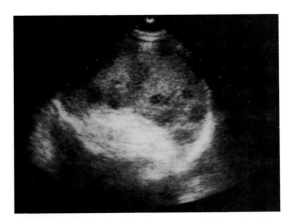

FIG. 6.23. Splenic lymphoma. Multiple small target lesions are seen in spleen in this patient with disseminated non-Hodgkin's lymphoma. Splenic metastases from other malignancies have a similar appearance, which may also be seen in microabscesses.

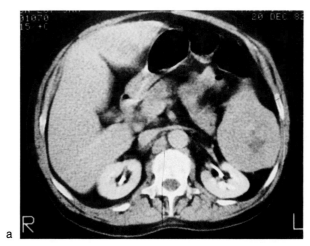
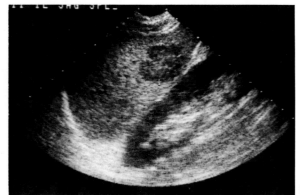

a R   L   b

FIG. 6.24. Splenic lymphoma. **a:** CT scan shows distortion of splenic contour and inhomogeneous densities in inferior tip of the spleen. **b:** Focal splenic lesion is better seen in this parasagittal scan.

Detection of focal lesions in the spleen is more helpful, because there is a higher correlation between focal defects and splenic lymphoma (43,44). In this regard, sonography, with its ability to identify subtle textural abnormality, performs better than CT and isotope scanning, claiming an accuracy rate of 75% (45,46). Focal disease may appear sonographically as areas of disorganized coarse echoes or as multiple small target lesions with an echogenic center surrounded by a hypoechoic rim (Fig. 6.23). Occasionally, a single large hypoechoic mass is seen (Fig. 6.24). The sonographic appearance, however, is not specific for lymphoma and may be seen in leukemic and metastatic deposits or abscesses (47). Tissue characterization of the lesions with MRI is not yet conclusive.

In summary, the role of ultrasound in splenic lymphoma is to (a) detect and monitor splenomegaly, (b) detect and monitor focal splenic lesions, (c) detect abnormalities that may occur elsewhere in the abdomen, and (d) guide percutaneous aspiration biopsies.

Splenic Metastases

Metastases to the spleen are relatively uncommon and are due to hematogenous spread. The most common primary sources are, in decreasing order of frequency, melanocarcinoma, bronchogenic carcinoma, and carcinoma of the breast (15).

Melanoma metastasizes to the spleen with an incidence of 8% to 50% in various autopsy series (48). They may be multiple and small, or they may be solitary and large. Metastases from lung and breast malignancies occur rarely as isolated findings; they are usually seen in the terminally ill patient, with widespread metastatic disease elsewhere (15).

Sonographically, focal metastases usually appear as hypoechoic solid masses, sometimes with a target appearance (Fig. 6.25). Diffuse infiltration results in enlargement and increased echogenicity of the spleen (48). Occasionally, a single large sonolucent metastasis may be seen (Fig. 6.26).

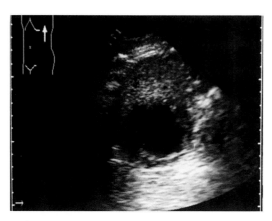

FIG. 6.25. Metastatic melanoma. There is a large lobulated solid mass with inhomogenous texture (*m*) compressing normal spleen (*s*) around it.

FIG. 6.26. Metastatic melanoma. This single splenic metastasis appears cystic.

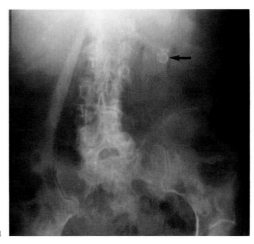
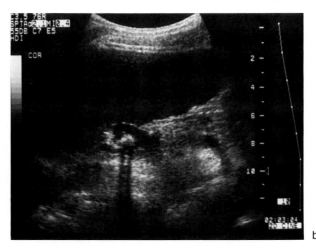

a   b

FIG. 6.27. Splenic artery aneurysm. **a:** Plain radiograph of abdomen shows a ring calcification in left upper quadrant (*arrow*). **b:** Coronal sonogram shows a small calcified aneurysm of splenic artery.

Vascular Abnormalities

Splenic Artery Calcification

Splenic artery calcification is commonly seen in older patients and in patients with severe arteriosclerotic disease. It appears as bright echoes along the course of the splenic artery. Correlation with a plain radiograph of the abdomen will establish the diagnosis.

Splenic Artery Aneurysm

Small aneurysms of the splenic artery are usually not detected by sonography. Larger aneurysms are saccular or fusiform. They are more common in women. Predisposing factors are multiparity, fibromuscular dysplasia, portal hypertension, splenomegaly, arteritis, and arteriosclerosis (49).

They may occur anywhere along the course of the splenic artery, but more frequently near the splenic hilus. Sonographically, they appear as round echo-free lesions with or without calcification in their wall (Fig. 6.27a,b). Pulsed Doppler or CDU can help to make the diagnosis by detecting flow within the aneurysm. However, the aneurysm may be thrombosed, in which case no flow is detected and the aneurysm may contain low-level echoes (49).

Complications are rare, consisting mainly of spontaneous rupture, which occurs most commonly into the peritoneal cavity. Rupture into the stomach, small bowel, colon, and pancreatic duct has been reported (50,51).

Splenic Vein Thrombosis

The splenic vein can be obstructed in pancreatitis and pancreatic carcinoma. Other causes include sepsis and hypercoagulatory states such as polycythemia, thrombo-cytosis, and myeloproliferative disorders (52). The obstruction may be due to narrowing by perivascular fibrosis or due to blood or tumor thrombosis. Isolated obstruction of the splenic vein results in the development of gastric varices, which can also be detected by ultrasound. The diagnosis should be suspected in patients with variceal bleeding in the absence of significant liver disease and with normal spleen size (52,53).

The thrombus typically contains low-level echoes and it may expand the splenic vein (Fig. 6.28) (54). Color Doppler ultrasound and PWD are very useful in assessing for blood flow in these situations.

Splenic Infarcts

Splenic infarcts are infrequently seen in ultrasound practice. They are most often due to embolic occlusion

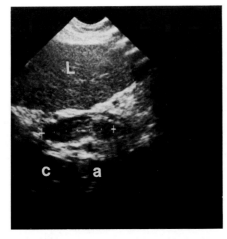

FIG. 6.28. Splenic vein thrombosis: transverse sonogram. Echogenic material representing thrombus is seen in splenic vein in this patient with polycythemia vera. *L*, liver; *a*, aorta; *c*, vena cava.

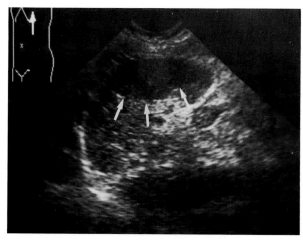
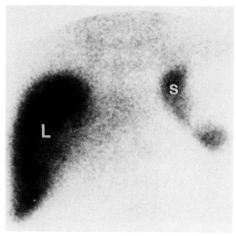

a b

FIG. 6.29. Splenic infarct. **a:** parasagittal sonogram. Note area of abnormal texture in periphery of spleen (*arrows*). **b:** isotope scan. Photopenic area corresponds to the lesion seen on sonography. *L*, liver; *S*, spleen.

of the splenic artery or one of its branches and less often caused by thrombosis. A frequent clinical presentation is sudden left upper quadrant pain in a patient with bacterial endocarditis (55,56).

In the initial stage, the spleen appears normal. Over the next 24 hr, a wedge-shaped peripheral lesion with low-amplitude echoes may be seen (Fig. 6.29a,b). This is fairly characteristic for a splenic infarct (55). In the healing phase, the lesion may become echogenic because of fibrosis and scarring or may become cystic (pseudocyst). Possible complications include infection, hemorrhage, and formation of pseudocyst, which may rupture spontaneously (56). They can be detected and monitored by sonography.

Isotope scans, CT, ultrasound, and angiography have been used in the investigation of splenic infarcts. Isotope scanning is sensitive but not specific. Ultrasound or CT is now the screening modality of choice. Angiography is

rarely if ever performed, because splenic infarcts are usually of little clinical significance if they remain free of complications (56).

6.4 PITFALLS, ARTIFACTS, AND PRACTICAL TIPS

1. A few normal patients have clefts or lobulations in the spleen. These should not be mistaken for splenic lacerations or tumors (Figs. 6.3 and 6.4).

2. A wandering spleen and posttraumatic splenosis appear as solid masses in the abdomen. They have sonographic appearances similar to normal spleen. Diagnosis is confirmed by a sulfur colloid isotope scan.

3. Some normal patients have an elongated left lobe of the liver, extending across the midline to cover the spleen (Fig. 6.30a,b). If the gain setting is too low, this

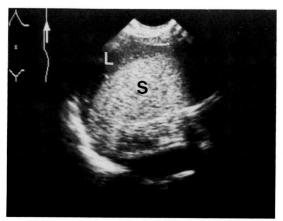
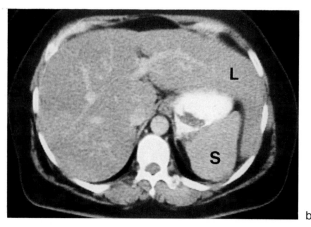

a b

FIG. 6.30. Elongated left lobe of liver. **a:** There is hypoechoic collection (*L*) suggesting perisplenic hematoma in this parasagittal scan of spleen (*S*). **b:** CT scan shows that "collection" is, in fact, an elongated left lobe of liver (*L*) covering the spleen (*S*).

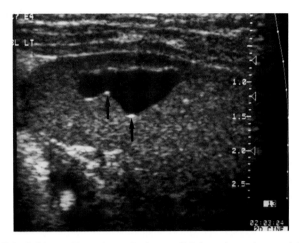

FIG. 6.31. Artifacts in wall of cyst. Bright echoes (*arrows*) in wall of this splenic cyst are reflection artifacts and not calcification.

appears as a sonolucent collection that may be confused with a perisplenic or subcapsular hematoma (57,58). Care must be taken to use the appropriate gain setting and focusing.

4. Some people have a very small spleen lying high up under the costal margin. If it is critical to visualize the spleen, isotope or CT scanning should be used in this situation.

5. In patients with ascites who are also investigated for blunt abdominal trauma, it is difficult to distinguish perisplenic ascites from subcapsular hematoma. One should carefully look for parenchymal abnormalities that may give a clue to the diagnosis. A subcapsular hematoma may indent on the contour of the spleen (Fig. 6.16).

6. A few nonparasitic splenic cysts may be entirely echogenic, simulating a solid mass, hydatid disease, or abscess. In case of doubt, a percutaneous fine needle aspiration is often useful. This, of course, should be performed after appropriate correlation with clinical and laboratory data.

7. Bright echoes simulating calcification may be seen in the wall of a cyst (Fig. 6.31). They are reflection artifacts, which occur when the sound beam hits the wall of the cyst at right angle.

REFERENCES

Normal Anatomy and Normal Variants

1. Perlmutter GS. Ultrasound measurements of the spleen. In: Goldberg B, Kurtz AB, eds. *Atlas of ultrasound measurements.* Chicago: Yearbook Medical Publishers; 1990:126–138.
2. Hine AL, Wilson R. Ultrasonography of splenic variants. *J Can Assoc Radiol* 1989;40:25–27.
3. Downey MT. Ultrasound estimation of spleen autopsy weight. Paper presented at the Canadian Association of Radiologists Con-

4. Dittrich M, Milde S, Dinkel E, Baumann W, Weitzel D. Sonographic biometry of liver and spleen size in childhood. *Pediatr Radiol* 1983;13:206–211.
5. Rosenberg HK, Markowitz RI, Kolberg H, Park C, Hubbard A, Bellah RD. Normal splenic size in infants and children: sonographic measurements. *AJR* 1991;157:119–121.
6. Taylor KJW, Burns PN, Woodcock JT, Wells PNT. Blood flow in deep abdominal and pelvic vessels: ultrasonic pulsed-Doppler analysis. *Radiology* 1985;154:487–493.
7. Doust BD, Pearce JD. Gray-scale ultrasonic properties of the normal and inflamed pancreas. *Radiology* 1976;120:653–658.
8. Bolondi L, Gandolfi L, Arienti V, et al. Ultrasonography in the diagnosis of portal hypertension: diminished response of portal vessels to respiration. *Radiology* 1982;142:167–172.
9. Subramanyam BR, Balthazar EJ, Harii SC. Sonography of the accessory spleen. *AJR* 1984;143:47–49.
10. Bollinger B, Lorentzen T. Torsion of a wandering spleen: ultrasonographic findings. *JCU* 1990;18:510–511.

Pathology

11. Hernanz-Schulman M, Ambrosino MM, Geniesen NB, et al. Current evaluation of the patient with abnormal viscero-atrial situs. *AJR* 1990;154:797–802.
12. Dodds WJ, Taylor AJ, Erickson SJ, Stewart ET, Lawson TL. Radiologic imaging of splenic anomalies. *AJR* 1990;155:805–810.
13. Nyberg DA. Intraabdominal abnormalities. In: Mahony BS, Pretorius DH, eds. *Diagnostic ultrasound of fetal anomalies.* Chicago: Yearbook Medical Publishers; 1990:342–394.
14. Strijk SP, Wagener DJT, Bogman MJJT, de Pauw BE, Wobbes T. The spleen in Hodgkin disease: diagnostic value of CT. *Radiology* 1985;154:753–757.
15. Robbins SL, Cotran RS. The spleen. In: Robbins SL, ed. *Pathologic basis of disease.* Philadelphia: WB Saunders; 1979:803–813.
16. Rosoff LR, Cohen JL, Telfer NT, Halpern M. Injuries of the spleen. *Surg Clin North Am* 1972;52:667–684.
17. Stark D. The liver, pancreas and spleen. In: Higgins CB, Hricak H., eds. *Magnetic resonance imaging of the body.* New York: Raven Press; 1987:347–372.
18. Weill F, Rohmer P, Didier D, Coche G. Ultrasound of the traumatized spleen: left butterfly sign in lesions masked by echogenic blood clots. *Gastrointest Radiol* 1988;13:169–172.
19. Asher WM, Parvin S, Virgilio RW, Haber K. Echographic evaluation of splenic injury after blunt trauma. *Radiology* 1976;118:411–415.
20. Lupien C, Sauerbrei EE. Healing in the traumatized spleen: sonographic investigation. *Radiology* 1984;151:181–185.
21. Jeffrey RB Jr. CT diagnosis of blunt hepatic and splenic injuries: a look to the future. *Radiology* 1989;171:17–18.
22. Umlas S-L, Cronan JJ. Splenic trauma: can CT grading systems enable prediction of successful non-surgical treatment? *Radiology* 1991;178:481–487.
23. Filiatrault D, Longpré D, Patriquin H, et al. Investigation of childhood blunt abdominal trauma: a practical approach using ultrasound as the initial diagnostic modality. *Pediatr Radiol* 1987;17:373–379.
24. Maillard JC, Menu Y, Scherrer A, Witz MO, Nahum H. Intraperitoneal splenosis: diagnosis by ultrasound and computed tomography. *Gastrointest Radiol* 1989;14:179–180.
25. Pawar S, Kay CJ, Gonzalez R, Taylor KJW, Rosenfield AT. Sonography of splenic abscess. *AJR* 1982;138:259–262.
26. Caslowitz PL, Labs JD, Fishman EK, Siegelman SS. The changing spectrum of splenic abscess. *Clin Imaging* 1989;13:201–207.
27. Niederman JC. Infectious mononucleosis. In: Isselbacker KJ, Adams RD, Braunwald E, et al., eds. *Harrison's principles of internal medicine.* New York: McGraw-Hill; 1980:854–857.
28. Ishibashi H, Okumura Y, Higuchi N, et al. Differentiation of mononucleosis from hepatitis by sonographic measurements of spleen size. *JCU* 1987;15:313–316.
29. Hoagland RJ, Henson HM. Splenic rupture in infectious mononucleosis. *Ann Int Med* 1957;46:1184–1191.

vention, October 1990, Vancouver, BC, Canada. *J Can Assoc Radiol* 1991 (*in press*).

30. Dachman AH, Ros PR, Murari PJ, Olmsted WW, Lichtenstein JE. Nonparasitic splenic cysts: a report of 52 cases with radiologic–pathologic correlation. *AJR* 1986;147:537–542.
31. Glancy JJ. Fluid-filled echogenic epidermoid cyst of the spleen. *JCU* 1979;7:301–302.
32. Goldfinger M, Cohen MM, Steinhardt MI, Rothberg R, Rother I. Sonography and percutaneous aspiration of splenic epidermoid cyst. *JCU* 1986;14:147–149.
33. Lichman JP, Miller EI. Prenatal ultrasonic diagnosis of splenic cyst. *J Ultrasound Med* 1988;7:637–638.
34. Rathaus V, Zissin R, Goldgerg E. Spontaneous rupture of an epidermoid cyst of the spleen: preoperative ultrasonographic diagnosis. *JCU* 1991;19:235–237.
35. Franquet T, Montes M, Lecumberri FJ, Esparza J, Bescos JM. Hydatid disease of the spleen: imaging findings in nine patients. *AJR* 1990;154:525–528.
36. Bret PM, Fond A, Bretagnolle M, et al. Percutaneous aspiration and drainage of hydatid cysts in the liver. *Radiology* 1988;168:617–620.
37. Ros PR, Moser RP, Dachman AH, Murari PJ, Olmsted WW. Hemangioma of the spleen: radiologic–pathologic correlation in 10 cases. *Radiology* 1987;162:73–77.
38. Manor A, Starynsky R, Garfinkel D, Yona E, Modai D. Ultrasound features of a symptomatic splenic hemangioma. *JCU* 1984;12:95–97.
39. Meyer JE, Harris NL, Elman A, Stomper PC. Large cell lymphoma of the spleen: CT appearance. *Radiology* 1983;148:199–201.
40. Marti-Bonmati L, Ballesta A, Chirivella M. Unusual presentation of non-Hodgkin lymphoma of the spleen. *J Can Assoc Radiol* 1989;40:49–50.
41. Osborne BM. Contextual diagnosis of Hodgkin's disease and non-Hodgkin's lymphoma. *Radiol Clin North Am* 1990;28:669–680.
42. Glatsein E, Guernsey JM, Rosenberg SA, Kaplan HS. The value of laparotomy and splenectomy in the staging of Hodgkin's disease. *Cancer* 1969;4:709–718.
43. Thomas JL, Bernardino ME, Vermesa M, et al. EOE-13 in the detection of hepatic splenic lymphoma. *Radiology* 1982;145:629–634.
44. Goerg C, Schwerk WB, Goerg K. Sonography of focal lesions of the spleen. *AJR* 1991;156:949–953.
45. Glees JP, Taylor KJW, Gazet JC, Peckham MJ, McCready VR. Accuracy of grey-scale ultrasonography of liver and spleen in Hodgkin's disease and the other lymphomas compared with isotope scans. *Clin Radiol* 1977;28:233–238.
46. Marghin SI, Castellino RA. Selection of imaging studies for the newly presenting patients with non-Hodgkin's lymphoma. *Semin Ultrasound CT MR* 1986;7:2–8.
47. Wernecke K, Peters PE, Krüger KG. Ultrasound patterns of focal hepatic and splenic lesions in Hodgkin's and non-Hodgkin's lymphoma. *Br J Radiol* 1987;60:655–660.
48. Murphy JF, Bernardino ME. Sonographic findings of splenic metastases. *JCU* 1979;7:195–197.
49. Derchi LE, Biggi E, Cicio GR, Bertoglio C, Neumaier CE. Aneurysms of the splenic artery: non-invasive diagnosis by pulsed Doppler sonography. *J Ultrasound Med* 1984;3:41–44.
50. Bishop NL. Splenic artery aneurysm rupture into the colon diagnosed by angiography. *Br J Radiol* 1984;57:1149–1150.
51. Harper PC, Garnelli RL, Kayle MD. Recurrent hemorrhage into the pancreatic duct from a splenic artery aneurysm. *Gastroenterology* 1984;87:417–420.
52. Itzchak Y, Glickman MG. Splenic vein thrombosis in patients with a normal size spleen. *Invest Radiol* 1977;12:158–163.
53. Sutton JP, Yarborough DY, Richards JT. Isolated splenic vein occlusion. *Arch Surg* 1979;100:623–626.
54. Weinberger G, Mitra SK, Yoeli G. Ultrasound diagnosis of splenic vein thrombosis. *JCU* 1982;10:345–346.
55. Shirkhoda A, Wallace S, Sokhandan M. Computed tomography and ultrasonography in splenic infarction. *J Can Assoc Radiol* 1985;36:29–33.
56. Goerg C, Schwerk WB. Splenic infarction: sonographic patterns, diagnosis, follow-up and complications. *Radiology* 1990;174;803–807.

Pitfalls, Artifacts, and Practical Tips

57. Crivello MS, Peterson IM, Austin RM. Left lobe of the liver mimicking perisplenic collections. *JCU* 1986;14:697–701.
58. Jacobs S, Kirsch J, Goldfinger M, Rosen I. Pitfall in the investigation of splenic trauma. *J Assoc Can Radiol* 1984;35:378–379.

CHAPTER 7

The Pancreas

INTRODUCTION

The pancreas is a retroperitoneal structure lying usually at a plane about 5 to 6 cm from the anterior abdominal wall (1). It has an endocrine function, secreting insulin and glucagon, which regulate sugar metabolism. Its exocrine function participates in the digestion of foods by producing a highly protolytic juice containing multiple enzymes.

Real-time sonography assumes a dominant role in the screening for and investigation of pancreatic diseases.

7.1 SCANNING TECHNIQUES

No single best scanning method is recognized universally, but a few basic concepts should be followed. A probe with the highest frequency possible is used, focused at the appropriate depth. Proper output and gain setting are important to display the internal characteristics of the gland.

Successful identification of the pancreas by ultrasound depends heavily on two factors:

1. patient's bodily build: In the heavily built or obese patient, visualization is often poor. CT scanning is more appropriate in this situation.

2. presence of bowel gas: This is one major limitation that may be overcome by certain maneuvers. Some authors have advocated the use of simethecone and other drugs. Others use the stomach filled with water as an acoustic window. Some limited success has been obtained. If bowel gas prevents adequate visualization, the patient should be rescanned at a later date or alternate imaging techniques should be considered (e.g., CT scan, ERCP).

The patient is scanned in the supine position, in quiet respiration. Other positions such as oblique, posterior, or erect may be used to displace gas-filled bowel away from the pancreas. The tail of the pancreas may be better visualized by scanning from the back with the patient lying prone. Other helpful maneuvers include applying gentle pressure on the abdomen with the probe to express the gas from bowel overlying the area of interest, or scanning the patient in deep inspiration, or by instructing the patient to perform the "belly out" maneuver (i.e., pushing the upper abdomen out by contracting the diaphragm). Better visualization of the gland may also be obtained by scanning through a fluid-filled stomach (Fig. 7.1a,b).

The pancreas is recognized by its vascular neighbors, which should be first identified. The planes of scanning are shown in Fig. 7.2. The corresponding sonograms with the vascular landmarks are shown in Fig. 7.3a–e. In the transverse scan, the main portal vein appears in cross section as a round sonolucent structure on the right side, anterior to the inferior vena cava. It is connected to the splenic vein, which runs from right to left across the upper abdomen. The body and tail of the pancreas lie anterior to these vessels, as visualized in transverse and para-

---

Abbreviations: **APUD,** amine precursor uptake and decarboxylation; **CF,** cystic fibrosis; **cm,** centimeter; **CT,** computed tomography; **DNA,** deoxyribonucleic acid; **ERCP,** endoscopic retrograde cholangiopancreatography; **ES,** endoscopic ultrasound; **MEN,** multiple endocrine neoplasia; **mm,** millimeter; **MRI,** magnetic resonance imaging; **ZE,** Zollinger-Ellison syndrome.

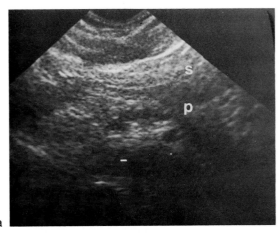
a

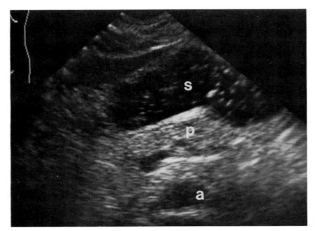
b

FIG. 7.1. Normal pancreas—scanning technique. **a:** pancreas (*p*) is vaguely seen, being obscured by gas in stomach (*s*). **b:** Better detail of the gland is obtained by scanning through fluid-filled stomach. *a*, aorta.

sagittal scans. Scanning toward the feet from this level, one encounters the head of the pancreas, which is usually seen anterior to the junction of the left renal vein and inferior vena cava. In the parasagittal scan, slightly to the right of the midline, the uncinate process is seen sandwiched between the superior mesenteric vein anteriorly and the inferior vena cava posteriorly.

The superior mesenteric vessels lie posterior to the neck of the pancreas, that is the junction between the head and body, which lies just posterior to the gastric

antrum. On transverse scans they are normally surrounded by a small echogenic space that is filled with perivascular fat. This space is nearly always identified unless it is infiltrated by disease.

7.2 NORMAL ANATOMY

Usual Normal Anatomy

The most common configuration of the gland is like a "J" lying on its side (⌐). There is usually gradual, smooth tapering from the head to the tail. Four parts are recognized: the head, neck, body, and tail. The pancreatic head lies on the right side of the spine within the "C" loop of the duodenum. Its medial extension, called the uncinate process, projects slightly posterior to the superior mesenteric vessels. The body runs anterior to the main portal vein and splenic vein. The tail extends across the left adrenal and the upper pole of the left kidney toward the splenic hilus. It is located at a more cephalad plane than the head. Although there is a wide variation in the normal course, there is a remarkably constant relationship with the vascular landmarks.

The pancreatic size has been measured by many authors using CT and ultrasound. Values obtained with CT are higher than the ones obtained with ultrasound. It is accepted that CT measurements are more accurate (2). It should be mentioned that absolute measurements are often misleading and should be interpreted with caution as indicators of disease. The mean weight has been estimated at 85 g in females and 100 g in males (2).

In our practice, we use the method and values described by Coleman et al. in 1983 (3). The head and body are measured in the maximal anteroposterior dimension. The tail is measured in a diameter perpendicular to the anterior wall of the gland (anatomic dorsal–ventral axis) (Fig. 7.4). Measurements are given in Table 7.1.

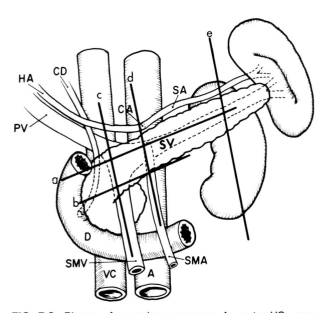

FIG. 7.2. Planes of scanning pancreas. *A*, aorta; *VC*, vena cava; *SMA*, superior mesenteric artery; *SMV*, superior mesenteric vein; *SV*, splenic vein; *CD*, common bile duct; *L*, liver; *s*, stomach; *SA*, splenic artery; *CA*, celiac axis; *HA*, hepatic artery; *PV*, portal vein; *D*, duodenum; *gd*, gastroduodenal artery; *rv*, renal vein. (Modified from Skolnick ML. *Real-time ultrasound imaging in the abdomen.* New York: Springer-Verlag; 1981, with permission.)

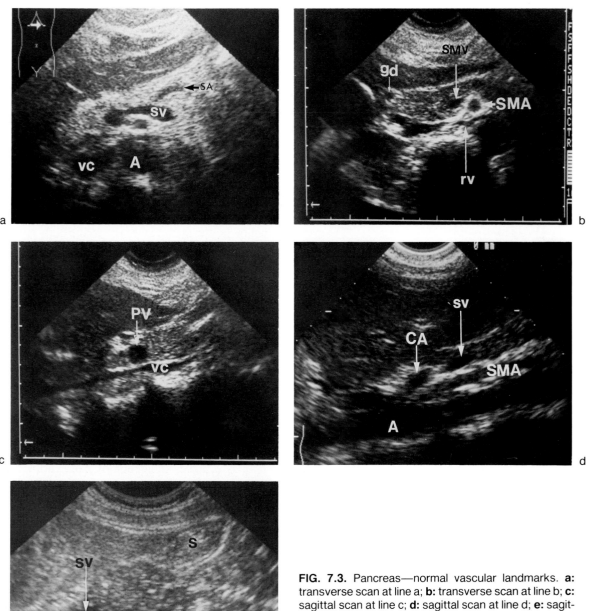

FIG. 7.3. Pancreas—normal vascular landmarks. **a:** transverse scan at line a; **b:** transverse scan at line b; **c:** sagittal scan at line c; **d:** sagittal scan at line d; **e:** sagittal scan at line e. See diagram (Fig. 7.2) for abbreviations and locations of lines **a–e.** Note clean echogenic space around superior mesenteric artery.

The normal texture of the gland varies widely, the most common pattern being similar to the texture of the normal liver (Fig. 7.5a). However, in children and adolescents, the gland usually appears less echogenic than the liver (Fig. 7.5b). In the obese and in the elderly, it appears more echogenic (Fig. 7.5c). This is thought to result from fatty infiltration and fibrosis.

With modern transducers, it is common to see the normal pancreatic duct, which can be detected in more than 90% of cases (2). In the transverse scan, this appears either as a single linear echo or as a hairline tubular structure running in the body of the pancreas anterior to the splenic vein. Its maximum normal diameter should not exceed 2 mm as measured in the mid body of the

gland (Fig. 7.6). It opens into the duodenum at the ampulla of Vater.

The pancreas is vascularized by branches of the celiac axis, superior mesenteric artery, and splenic artery. Venous drainage is by way of the splenoportal system.

Normal Variants

Prominent Pancreatic Tail

In some patients, the normal pancreatic tail appears more prominent than the body, assuming occasionally the appearance of a focal mass (Fig. 7.7). Careful scan-

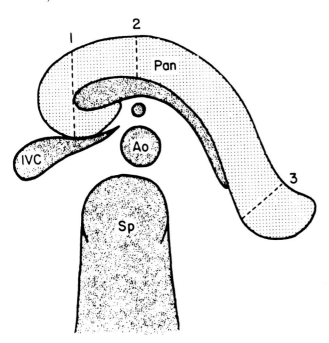

FIG. 7.4. Technique of measuring the pancreas (maximal anteroposterior diameters). *1*, head; *2*, body; *3*, tail; *Ao*, aorta; *IVC*, inferior vena cava; *Sp*, spine; *Pan*, pancreas. (From Shackelford GD. Adrenal glands, pancreas and other retroperitoneal structures. In: Siegel MJ, ed. *Pediatric sonography*. New York: Raven Press; 1991:213–256, with permission.)

ning should be performed in various patient positions to look for textural abnormality and other possible associated changes such as presence of stones or dilated ductal branches. As an isolated finding, a sonographically prominent pancreatic tail is most often a normal variant. In case of doubt, correlation with CT scanning is helpful.

Fatty Infiltration

In the obese and the elderly, the pancreas appears more echogenic than usual. This is presumed to be secondary to fatty infiltration of the gland (4,5). This usually does not need further investigation.

Uneven Lipomatosis

In a few patients, particularly the obese, there are focal areas of decreased echogenicity as compared with the rest of the gland, which is highly echogenic. This is often in the posterior aspect of the pancreatic head (Fig. 7.8a,b). These are thought to represent areas of focal sparing in a gland diffusely infiltrated by fat (6).

7.3 PATHOLOGY

Congenital Anomalies

There are two major developmental anomalies of the pancreas: pancreas divisum and annular pancreas.

The pancreas is normally formed by two separate anlages from the foregut. The dorsal anlage contains the duct of Santorini and gives rise to the body and tail. The ventral anlage is composed of two buds: the left bud, which normally atrophies, and the right ventral bud, which contains the duct of Wirsung and from which develops the head of the gland.

Pancreas Divisum

Pancreas divisium results from failure of fusion of the two anlages during development. This is seen in about 11% of necropsy specimens (7). The duct of Santorini draining the body and tail (dorsal anlage) opens at the minor papilla; the duct of Wirsung draining the head (ventral anlage) opens separately at the major papilla. There is a higher incidence of pancreatitis associated with this anomaly, which is usually diagnosed by ERCP.

Annular Pancreas

Annular pancreas develops from failure of regression of the left ventral bud, which should atrophy during development. The annular pancreas encircles the duodenum, causing duodenal obstruction or biliary obstruction. There is also a higher incidence of pancreatitis, which may affect only the annular portion. Diagnosis is usually made by ERCP. If this fails, a percutaneous transhepatic cholangiogram may be indicated to determine the level of biliary obstruction. In rare instances, CT may show the annular pancreas encircling the duodenum (8).

Neither pancreas divisum nor annular pancreas has been detected by ultrasound.

TABLE 7.1. *Normal measurements of pancreas*

Age group (years)	Head (cm)	Body (cm)	Tail (cm)
0–6	1.6 (1.0–1.9)	0.7 (0.4–1.0)	1.2 (0.8–1.6)
7–12	1.9 (1.7–2.0)	0.9 (0.6–1.0)	1.4 (1.3–1.6)
13–18	2.0 (1.8–2.2)	1.0 (0.7–1.0)	1.6 (1.3–1.8)
Adults			
(maximum anteroposterior)	2.5	2.0	2.0

From Perlmutter, ref. 2, and Coleman et al., ref. 3, with permission.

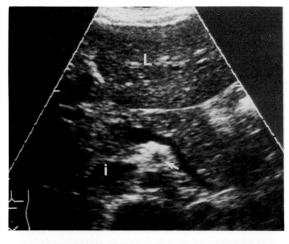

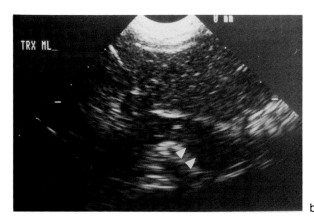

a

b

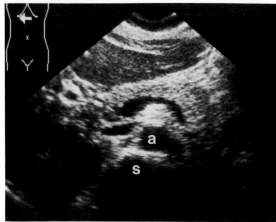

c

FIG. 7.5. Normal texture of pancreas: transverse scans. **a:** isoechoic—Echogenicity of this gland is similar to that of liver. **b:** hypoechoic—This gland is less echogenic than liver. This is more often seen in children than in adults. **c:** hyperechoic—This gland is more echogenic than liver. Some glands are much more echogenic than this, particularly in the obese and elderly. *a*, aorta; *i*, inferior vena cava; *s*, spine; *L*, liver; *arrowheads*, splenic vein; *small arrow*, superior mesenteric artery.

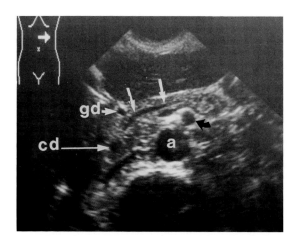

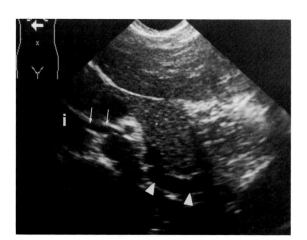

FIG. 7.6. Normal pancreatic duct: transverse sonogram. Pancreatic duct (*small arrows*) parallels course of splenic vein. It shows smooth tapering from head toward tail. *a*, aorta; *black arrow*, superior mesenteric artery; *cd*, common bile duct; *gd*, gastroduodenal artery.

FIG. 7.7. Prominent pancreatic tail: oblique scan. Smooth enlargement of pancreatic tail is often a normal variant when there is no textural abnormality. *Arrowheads* point to splenic vein. Note left renal vein (*small arrows*) draining into inferior vena cava (*i*).

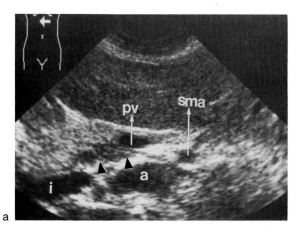
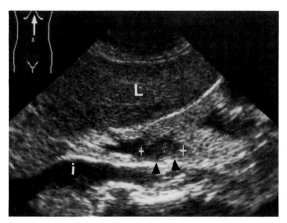

a

b

FIG. 7.8. Uneven lipomatosis. **a:** oblique scan; **b:** parasagittal scan. An irregular hypoechoic area (*arrowheads*) is seen in posterior aspect of pancreatic head in transverse and longitudinal planes. Remainder of gland is hyperechoic. Hypoechoic area represents focal sparing in a gland diffusely infiltrated by fat. *a*, aorta; *sma*, superior mesenteric artery; *L*, liver; *i*, inferior vena cava; *pv*, portal vein.

Cystic Fibrosis

Cystic fibrosis is a genetic disease inherited as an autosomal recessive trait affecting about 1 in 2,000 to 3,000 live births among whites. Recent investigations have identified the defective gene, which can be detected in 70% of carriers by current DNA analysis (9). The hereditary defect results in the secretion of sticky, dry serous and mucous fluid by exocrine glands and cells. Multiple organs are affected, including the sweat glands, salivary glands, lungs, liver, pancreas, and gut.

Inspissated meconium in the fetal gut causes meconium ileus, which is seen in 10% to 15% of infants with CF and which is complicated in 50% of cases by perforation or volvulus. Diagnosis of meconium ileus should be suspected when dilated bowel loops are demonstrated sonographically in the fetal abdomen (10).

Precipitates of concentrated viscous pancreatic secretions cause ductal obstruction, resulting in severe pancreatic fibrosis, loss of exocrine function, and malabsorption. Ultrasound shows changes similar to those seen in chronic pancreatitis (Fig. 7.9). The size of the gland may be increased or decreased (11,12). Swobodnik et al. (12) found a marked age-independent increase in tissue echogenicity in the pediatric age group. In advanced cases and in older patients, the pancreas is usually atrophic and strongly echogenic because of fatty replacement and dystrophic calcification (13,14). Small cysts measuring about 2 to 3 mm in diameter are commonly found, especially in the tail, but larger cysts, up to 5 cm in diameter, have occasionally been reported. These cysts are not associated with a history of trauma or pancreatitis but are thought to result from ductal obstruction (13,14). The pancreatic duct is rarely seen in patients with CF. There is no significant and reliable correlation between the morphological changes and pancreatic function.

Acute Pancreatitis

Acute pancreatitis represents a spectrum of inflammatory attacks of the gland, *not* associated with progressive glandular destruction nor pancreatic insufficiency, both of which are characteristic of chronic pancreatitis.

In North America, the most common cause is biliary tract disease, which accounts for 75% of cases of acute pancreatitis. The exact pathogenesis of gallstone pancreatitis is still unknown, but transient obstruction of the ampulla by migrating stones and reflux of bile into the pancreatic duct appear to play a prominent role. Another common cause is alcohol abuse, which in some series is the most common cause of acute pancreatitis in men. It is postulated that alcohol causes pancreatitis by altering the pancreatic enzyme concentration. This, in turn, results in protein precipitates plugging the ducts

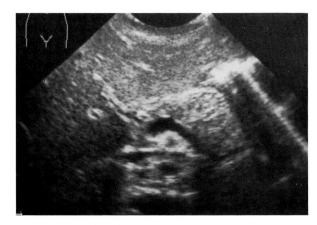

FIG. 7.9. Cystic fibrosis: transverse scan. Gland is irregular in contour and inhomogeneous in texture. This is seen in an 8-year-old child with CF. Occasionally, cysts are identified. Appearances simulate chronic pancreatitis.

(15). Other less common causes accounting for about 8% of cases include previous instrumentation (ERCP) and surgery (renal transplantation), trauma, structural abnormalities of the pancreatic and bile ducts, hyperparathyroidism, and hyperlipidemia (15).

Symptoms and signs are often not specific, consisting mainly of abdominal pain and fever. Helpful laboratory findings include elevation of serum amylase and lipase, and decreased serum calcium and magnesium concentrations. The clinical course is usually self-limited, lasting 3 to 5 days, but may become protracted in some patients, with high morbidity and mortality.

Pathologically, three forms are recognized:

1. acute edematous pancreatitis
2. acute phlegmonous pancreatitis
3. acute hemorrhagic necrotizing pancreatitis

Complications and sequelae include development of pancreatic and extrapancreatic fluid collections, pancreatic pseudocysts, pancreatic ascites, pancreatic abscess, fistulous communication with the gastrointestinal tract, biliary obstruction, hemorrhage, and arterial and venous occlusion. The role of sonography in acute pancreatitis is

1. to establish the diagnosis in the infrequent instances where clinical and laboratory findings are equivocal. This occurs in about 10% of cases (15)
2. to identify possible etiologies such as biliary stone or parasitic infestation of the bile ducts
3. to document and monitor complications, many of which can be detected by ultrasound

Acute Edematous Pancreatitis

Acute edematous pancreatitis is the mildest form of the disease, usually lasting 3 to 5 days. In the uncomplicated case, there is most often mild to moderate diffuse enlargement of the gland associated with textural abnormalities ranging from normal to decreased to increased echogenicity (16). The most common pattern seen in our practice is that of a heterogeneous texture composed of disorganized coarse echoes in a gland that appears overall hypoechoic (Fig. 7.10). A dilated pancreatic duct may be seen and may be the only sign of the disease. However, this is not specific for acute pancreatitis and will be discussed later in this chapter.

Choledocholithiasis can be detected by ultrasound and should be looked for in acute pancreatitis as a possible etiology. Please refer to Chapter 3 for further details.

Acute Phlegmonous Pancreatitis

A phlegmon is defined as an *indurated* inflammatory mass. In the past, before the age of ultrasound and CT, this had been mistaken for a pseudocyst (17).

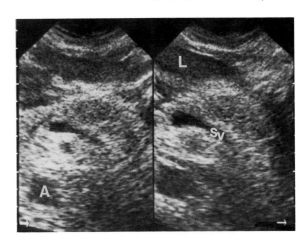

FIG. 7.10. Acute edematous pancreatitis: transverse sonograms. Gland is diffusely enlarged (anteroposterior diameter 3.5 cm). Its echogenicity is coarse but remains relatively hypoechoic. No focal fluid collection is seen. *A*, aorta; *L*, liver; *sv*, splenic vein.

The exact incidence of pancreatic phlegmon is unknown. They are more commonly seen in patients with a prolonged clinical course characterized by persistent pain and leukocytosis and complicated by volume depletion and respiratory and renal failure. In most cases, they resolve spontaneously with conservative and supportive management.

Sonography is crucial in demonstrating the *solid* nature of the diffuse glandular enlargement or of the focal mass that may occur in or outside the pancreas (Fig. 7.11a,b). In this respect, it performs better than CT, which is less reliable in differentiating a cystic from a solid lesion. Sonography can also be used to monitor the resolution of the phlegmon, which may be complicated by necrosis, infection, biliary obstruction, and pseudocyst formation.

Acute Necrotizing Pancreatitis

Acute necrotizing pancreatitis is the most severe form of acute pancreatitis, characterized by erosions of small blood vessels, interstitial hemorrhage, and parenchymal necrosis. It is more commonly due to alcohol abuse and is frequently complicated by secondary bacterial infection on the third or fourth day of the disease. Clinical course is often protracted, and mortality is high (15).

Hemorrhage and necrosis are better detected by contrast-enhanced CT scanning than by ultrasound (18), which still offers valuable information in the detection and monitoring of associated abnormalities such as presence of gallstones, biliary obstruction, and development of pseudocysts. Vascular complications such as narrowing or thrombosis may also be detected by Doppler interrogation.

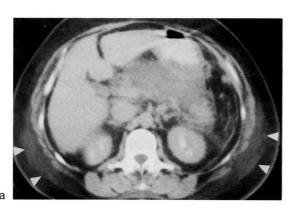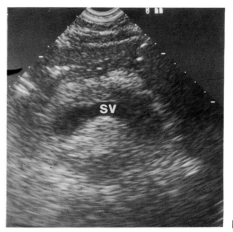

FIG. 7.11. Acute phlegmonous pancreatitis. **a:** CT scan; **b:** transverse sonogram. CT scan shows diffuse swelling of pancreas. Density suggests effusion in and around the gland. A palpable mass was felt, and a pseudocyst was suspected. Sonogram shows no fluid collection but only irregular thickening of the gland compatible with phlegmon. Note inflammatory changes in subcutaneous fat on CT (*arrowheads*). *sv*, splenic vein.

Pancreatic and Peripancreatic Effusions

Collections of pancreatic secretions seen in the acute stage should not be called pseudocysts because they are confined within a pre-existing anatomic space and not by a thick fibrous wall and because they usually resolve spontaneously within days or weeks. Effusions often develop within 7 to 10 days of the acute onset. The exact incidence is unknown but is estimated at about 60% of patients investigated by ultrasound or CT for pancreatitis (19).

The fluid comes from the large exudate associated with the severe inflammatory reaction and from leakage of pancreatic juice secondary to acinar and ductal disruption. It may remain confined within the gland (intrapancreatic fluid collection) or may break through the thin fibrous membrane covering the gland to collect in the lesser sac or anterior pararenal space (extrapancreatic collection) (Fig. 7.12). Tracking of pancreatic fluid may cause discoloration of the skin on the patient's back (Grey Turner's sign) or in the periumbilical region (Cullen's sign).

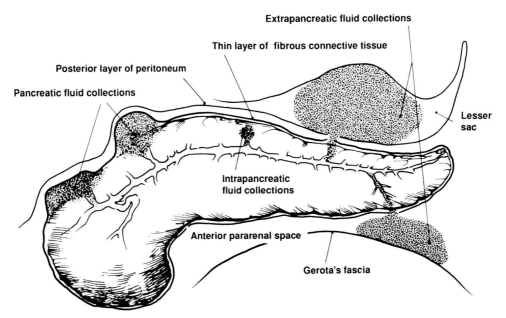

FIG. 7.12. Diagram illustrating sites of pancreatic effusions. (From Donovan et al., ref. 19, with permission.)

By the time the acute disease subsides, there is usually complete reabsorption of the fluid collections. Even large extrapancreatic collections disappear over time, usually within 6 weeks after formation (19).

Pancreatic ascites, more commonly seen in alcoholics, is thought to be caused by ductal disruption or by rupture of a pseudocyst. It is almost always associated with ductal abnormalities that include stenosis or calculi. These should be determined by ERCP or operative pancreatography, which also show the site of the leakage (20).

Real-time sonography is very sensitive in the detection of pancreatic and extrapancreatic fluid collections (7). Computed tomography is a better technique in detecting smaller fluid collections in the retroperitoneal spaces, especially in obese patients (19).

Pancreatic Abscess

Pancreatic abscess is defined as a collection of necrotic pancreatic tissue mixed with blood and pus. The most common organisms involved are *Escherichia coli* or other types of coliforms.

The overall incidence is about 10% of all patients hospitalized for acute pancreatitis. This is much higher, about 40%, in patients with acute necrotizing pancreatitis and postoperative pancreatitis (21). It often develops 2 to 4 weeks after the acute onset, either in or adjacent to the gland. Mortality is high if the disease is not diagnosed and treated early.

Sonography performs poorly in the early detection of pancreatic abscess, which in the acute and subacute phase often shows changes indistinguishable from edematous or phlegmonous pancreatitis or sterile fluid collections. It is also often limited by bowel gas associated with ileus. Computed tomography scanning is the modality of choice for imaging pancreatic abscess (22). The presence of tiny bubbles of gas in an inflammatory mass or fluid collection is better detected by CT (Fig. 7.13) and is often seen in a pancreatic abscess, although it may also be secondary to a noninfected fistula with the bowel (23). Diagnosis is usually established by fine needle aspiration under ultrasound or CT guidance.

Chronic Pancreatitis

Chronic pancreatitis is defined as a prolonged inflammatory disease of the gland associated with progressive parenchymal destruction and loss of endocrine and exocrine functions. It is not a sequela of recurrent acute pancreatitis. The most common cause in North America is chronic alcoholism, accounting for 60% to 90% of cases. Other causes include biliary tract disease (25% of cases) and CF. Hereditary pancreatitis is also a form of chronic pancreatitis inherited as an autosomal dominant

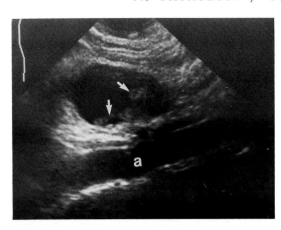

FIG. 7.13. Pancreatic abscess: sagittal scan. A fluid collection containing debris (*arrows*) is seen in body of pancreas. Pus was evacuated surgically. *a*, aorta.

trait. In about 10% to 40% of cases, no cause is found (15).

The role of ultrasound is

1. to document the morphological abnormalities of the gland. These include focal mass, ductal dilatation, and stones
2. to monitor the development and evolution of pseudocysts
3. to look for associated abnormalities that may occur elsewhere in the abdomen

Ultrasound claims a sensitivity close to 90% and a much lower specificity, in the range of 25% to 50%. Computed tomography is a more accurate technique, with a sensitivity approaching 95% to 100% and specificity of 85% (15).

Focal Mass

A focal mass is seen in about one third of patients with chronic pancreatitis. This results from proliferation of fibrous tissue and infiltration by inflammatory cells (24). Sonographically, the mass is usually small, measuring about 2 to 3 cm in diameter. It is usually hypoechoic, with a disorganized echo pattern. However, there is a wide range in size and texture. Some masses may be quite large and strongly echogenic. A few features favor the diagnosis of a benign inflammatory mass over a tumor: presence of small ductal stones and presence of dilated ductal side branches within the mass (Fig. 7.14).

In practice, however, it is difficult to distinguish a benign from a malignant focal pancreatic mass by imaging alone (25). A percutaneous aspiration biopsy under ultrasound or CT guidance is usually required. It should be stressed that a biopsy negative for malignancy does not exclude cancer. Clinical follow-up, imaging monitoring, and repeated biopsies may be necessary to make the diagnosis.

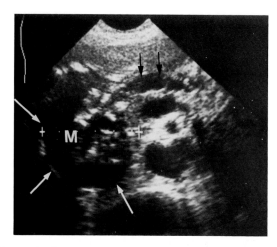

FIG. 7.14. Chronic pancreatitis—focal mass. This transverse sonogram shows a large mass (*arrows*) containing stones in pancreatic head in this patient with long-standing chronic alcoholic pancreatitis. Note dilated pancreatic duct (*thin black arrows*) measuring 9 mm in diameter.

Abnormalities in Size and Texture

The size of the pancreas in chronic pancreatitis varies from patient to patient and with the stages of the disease. In the early phase, it often appears diffusely enlarged; as the disease progresses, focal enlargement or atrophy is more commonly seen (24,25). In Luetmer's series of 56 patients (24), 7% had normal-sized gland, 30% had focal enlargement, and 54% had parenchymal atrophy; none had diffuse generalized enlargement. This is in contrast to the findings by Ferrucci et al. (26), who reported 16% with normal-sized gland, 36% with diffuse enlargement or mass, and 14% with glandular atrophy. The discrepancy probably reflects the difference in severity of the disease in the two patient populations. The contour of the gland may be normal or deformed by scarring or focal masses.

Nearly 90% of patients with chronic pancreatitis demonstrate abnormal pancreatic texture on sonography. Kunzman et al. (27), as well as Cotton et al. (28), identified four major patterns, which they described as faded, distorted, smudged (echogenic), and cystic. In practice, although the alterations in parenchymal texture constitute a sensitive indication of pancreatic disease, they are often operator-dependent and nonspecific and should be interpreted with caution. As a general rule, whereas carcinoma of the pancreas usually appears hypoechoic, chronic pancreatitis is usually associated with increased and disorganized echogenicity caused by a combination of fibrosis, fatty replacement, and ductal stones.

Pancreatic Ductal Dilatation and Stones

A pancreatic duct is considered dilated when its internal diameter exceeds 2 mm in the pancreatic body. This is detected in 60% to 90% of patients with chronic pancreatitis, either by ultrasound or CT scanning (29). Ductal dilatation results from a combination of glandular atrophy and ductal obstruction (29). A dilated pancreatic duct is also seen in acute pancreatitis and pancreatic neoplasms. This sign is therefore not specific for chronic pancreatitis.

Only the presence of ductal stones is pathognomonic of the disease. They are formed by calcified protein plugs filling the ducts and are composed of calcite, protein, and polysaccharide. They are seen in about 50% of patients with chronic pancreatitis (30). They may be tiny or quite large. On sonography, they appear as highly reflective echoes, with or without acoustic shadowing (Figs. 7.15 and 7.16). When multiple calculi or large calculi are present, the ultrasound scan may be difficult to interpret. Plain radiograph of the abdomen is helpful in this situation.

Pancreatic Pseudocyst

Simple Pseudocyst

A pancreatic pseudocyst is defined as a fluid collection surrounded by a thick fibrous capsule occurring in or outside the pancreas, beyond the usual 5 days of the acute attack and showing no significant change in appearance on serial scans for 1 month. Fluid collections seen in the acute episode should not be called pseudocysts, but "collections of pancreatic fluid or pancreatic effusions" (19).

The exact incidence of pseudocysts in acute and chronic pancreatitis is unknown, because of selection bias in published series. It has been estimated in one series at about 55% (31). Luetmer et al. (24) reported a 27% incidence in a series of 56 patients with chronic pancreatitis.

About 50% of pseudocysts are intrapancreatic. Fifty percent are found outside the gland (32). Intrapancreatic

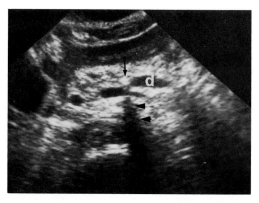

FIG. 7.15. Stone in pancreatic duct: transverse scan. Stone (*arrow*) casts posterior acoustic shadowing (*arrowheads*). Dilated pancreatic duct (*d*) should not be confused with a tortuous splenic artery or a dilated splenic vein.

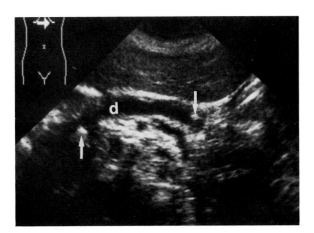

FIG. 7.16. Stones in pancreatic duct: transverse scan. Pancreatic duct (*d*) is grossly dilated. It contains two stones (*arrows*).

pseudocysts may be seen anywhere in the gland. They may be small, measuring only a few millimeters in diameter, or they may be quite large, attaining several centimeters in diameter (Fig. 7.17a,b). Extrapancreatic pseudocysts occur most commonly in the lesser sac (Fig. 7.18a,b) and in the anterior pararenal space. Infrequent locations include the mesentery adjacent to bowel, the porta hepatis, and the pelvic recesses (19,24,31).

It has been shown that CT is more sensitive than ultrasound in detecting pancreatic pseudocysts, especially in the anterior pararenal space. However, sonography still contributes important information in monitoring the evolution of documented pseudocysts and in demonstrating their internal characteristics (33).

Sonographically, uncomplicated pseudocysts appear as well-defined cystic collections with good through transmission. A capsule of variable thickness may be seen in mature pseudocysts. Spontaneous resolution of pancreatic pseudocysts has been documented by serial CT or ultrasound scanning. This occurs in about 20% of

cases and frequently within 6 weeks and only rarely after 7 to 12 weeks after formation (34).

Complicated Pseudocyst

Pancreatic pseudocysts may be complicated by hemorrhage, infection, or spontaneous rupture. They may also extend into locations remote from their original site such as the mediastinum, lumbar, pelvic, or inguinal regions, causing unusual clinical manifestations. The exact incidence of these complications is not yet determined.

Erosion of blood vessels by the pancreatic enzymes may result in the formation of a pseudoaneurysm, which may rupture into the pseudocyst, causing massive hemorrhage (Fig. 7.19a,b). Only a few cases of vascular complications of pseudocyst identified by ultrasound have been reported (35,36). It is expected that the increasing use of Doppler will help to detect these serious complications, obviating the need for angiography in some cases.

Infected pseudocysts may contain septations or bubbles of gas, which can be seen as highly reflective echoes (Fig. 7.20a,b). However, deeply located abscesses may be missed by ultrasound. Computed tomography scanning, if available, should be performed in the presence of persistent fever and leukocytosis. It should be noted that presence of gas bubbles in the pseudocyst may not be due to infection but to fistulous communication with the bowel. However, most infected pseudocysts do not contain gas (37).

Acute pain associated with increase in size of the pseudocyst on serial scans may herald impending rupture (5–10% of the pseudocysts rupture). Fifty percent of ruptured pseudocysts drain intraperitoneally. This is associated with a 70% mortality rate. The remainder rupture into the gastrointestinal tract, some without ill effects (38).

A rare but well-recognized complication of a pancreatic pseudocyst is its extension into the mediastinum

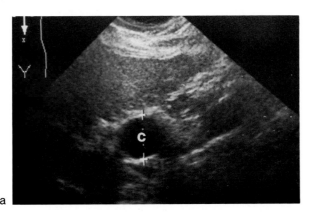

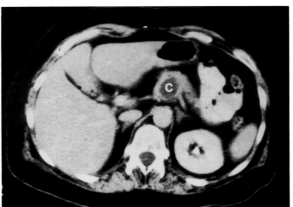

a   b

FIG. 7.17. Pancreatic pseudocyst. **a:** sagittal sonogram; **b:** CT scan. This small round fluid collection (*c*) is confined within mid body of pancreas.

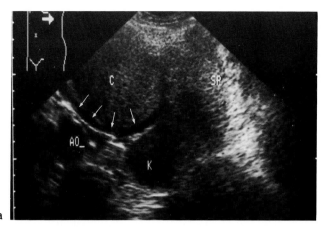
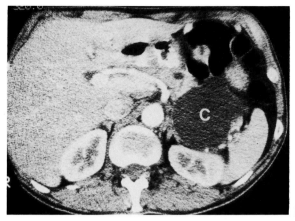

FIG. 7.18. Pseudocyst in lesser sac. a: transverse sonogram; b: CT scan. This echogenic pseudocyst is located in region of anterolateral recess of lesser sac. Splenic vessels (*thin arrows*) are compressed around the pseudocyst, which yields thick viscous fluid at percutaneous aspiration. Patient has well-documented alcoholic chronic pancreatitis. *Ao*, aorta; *K*, kidney; *SP*, spleen; *C*, pseudocyst.

(Fig. 7.21a,b). About 30 cases have been reported in the literature. The fluid collection extends into the mediastinum by way of the aortic/esophageal hiatus, often causing cardiorespiratory symptoms and rarely esophageal obstruction (39). Dissection of a pseudocyst into the liver and spleen and extension into the neck, pelvis, and scrotum have been described (15).

Complicated pseudocysts may be aspirated or drained percutaneously under CT or ultrasound guidance (40).

Pancreatic Neoplasms

Pancreatic Adenocarcinoma

Pancreatic adenocarcinoma is the most common type of pancreatic cancer, accounting for 75% of all pancre-

atic carcinoma of ductal cell origin. It is more commonly seen in men, in blacks, and in diabetic patients. Cigarette smoking is also a risk factor. The 5-year survival rate is only 1%. The mean and median survival is only 4 months from the time of diagnosis. Pancreatic carcinoma is the fourth leading cause of death from cancer in men and the fifth in women. The location of the tumor in the gland is as follows: head, 60%; body, 16%; tail, 5%; combination of above, 20%. At clinical presentation, tumors in the tail are usually larger (average diameter 10 cm) than those in the head (average diameter 5 cm). The most common symptom is epigastric pain, which frequently radiates to the back. Common physical findings include jaundice, which is seen with carcinoma of the pancreatic head, steatorrhea, venous thrombosis, and skin lesions resembling erythema nodosum (41,42).

The role of ultrasound is:

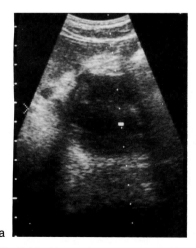
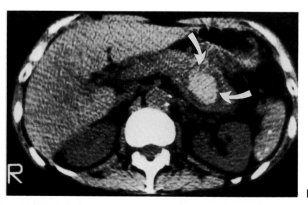

FIG. 7.19. Hemorrhage in pseudocyst. a: sonogram; b: CT scan. Irregular echoes are seen in this pseudocyst. Unenhanced CT scan demonstrates blood density in pseudocyst (*arrows*). Patient had a protracted clinical course. Doppler scans may help to demonstrate active bleeding in a pseudocyst.

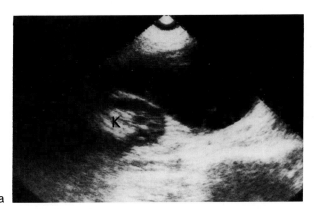
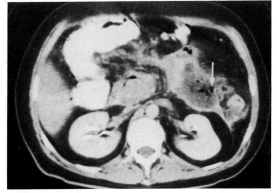

FIG. 7.20. Infected pseudocyst. **a:** sagittal sonogram; **b:** CT scan. Sonogram identifies a septated fluid collection (*C*) on left side of abdomen, anterior to kidney (*K*). CT scan shows gas bubbles in pseudocyst (*arrow*). Pus was aspirated percutaneously.

1. to establish the diagnosis by identifying a pancreatic mass and assisting in percutaneous biopsy
2. to determine the extent of the disease for assessing resectability of the tumor
3. to assist in palliative procedures such as percutaneous biliary drainage

Most tumors are hypoechoic (Figs. 7.22a,b and 7.23), but some are hyperechoic, and a few are isoechoic as compared with the normal gland. Some masses contain small cystic spaces representing either retention cysts, obstructive pseudocysts, or areas of necrosis. In most cases, a diagnosis cannot be made without a biopsy (41–43).

Ancillary abnormalities that can be detected by ultrasound include

1. *ascites*: This is not seen commonly in pancreatic carcinoma. Its presence often implies peritoneal metastases, but it may also be due to pancreatitis associated with carcinoma. As an isolated finding, it should not be considered a contraindication to surgical resection.

2. *dilated bile ducts*: Carcinoma of the head of the pancreas causes obstructive jaundice in about 90% of cases. Sonography is the best noninvasive technique in the detection of dilated bile ducts.

3. *dilated pancreatic duct* (Fig. 7.22a,b): This is also easily detected by ultrasound. However, this is not specific for carcinoma and is commonly seen in chronic pancreatitis.

4. *lymph node metastases and invasion of adjacent organs*: Lymphadenopathy is seen in about one third of patients with pancreatic cancers. However, CT scan performs better in detecting retrocrural nodes and invasion of surrounding organs such as the stomach and duodenum (42).

5. *liver metastases*: They are seen in 36% to 50% of

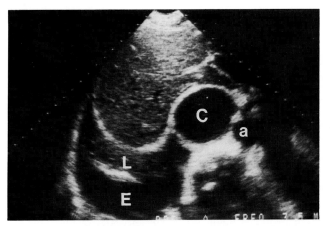
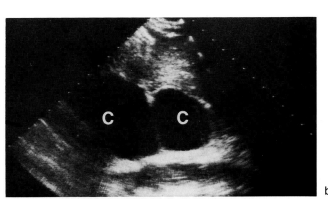

FIG. 7.21. Mediastinal pseudocyst. **a:** transverse sonogram; **b:** sagittal sonogram. Sonograms show a bilobated fluid collection (*C*) extending from upper abdomen into lower thorax in the midline, compressing lower esophagus. Patient presented with progressive dysphagia after an attack of acute pancreatitis a few months earlier. Note right pleural effusion (*E*) surrounding collapsed lung (*L*). *a*, aorta. (From Nguyen et al., ref. 39, with permission.)

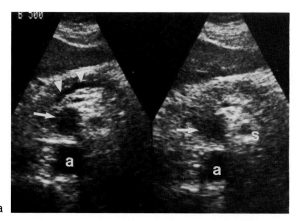

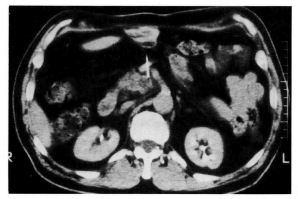

a

b

FIG. 7.22. Pancreatic carcinoma. **a:** transverse sonogram; **b:** CT scan. There is a small echo-poor mass (*arrow*) in uncinate process of pancreas. Pancreatic duct is dilated (*arrowhead*). The mass was biopsied percutaneously under CT guidance. Note tip of needle in mass. *a*, aorta; *s*, superior mesenteric artery.

patients with pancreatic carcinoma at presentation (42,43).

6. *vascular invasion* (Fig. 7.24a,b): This is considered a sign of tumor nonresectability. Ultrasound appears to compete well with angiography in detecting vascular involvement (43–45). Its capacity will be enhanced with the increasing use of Doppler technique. Encasement of the superior mesenteric artery and invasion of the splenic vein are frequent findings (42).

In summary, in the diagnosis of pancreatic carcinoma, it has been estimated that ultrasound has an accuracy of 88% in nine large series (41).

Pancreatic-Cystic Neoplasms

Cystic neoplasms constitute 2.5% to 6% of all nonendocrine pancreatic neoplasms and 5% to 15% of all pancreatic cystic lesions. Two types are recognized: 50% are microcystic adenoma and 50% are mucinous cystic neoplasms. They have been extensively evaluated by ultrasound, CT, and MRI (46–51).

Microcystic Adenomas (serous cystadenomas; glycogen-rich cystadenomas)

These are benign neoplasms that occur more commonly in women older than 60 years of age, in diabetics, and in patients with von Hippel-Lindau disease. They affect more commonly the pancreatic head and body. They tend to be lobulated and large, with an average diameter of 11 cm at the time of diagnosis. They are composed of multiple small cysts that contain a clear serous fluid and that are lined by epithelial cells rich in glycogen. A calcified fibrous stellate scar may be seen in the center of the mass (46,49).

Sonography demonstrates a highly echogenic mass caused by the myriad of interfaces between the cysts (Fig. 7.25a,b). Bright echoes in the center of the mass may represent calcified fibrous scars.

Mucinous Cystic Neoplasms (mucinous cystadenomas; mucinous cystadenocarcinomas)

These potentially malignant tumors occur almost always in women in their fifth or sixth decades. They arise more commonly from the body and tail of the pancreas. They may invade adjacent organs and vessels. However, they have a more favorable prognosis than ductal adenocarcinoma after total surgical excision (47). Sonographically, they typically appear as a lobulated mass with unilocular or multilocular large cystic cavities that contain thick, mucoid brown fluid (Fig. 7.26a,b). Septations, dystrophic calcification, and papillary solid excrescences in the wall are often seen (48,50,51).

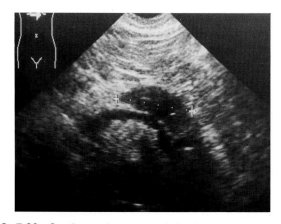

FIG. 7.23. Carcinoma in pancreatic body. Pancreatic carcinomas are often hypoechoic like this one. +---+ demarcates medial and lateral borders of the tumor.

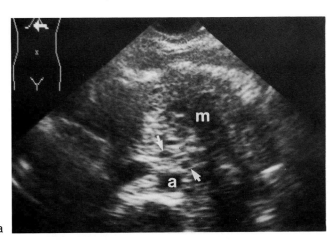
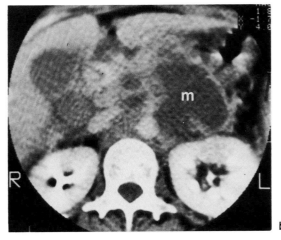

FIG. 7.24. Pancreatic carcinoma—vascular encasement. **a:** transverse sonogram; **b:** CT scan. Echogenic material is seen surrounding the aorta (*a*) and superior mesenteric vessels (*arrows*). A hypoechoic mass (*m*) is in posterior aspect of pancreatic body. Findings correlate well with those seen on CT scan.

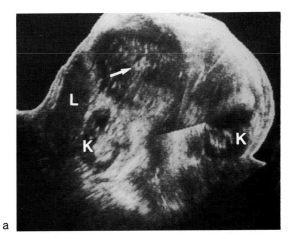
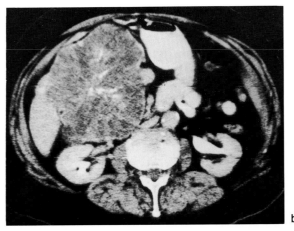

FIG. 7.25. Microcystic adenoma. **a:** transverse sonogram; **b:** CT scan. A large echogenic mass is seen in head of pancreas. Note central stellate scar (*arrow*). Echogenicity of the tumor is due to interfaces of multiple tiny cysts. *K*, kidney; *L*, liver.

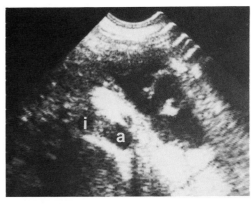
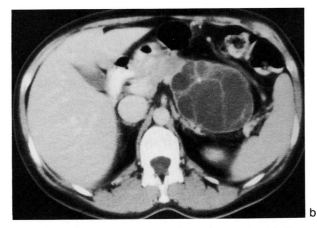

FIG. 7.26. Mucinous cystic neoplasm. **a:** transverse sonogram; **b:** CT scan. Tumor is composed of multiple large cystic cavities separated by septa. Appearances simulate a complicated pseudocyst or loculated ascites. Mucinous cystic neoplasms typically occur in body and tail of pancreas. *a*, aorta; *i*, inferior vena cava.

TABLE 7.2. *APUDomas of pancreas*

Cells	Hormone produced	Neoplasm	Clinical syndrome
A	Glucagon	Glucagonoma	Diabetogenic-pemphigoid
B	Insulin	Insulinoma	Whipple's triad
D	Somatostatin	Somatostatinoma	
D₁	VIP (vasoactive intestinal polypeptide)	VIPoma	Verner-Morrison (WDHH)
G	Gastrin	Gastrinoma	ZE

APUD, amine precursor uptake and decarboxylation; WDHH, watery diarrhea and hypokalemia and hypovolemia.

Differential diagnosis with microcystic adenoma is usually not difficult. However, differentiation with loculated ascites, ductal cell adenocarcinoma, and islet cell neoplasms often requires percutaneous aspiration or surgical biopsies (50).

Endocrine Neoplasms of Pancreas (APUDomas)

Endocrine neoplasms of pancreas arise from APUD cells, which are islet cells originating from the neural crest, capable of secreting a specific hormone, hence their name APUDomas (Table 7.2) (52,53).

Insulinomas and gastrinomas account for 90% to 95% of all endocrine pancreatic neoplasms.

Insulinomas are the most common apudomas. Typically, the patients exhibit symptoms and signs related to hyperinsulinism, which consist of spontaneous hypoglycemic attacks relieved by oral or intravenous glucose administration; the fasting blood sugar concentration is less than 50 mg/ml. Nearly 90% of insulinomas are solitary, benign, and small (<2 cm). The remainder (10%) are malignant or multiple (54). Multiple insulinomas are almost always seen in MEN type 1. Preoperative localization can be made by CT, ultrasound, angiography, and pancreatic venous sampling. Real-time sonography can

detect 60% of solitary insulinoma (Fig. 7.27a,b). Intraoperative ultrasound claims a higher sensitivity (84% detection rate), identifying lesions less than 1 cm in diameter (54).

Gastrinomas are associated with the ZE syndrome, which is characterized by recurrent gastric and duodenal ulceration and elevated serum gastrin. In about one third of the cases, they are associated with the MEN type 1 syndrome. Medical control of gastric acid hypersecretion is now possible with histamine receptor antagonists (Cimetidine) and with H^+, P^+, ATPase inhibitor (Omeprazole). Surgery is reserved for resection of localized gastrinoma without evidence of metastatic disease. Preoperative localization is usually achieved by CT, ultrasound, angiography, pancreatic venous samplings, and recently, MRI. It appears from some series (55) that both ultrasound and MRI are less sensitive than CT scanning in the detection of gastrinoma, which are often multiple, small (less than a few millimeters in diameter), and sometimes ectopic, occurring in locations other than the pancreas. A recent report claims, however, that CT and ultrasound are equally effective for the detection of extrahepatic gastrinomas and that angiography is superior than both (56). Nearly 70% of gastrinomas are malignant.

Other types of APUDomas are exceedingly rare.

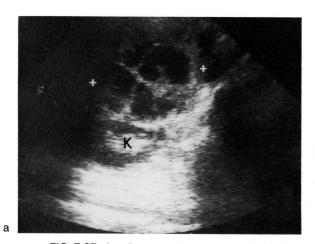 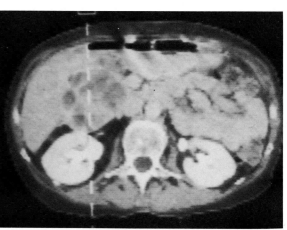

a   b

FIG. 7.27. Insulinoma. **a:** transverse sonogram; **b:** CT scan. A large solid mass with multiple small cystic cavities is seen in head of pancreas. This appearance is unusual for an insulinoma, which is usually small and echogenic. Multiple small insulinomas are often found in MEN type 1 syndrome. *K*, kidney.

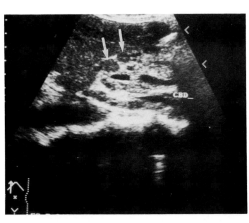

FIG. 7.28. Peripancreatic nodes: sagittal scan. Enlarged lymph nodes (*arrows*) are seen surrounding head of pancreas in this patient with non-Hodgkin's lymphoma. Lymphomatous nodes are usually hypoechoic but may be hyperechoic.

Pancreatic Lymphoma

Primary lymphoma of the pancreas is a rarity. However, the pancreas is affected in 35% of lymphoma patients at autopsy. The percentage is much higher with Burkitt's lymphoma, reaching 80% of these cases (57). Involvement most often occurs within peripancreatic nodes along the superior and anterior surface of the gland and around the pancreatic head (Fig. 7.28). Less frequently, intrapancreatic masses are found (57). Sonographically, lymphomatous pancreatic and peripancreatic masses are indistinguishable from other types of pancreatic neoplasms. Diagnosis should be established by biopsies whenever indicated.

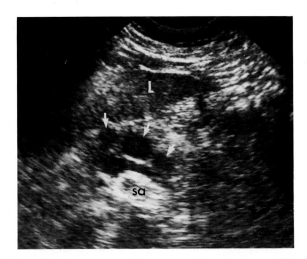

FIG. 7.29. Metastases to pancreas: transverse scan. Hypoechoic masses (*arrows*) are seen in body of pancreas in this patient with bronchogenic carcinoma. *L,* liver; *sa,* superior mesenteric artery.

Metastases to Pancreas

Metastases to the pancreas may originate from melanocarcinoma, carcinoma of the lung, breast, ovary, prostate, liver, or kidney, and various types of sarcoma (58). They occur rarely as an isolated finding; they are most often found in patients with widespread metastatic disease elsewhere. Sonographically, they are usually hypoechoic. They may be small or large, single or multiple (Fig. 7.29). They may undergo rapid lysis during chemotherapy, causing tumor lysis pancreatitis (58).

7.4 SPECIAL TECHNIQUES

Endoscopic Ultrasound

Endoscopic ultrasound is a relatively recent advance in imaging, performed only in a few specialized centers in North America, Japan, and Europe. There are commercially available echoendoscopes using 7.5- to 12-MHz transducers with built-in channel for ES-guided cytologic puncture or biopsy needles. Endoscopic ultrasound plays an important role in the preoperative evaluation of malignancy occurring at the hepatico-pancreatico-ampullary region (i.e., at the confluence of the bile duct, pancreatic duct, and duodenum). Endoscopic ultrasound can differentiate an ampullary carcinoma from a pancreatic carcinoma. Depth of tumor infiltration and local invasion of surrounding vessels and nodes are readily detected by ES. Preoperative ES staging may obviate the need for exploratory surgery in the future (59).

Intraoperative Ultrasound

This technique is particularly useful in identifying or localizing small focal masses that escape detection by other imaging methods and by direct palpation of the gland at surgery. A 5- or 7.5-MHz transducer is commonly used. Scanning is performed in the operating room after appropriate aseptic precautions. Small carcinoma, gastrinoma, and insulinoma with an average diameter less than 1 cm have been identified. Pancreatic stones and small pseudocysts are also more easily detected by this technique (60).

7.5 PITFALLS, ARTIFACTS, AND PRACTICAL TIPS

1. Care must be taken not to confuse a pancreatic duct with the splenic vein when the duct is dilated. One way to avoid this mistake is to obtain a transverse scan in which both structures are visualized simultaneously. Another way is to use color Doppler ultrasound. The splenic vein lies posterior to the pancreatic duct. Seg-

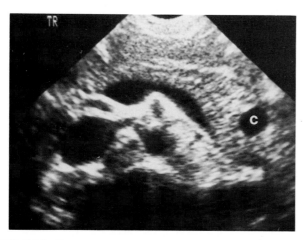

FIG. 7.30. Pancreatic cyst in adult polycystic kidney disease. This small cyst (c) is seen in tail of pancreas. Patient has documented adult polycystic kidney disease. In this inherited condition, cysts may also be seen in liver and spleen. They are thought to be developmental.

ments of a tortuous splenic artery may simulate a small cyst within the gland. Scanning at a different angle and in a different plane or color Doppler ultrasound will help to eliminate this confusion.

2. Occasionally, the posterior wall of the collapsed stomach may be mistaken for the pancreatic duct. In case of doubt, scanning through a fluid-filled stomach will eliminate this confusion.

3. Small cysts may be seen in the pancreas in patients with adult polycystic kidney disease (Fig. 7.30). They are developmental and not related to pancreatitis.

4. It may be difficult to differentiate a large mass in the pancreatic tail from a large left adrenal mass. In this situation, identification of the splenic vein is crucial. If the mass lies anterior to the splenic vein, it is a pancreatic lesion.

5. A pseudocyst often has a similar sonographic appearance as loculated ascites, a lymphocele, or a mesenteric cyst. Diagnosis usually requires fine needle aspiration.

6. Focal pancreatitis is difficult to distinguish from carcinoma. In most instances, follow-up scans or biopsies, or both, are required.

7. The pancreatic head is a rather long structure in the cranio-caudad dimension. If only the top of the head is scanned in the transverse plane, a tumor in the distal uncinate process may be overlooked. Sagittal scanning in the plane of the inferior vena cava will avoid this problem.

REFERENCES

Normal Anatomy

1. Weill F, Schraub A, Eisenscher A, Bourgoin A. Ultrasonography of the normal pancreas. Success rate or criteria for normality. *Radiology* 1977;123:417–423.

2. Perlmutter GS. Ultrasound measurements of the pancreas. In: Goldberg B, Kurtz AB, eds. *Atlas of ultrasound measurements.* Chicago: Yearbook Medical Publishers; 1990:113–125.

3. Coleman BG, Arger PH, Rosenberg HK, Mulhern CB, Ortega W, Stauffer D. Gray-scale sonographic assessment of pancreatitis in children. *Radiology* 1983;146:145–150.

4. Kreel L, Sandin B. Changes in pancreatic morphology associated with aging. *GUT* 1973;14:962–970.

5. Heuck A, Maubach PA, Reiser M, et al. Age-related morphology of the normal pancreas on computed tomography. *Gastrointest Radiol* 1987;12:18–22.

6. Marchal G, Verbeken E, Van Steenbergen W, Baert A, Lauwereyns J. Uneven lipomatosis: a pitfall in pancreatic sonography. *Gastrointest Radiol* 1989;14:233–237.

Pathology

7. Zeman RK, McVay LV, Silverman PM, et al. Pancreas divisum: thin-section CT. *Radiology* 1988;169:395–398.

8. Nguyen KT, Pace R, Groll A. CT appearance of annular pancreas: a case report. *J Can Assoc Radiol* 1989;40:322–323.

9. Feldman W. Screening for cystic fibrosis. In: Periodic health examination, 1991 update. Canadian Task Force on the Periodic Health Examination. *Can Med Assoc J* 1991;145:629–635.

10. Goldstein RB, Filly RA, Callen PW. Sonographic diagnosis of meconium ileus *in utero. J Ultrasound Med* 1987;6:663–666.

11. Willi UV, Reddish JM, Teele RL. Cystic fibrosis: its characteristic appearance on abdominal sonography. *AJR* 1980;134:1005–1010.

12. Swobodnik W, Wolf A, Wechsler JG, Kleihauer E, Ditschuneit H. Ultrasound characteristics of the pancreas in children with cystic fibrosis. *JCU* 1985;13:469–474.

13. Liu P, Daneman A, Stanger DA, Durie PR. Pancreatic cysts and calcification in cystic fibrosis. *J Can Assoc Radiol* 1986;37:279–282.

14. Daneman A, Gaskin K, Martin DJ, Cutz E. Pancreatic changes in cystic fibrosis: CT and sonographic appearances. *AJR* 1983;141:653–655.

15. Freeny PC, Lawson TL. Acute pancreatitis. In: Freeny PC, Lawson TL, eds. *Radiology of the pancreas.* New York: Springer-Verlag; 1982:169–222.

16. Simeone JF, Wittenberg J, Ferrucci JT Jr. Modern concepts of imaging the pancreas. *Invest Radiol* 1980;15:6–18.

17. Shafer RB, Silvis SE. Pancreatic pseudo-pseudocysts. *Am J Surg* 1974;127:320–325.

18. Balthazar EJ, Robinson DL, Megibow AJ, Rawson JHC. Acute pancreatitis: value of CT in establishing prognosis. *Radiology* 1990;174:331–336.

19. Donovan PS, Sanders RC, Siegelman SS. Collections of fluid after pancreatitis: evaluation by CT and ultrasound. *Radiol Clin North Am* 1982;4:653–665.

20. Rawlings W, Bynum TE, Pasternak G. Pancreatic ascites: diagnosis of leakage site by endoscopic pancreatography. *Surgery* 1977;81:363–365.

21. Tylen V, Dewncker H. Roentgenologic diagnosis of pancreatic abscess. *Acta Radiol* 1973;14:9–16.

22. Vernacchia FS, Jeffrey RB Jr, Federle MP, et al. Pancreatic abscess: predictive value of early abdominal CT. *Radiology* 1987;162:435–438.

23. Saha SP, Stephenson SE Jr. Gastrocolic fistula secondary to pancreatic abscess. *South Med J* 1974;67:367–368.

24. Luetmer PH, Stephens DH, Ward EM. Chronic pancreatitis: reassessment with current CT. *Radiology* 1989;171:353–357.

25. DelMaschio A, Vanzulli A, Sironi S, et al. Pancreatic cancer versus chronic pancreatitis: diagnosis with CA 19-9 assessment, US, CT and CT-guided fine-needle biopsy. *Radiology* 1991;178:95–99.

26. Ferrucci JT Jr, Wittenberg J, Black EB, Kirkpatrick RH, Hall DA. Computed body tomography in chronic pancreatitis. *Radiology* 1979;130:175–182.

27. Kunzman A, Bowie JD, Rochester D. Texture patterns in pancreatic sonograms. *Gastrointest Radiol* 1980;134:185–189.

28. Cotton PB, Lees WR, Vallon AG, Coltone M, Crocker JR, Chapman M. Gray-scale ultrasonography or endoscopic pancreatography in pancreatic diagnosis. *Radiology* 1980;134:453–459.

29. Weinstein DP, Weinstein BJ. Ultrasonic demonstration of the pancreatic duct: an analysis of 41 cases. *Radiology* 1979;130:729–734.
30. Ring EJ, Eaton SB Jr, Ferrucci JT Jr, Short WF. The differential diagnosis of pancreatic calcification. *AJR* 1973;117:446–452.
31. Siegelman SS, Copeland BE, Saba GP, Cameron JL, Sanders RC, Zerhouni EA. CT of fluid collections associated with pancreatitis. *AJR* 1980;134:1121–1132.
32. Gonzalez AC, Bradley EL, Clements JL Jr. Pseudocyst formation in acute pancreatitis: ultrasonic evaluation of 99 cases. *AJR* 1976;127:315–317.
33. Kressel HY, Margulis AR, Booding GW, Filly RA, Moss AA, Korobkin M. CT scanning or ultrasound in the evaluation of pancreatic pseudocysts: a preliminary comparison. *Radiology* 1978;126:153–157.
34. Sarti DA. Rapid development or spontaneous regression of pancreatic pseudocysts demonstrated by ultrasound. *Radiology* 1977;125:789–793.
35. Vujic I, Seymour EQ, Meredith HL. Vascular complications associated with sonographically demonstrated cystic epigastric lesions: an important indication for angiography. *N Engl J Med* 1972;287:72–75.
36. Ates KB, Boyacioglu S, Tas I, Gencer A, Temucin G, Sahin B. The ultrasonographic diagnosis of bleeding into a pancreatic pseudocyst. *Gastrointest Radiol* 1991;16:178–180.
37. Warshaw AL. Inflammatory masses following acute pancreatitis: phlegmon, pseudocyst and abscess. *Surg Clin North Am* 1974;54:621–636.
38. Hanna WA. Rupture of pancreatic cysts: report of a case or review of the literature. *Br J Surg* 1960;47:495–498.
39. Nguyen KT, Kosiuk J, Place C, Winton TH, Sauerbrei EE. Two unusual causes of dysphagia: a pictorial essay. *J Can Assoc Radiol* 1987;38:42–44.
40. vanSonnenberg E, Wittich GR, Casola G, et al. Percutaneous drainage of infected or non-infected pancreatic pseudocysts: experience in 101 cases. *Radiology* 1989;170:757–761.
41. Freeny PC, Lawson TL. Adenocarcinoma of the pancreas. In: Freeny PC, Lawson TL, eds. *Radiology of the pancreas.* New York: Springer-Verlag; 1982:397–496.
42. Freeny PC, Mark WM, Ryan JA, Traverso LW. Pancreatic ductal adenocarcinoma: diagnosis or staging with dynamic CT. *Radiology* 1988,166:125–133.
43. Campbell JP, Wilson SR. Pancreatic neoplasms. How useful is evaluation with ultrasound? *Radiology* 1988;167:341–344.
44. Garra BS, Shawker TH, Doppman JL, Sindilar WF. Comparison of angiography or ultrasound in the evaluation of the portal venous system in pancreatic carcinoma. *JCU* 1987;15:83–93.
45. Kosuge T, Makuuchi M, Takayama T, Yamamoto J, Kinoshita T, Ozaki H. Thickening at the root of the superior mesenteric artery on sonography: evidence of vascular involvement in patients with cancer of the pancreas. *AJR* 1991;156:69–72.
46. Moser RP, Buck JL, Hayes WS. Microcystic adenoma of the pancreas. *Radiographics* 1990;10:313–322.
47. Compagno J, Oertel JE. Mucinous cystic neoplasms of the pancreas with overt or latent malignancy (cystadenocarcinoma or cystadenoma): a clinico-pathologic study of 41 cases. *Am J Clin Pathol* 1978;69:573–580.
48. Fugazzola C, Procacci C, Andreis IAB, et al. Cystic tumours of the pancreas: evaluation by ultrasonography and computed tomography. *Gastrointest Radiol* 1991;16:53–61.
49. Padovani B, Neuveut P, Chanalet S, et al. Microcystic adenoma of the pancreas: report on four cases and review of the literature. *Gastrointest Radiol* 1991;16:62–66.
50. Johnson CD, Stephens DH, Charboneau JW, Carpenter HA, Welch TJ. Cystic pancreatic tumors: CT and sonographic assessment. *AJR* 1988;151:1133–1138.
51. Minami M, Itai Y, Ohtomo K, Yoshida H, Yoshikawa K, Iio M. Cystic neoplasms of the pancreas: comparison of MR imaging with CT. *Radiology* 1989;171:53–56.
52. Pearse AGE. The APUD concept or its implications in pathology. *Pathol Annu* 1974;9:27–42.
53. Greider MH, Rosai J, McGuigan JE. The human pancreatic islet cells or their tumors. Ulcerogenic or diarrheogenic tumors. *Cancer* 1974;33:1423–1443.
54. Galiber AK, Reading CC, Charboneau JW, et al. Localization of pancreatic insulinoma: comparison of pre- or intra-operative ultrasound with CT and angiography. *Radiology* 1988;166:405–408.
55. Frucht H, Doppman JL, Norton AJ, et al. Gastrinomas: comparison of MR imaging with CT, angiography and ultrasound. *Radiology* 1989;171:713–717.
56. London JF, Shawker TH, Doppman JL, et al. Zollinger-Ellison syndrome: prospective assessment of abdominal ultrasound in the localization of gastrinomas. *Radiology* 1991;178:763–767.
57. Shirkhoda A, Ros PR, Farah J, Staab E. Lymphoma of the solid abdominal viscera. *Radiol Clin North Am* 1990;28:785–799.
58. Levine M, Danovitch S. Metastatic carcinoma to the pancreas: another cause for acute pancreatitis. *Am J Gastroenterol* 1973;60:290–294.

Special Techniques

59. Tio TL, Tygat GN, Cikot RJL, Houthoff HJ, Sars PRA. Ampullopancreatic carcinoma: preoperative TNM classification with endosonography. *Radiology* 1990;175:455–461.
60. Rifkin MD, Weiss SM. Intraoperative sonographic identification of nonpalpable pancreatic masses. *J Ultrasound Med* 1984;3:409–411.

CHAPTER 8

The Kidney

INTRODUCTION

Ultrasound permits the examining technologist/physician to examine the kidney and proximal ureter for most important pathologic entities. It may not be sensitive with small focal masses (particularly if they are isoechoic) or small areas of calcification (e.g., calculus). The sensitivity will be determined by the patient's body habitus, transducer frequency, focal zone characteristics, acoustic window, scan technique, and time spent on the examination by the scanner.

Abbreviations: **ATN**, acute tubular necrosis; **AVM**, arteriovenous malformation; **CT**, computed tomography; **DSR**, diastolic/systolic ratio; **MCDK**, multicystic dysplastic kidney; **MRI**, magnetic resonance imaging; **PI**, pulsatility index; **PW**, pulsed wave Doppler; **RI**, resistive index; **SDR**, systolic/diastolic ratio; **Tc^{99m}DMSA**, Technetium 99^m–dimethyldimercapto succinic acid; **TCC**, transitional cell carcinoma; **UPJ**, ureteropelvic junction; **XGP**, xanthogranulomatous pyelonephritis.

Most of the information derived will be anatomic or anatomic–pathologic. Pulsed wave or color Doppler permits some physiologic assessment of vascularity of the kidney or mass. Renal function is usually better assessed by nuclear medicine techniques. Computed tomography and MRI are valuable in the assessment of renal masses.

8.1 SCANNING TECHNIQUES

The kidneys should be scanned in at least two planes to adequately visualize all the parenchyma and collecting system. The kidneys may be scanned in coronal, sagittal, transverse, and occasionally oblique planes. Kidneys that are anatomically cephalad in the retroperitoneal space will be better visualized during sustained inspiration. The liver and spleen can be used as an acoustic window to visualize the kidneys. The kidneys may be obscured by bowel gas or may be difficult to visualize in obese patients. Various maneuvers may improve the vi-

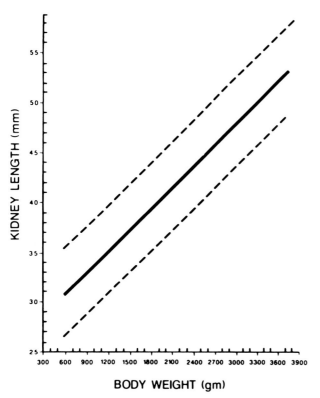

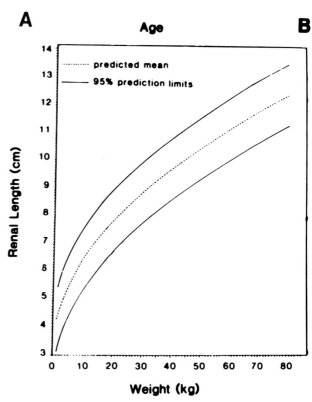

FIG. 8.1. Nomogram for kidney length versus body weight for infants. *Solid line* represents mean, and *dotted lines* denote 95% confidence limits. (From Schlesinger et al., ref. 1, with permission.)

FIG. 8.2. Nomogram for kidney length versus body weight for children. *Dotted line* represents mean, and *solid lines* denote 95% confidence limits. (From Han et al., ref. 2, with permission.)

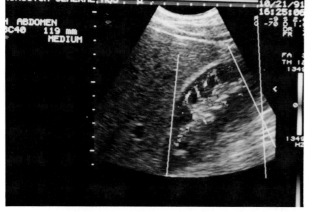

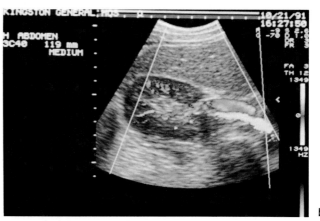

FIG. 8.3. Color Doppler of kidney in sagittal axis (**a**) and transverse axis (**b**). (*See color images for parts a and b in color plate section B, which follows page 242.*) Color assignment is dependent on direction of flow and is indicated in color bar to right. Flow toward transducer is red, whereas flow away from transducer is blue. Note that arterial or venous structures may be red or blue on the same color Doppler picture depending on whether flow is toward or away from transducer. Arterial flow toward transducer will be depicted as red, whereas arterial flow away from transducer will be depicted as blue. The same is true of venous flow. One can discriminate between arterial and venous structures by PW spectral analysis and the pattern of pulsation. (Courtesy of Dr. Patrick Llewellyn).

TABLE 8.1. *Kidney size—adult*

	Right (mm)		Left (mm)	
	Mean	SD	Mean	SD
Length	106.5	13.5	101.3	11.7
Width	49.2	6.4	53.0	7.4
Anteroposterior (depth)	39.5	8.1	35.8	9.1

From Brandt et al., ref. 3, with permission.

sualization. Cooperative patients can be placed in various positions (e.g., right anterior oblique, left anterior oblique, decubitus, prone) in addition to the usual supine position.

The highest frequency transducer permitting adequate penetration is usually used. Sector or convex transducer configurations are usually preferable.

The maximum renal length should be recorded on sagittal or coronal scans (1–3). The maximum anterior–posterior diameter and width measurement should be recorded on transverse scans through the renal hilum (3). The measurements represent one set of parameters by which the kidney is evaluated. Normal measurements are presented in Figs. 8.1 and 8.2 and Table 8.1 (1–3).

Doppler (PW and color) should be performed for suspected vascular abnormalities in renal allographs and in renal tumors. Vessel patency is most easily identified by color Doppler (Fig. 8.3). It will also identify significant focal stenosis and vascular malformations. These can be analyzed in greater detail by spectral analysis. One should attempt to obtain Doppler signals from the main renal artery, segmental branches, interlobar arteries, and arcuate arteries (Fig. 8.4). Doppler samples should be obtained at several sites in the cortex if segmental vascular disease is suspected (e.g., emboli, small vessel disease, renal allograph). These are usually easily obtained in the renal allograph but are more difficult in native kidneys.

Doppler sampling of the renal vein should be obtained in renal allographs and in renal tumors. The inferior vena cava should also be assessed with renal tumors.

The Doppler angle (i.e., angle of insonation of the vessel) should ideally be 30° to 60°. The more perpendicular the Doppler angle is to the vessel the less optimal will be the resultant Doppler signal (4). The direction of flow should be noted in all cases.

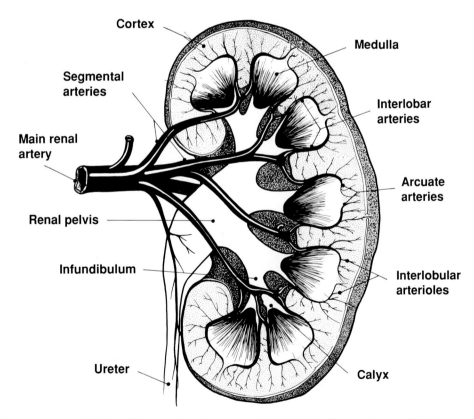

FIG. 8.4. Anatomy of kidney. Venous structures are not included in diagram to permit better appreciation of other structures. Venous structures parallel arterial structures. Parenchyma consists of outer cortex and inner medulla. Vascular structures show sequential branching of main renal artery into segmental arteries, interlobar arteries, arcuate arteries, and intralobular arteries. Pelvicalyceal collecting system consists of calyces, infundibula, renal pelvis, and ureter. (Modified from Netter, ref. 6, with permission.)

8.2 NORMAL ANATOMY, VARIANTS, AND CONGENITAL ANOMALIES

The kidneys (Fig. 8.4) are normally located within the perirenal space of the retroperitoneum. They lie at an oblique angle to the spine, with the lower poles more lateral than the upper poles.

The renal cortex consists of glomeruli and convoluted tubules. It occupies the outer one third of the renal parenchyma and projects deeper into the parenchyma between the renal pyramids as *columns of Bertin*. The *medulla* represents collecting tubules and loops of Henle. It occupies the inner two thirds of the parenchyma except where cortical tissue (columns of Bertin) projects between the pyramids. The *central sinus* contains fat, vascular structures, lymphatics, and the pelvicalyceal collecting system (5,6).

There is usually one renal artery to each kidney, but up to 25% of kidneys have accessory renal arteries. The *main renal artery* usually divides into five *segmental arteries* in the region of the hilum. The segmental arteries divide into *interlobar arteries,* which pass through the parenchyma adjacent to the renal pyramids. These become the *arcuate arteries* peripherally and run between the cortex and medulla. The interlobar and arcuate arteries give rise to small *interlobular arteries* that supply the cortex. Smaller branches supply the medulla and glomeruli. The veins run parallel with the arteries (5,6).

Newborn Kidney

The renal cortex is more hyperechoic than in older children and may be equal to that of the adjacent liver and spleen. The medullary pyramids are triangular-shaped. They are relatively hypoechoic and therefore appear prominent (Fig. 8.5). This pattern may persist up to

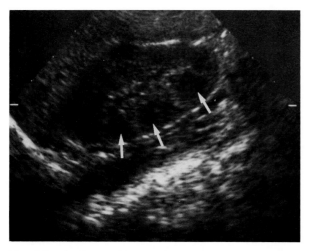

FIG. 8.5. Newborn kidney. Hypoechoic renal pyramids (*arrows*) of medulla are surrounded by relatively hyperechoic renal cortex.

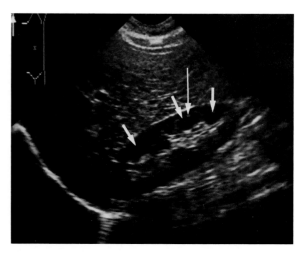

FIG. 8.6. Pediatric and adult kidney. Medullary pyramids (*arrows*) are hypoechoic relative to cortex. *Long thin arrow* indicates an arcuate artery.

approximately 6 months of age. A proportionately greater volume of the renal cortex is occupied by glomeruli, resulting in more acoustic interfaces than in the older child and adult (7), resulting in the hyperechoic cortex. The central sinus is usually isoechoic with the cortex, caused by a paucity of central sinus fat.

Pediatric and Adult Kidney

The renal cortex is hypoechoic relative to the adjacent liver and spleen. The medullary pyramids are triangular-shaped and hypoechoic relative to the renal cortex (Fig. 8.6). In adults, the renal pyramids are not as easily appreciated as in infant kidneys. The medulla (pyramids), as defined on ultrasound, occupies 50% or less of the parenchymal thickness. The ultrasound–defined medulla represents only a portion of the anatomic medulla. The central sinus contains a variable amount of fat, vascular structures, lymphatics, and the pelvicalyceal collecting system. The central sinus is hyperechoic relative to the renal cortex.

Renal Doppler

Arterial Doppler

Renal Doppler demonstrates a peak in frequency shift in systole with a gradual decrease in flow throughout diastole (Fig. 8.7). There is persistent antegrade flow, which is gradually dampened in peripheral vessels throughout the cardiac cycle (8). There is a spectral window in the sample from the main renal artery of the native kidney. In the renal allograph, the spectral window is lost because of turbulence at the site of the vascular anastomosis (9).

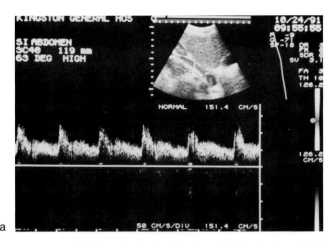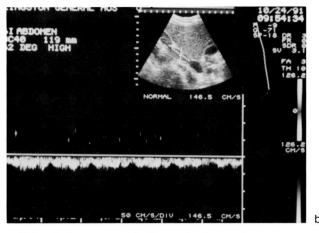

a   b

FIG. 8.7. Triplex (PW, color, real-time) scan of right renal hilum in transverse axis. (*See color images for parts a and b in color plate section B, which follows page 242.*) **a:** PW sample is placed on renal artery. Renal artery flow is toward transducer and is red. **b:** PW sample is placed on renal vein. Renal vein flow is away from transducer and is blue. (Courtesy of Dr. Patrick Llewellyn.)

Quantitation of Flow by PW Doppler

Renal doppler flow can be quantified (10) by measurements taken at the peak systolic frequency shift (Fig. 8.8a) and at the minimum diastolic frequency shift (Fig. 8.8b). Calculation of the mean frequency shift requires appropriate software in the duplex unit or a digitizing board.

Table 8.2 lists the calculations that can be performed using these measurements (11,12).

Venous Doppler

The renal vein flow is continuous throughout the cardiac cycle and may show slight variation caused by phase of respiration and cardiac cycle (Fig. 8.7). The patterns are similar in native and allograph kidneys, and the flow is opposite in direction to the arterial flow (8).

Renal Duplication Artifact

Refraction of the sound beam at the lower pole of the spleen or edge of liver can cause a duplication artifact of the upper pole of the kidney (13). It is more common on the left side. On ultrasound it may appear as (Fig. 8.9)

1. duplication of the collecting system
2. suprarenal mass
3. upper pole cortical thickening

Renal Agenesis

Renal agenesis occurs as a result of failure of the ureteric bud to develop or from failure of the ureteric bud to grow into the metanephric mass of mesoderm (14). Ultrasound will show bowel prolapsed into the renal fossa but no evidence of a kidney. The contralateral kidney may be hypertrophied. This should initiate a careful

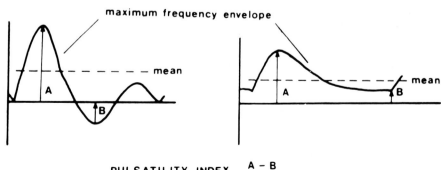

$$\text{PULSATILITY INDEX} = \frac{A - B}{\text{mean}}$$

FIG. 8.8. Pulsatility index. Pulsatility index is ratio of peak systolic frequency shift (*a*) minus minimum diastolic frequency shift (*b*) divided by mean frequency shift (mean). (From Rigsby et al., ref. 8, with permission.)

TABLE 8.2. *Calculations derived from PW frequency shifts*

	Normal calculations mean ± 2 SD	
	Native kidney	Allograph kidney
Pulsatility Index (PI) = $\dfrac{A - B}{mean}$		1.56 ± 0.82
Resistive Index (RI) = $\dfrac{A - B}{A}$	0.64 ± 0.8	0.69 ± 0.16
Diastolic/systolic ratio (DSR) = A/B		0.31 ± 0.16
Systolic/diastolic ratio (SDR) = B/A		3.6 ± 3.4

search for an ectopic kidney, crossed renal ectopia, and pancake or discoid kidney (i.e., fused unascended kidney).

The differential diagnosis should include hypoplastic kidney, atrophic kidney, and a normally located kidney with hyperechoic renal cortex. A Tc^{99m}-DMSA or TC^{99m} glucoheptonate radioisotope scan is an excellent method to demonstrate functioning renal tissue in an ectopic location.

Hypoplastic Kidney

Hypoplastic kidney is regarded as incomplete development of the metanephros, which was embryologically arrested at an early stage.

The kidney will appear small but otherwise have a normal appearance. It may be impossible to differentiate from atrophy of any etiology (e.g., infection, vascular). A Tc^{99m}-DMSA or Tc^{99m} glucoheptonate radioisotope scan can demonstrate functioning renal tissue.

Abnormal Rotation of the Kidney

With "incomplete rotation" the renal pelvis is directed anteriorly. This is a common isolated anomaly of no clinical significance. It is also common with ectopic kidneys and horseshoe kidneys (see Fig. 8.18).

Lobation/Junctional Parenchymal Defect

The kidney develops from the metanephric diverticulum (or ureteric bud) and the metanephric mass of mesoderm, which develops into the parenchyma. The metanephric diverticulum develops into the ureter, renal pelvis, calyces, and collecting tubules. The metanephric mass develops into the cortex and medulla (14). A lobe of parenchyma develops in relation to each branch of the metanephric diverticulum. These lobes start to fuse late in the second trimester of pregnancy, and fusion continues into early childhood. Some grooves or sulci on the surface of the kidney persist (15).

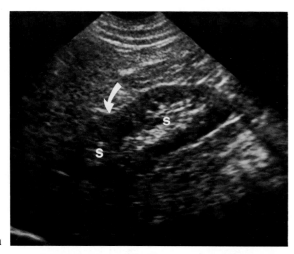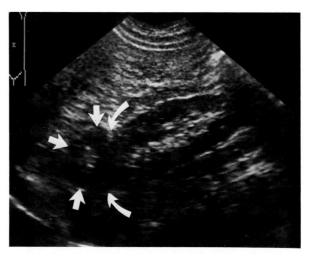

a   b

FIG. 8.9. Renal duplication artifact. Normal left kidney is scanned in coronal axis. **a:** apparent contour change (*curved arrow*) at upper pole of kidney. There is also an apparent duplication of central sinus (*s*) separated by parenchyma. **b:** apparent separate mass (*arrows*) with a hyperechoic center separate from upper pole of kidney. *Curved arrows* indicate interface between apparent mass and kidney. In both examples, findings were artifactual.

The indentations on the surface of the kidney are sometimes called *fetal lobation* (Fig. 8.10). Occasionally one of the interlobar grooves may extend through the cortex partly or completely to the hilum (Fig. 8.11). This has been called the *junctional parenchymal defect* (16). These should not be mistaken for renal cortical masses or focal areas of cortical scarring.

Splenic Hump

Splenic hump is a focal flattening of the lateral aspect of the upper pole with smooth convexity of the mid portion of the left kidney caused by extrinsic compression by a normal spleen (Fig. 8.12). This is of no clinical significance. If there is a questionable mass, contrast-enhanced CT or Tc^{99m} glucoheptonate or Tc^{99m}-DMSA radioisotope scan is recommended.

Column of Bertin

The column of Bertin represents the fusion of the medial portions of the cortex of contiguous lobes of metanephric mesoderm. Therefore this appears as cortical tissue interposed between contiguous medullary pyramids. They may be large enough to bulge into the central sinus (Fig. 8.13). These are common normal findings. The column of Bertin is isoechoic with the renal cortex, and the kidney has a smooth cortical outline superficial to it (17).

It is a common cause of renal "pseudotumor" and should not be mistaken for a renal tumor. When in doubt, CT with contrast enhancement or nuclear medicine scan with Tc^{99m}-DMSA or Tc^{99m} glucoheptonate will demonstrate functioning renal tissue at the site of apparent mass (column of Bertin).

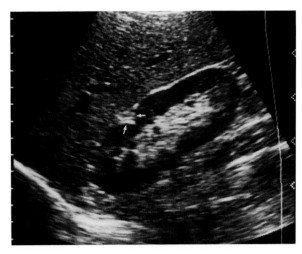

FIG. 8.11. Junctional parenchymal defect. This is a deep focal interlobular groove (*arrows*). Hyperechoic perinephric fat extends into groove. (Courtesy of Dr. Steve Valentine.)

Ectopic Kidney

One or both kidneys may fail to ascend, resulting in an ectopic position. Most are in the pelvis, but some are in the lower abdomen. They are usually malrotated. Rarely, the kidneys are fused, resulting in a round single renal mass called a discoid or pancake kidney (14). A normally ascended kidney may rarely be abnormally high in position as a result of herniation through a congenital diaphragmatic hernia (Fig. 8.14). Ultrasound may show a typical kidney in an ectopic location (Fig. 8.15), absence of the kidney in the normal location, and malrotation.

The differential diagnosis includes supranumerary kidney and the pseudokidney sign associated with a gastrointestinal tumor.

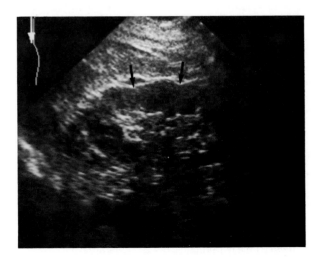

FIG. 8.10. Fetal lobation. Renal contour demonstrated indentations (*arrows*) at points of fusion of embryonic lobes.

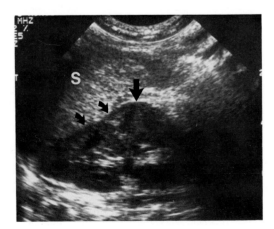

FIG. 8.12. Splenic hump. Spleen (*s*) causes indentation on lateral aspect of upper pole of kidney (*curved arrows*) with a smooth convexity (*arrow*) in mid portion of kidney.

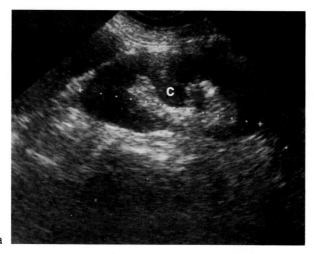
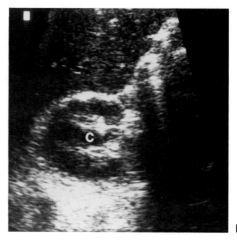

FIG. 8.13. Column of Bertin. Coronal scan of left kidney (**a**) and transverse scan of right kidney (**b**) show a column of parenchyma (*c*), which extends into central sinus complex.

Crossed Renal Ectopia/Crossed-fused Renal Ectopia

Occasionally, a kidney may cross the midline during ascent from the pelvis. It may fuse with the other kidney, producing a single large kidney with two ureters descending to either side of the midline (14). Ultrasound will show two kidneys on one side (crossed renal ectopia), which must be distinguished from supranumerary kidney. Ultrasound may show a single large kidney (crossed-fused renal ectopia), which must be distinguished from a hypertrophied kidney. Other investigations including intravenous urograms, retrograde pyelograms, CT, and radioisotope studies may be necessary to define the renal and ureteric anatomy.

Horseshoe Kidney

This relatively common anomaly results from fusion of the metanephros across the midline (14). There may be a fibrous band or parenchymal fusion of the lower poles. This results in an abnormal axis of the "kidney," with the upper poles more lateral than the fused lower poles. The kidney will be low in position, as complete ascent is impeded by the root of the inferior mesenteric artery. There is often an element of stasis with increased incidence of infection and nephrolithiasis. Ultrasound will show abnormal axis of the kidneys, low position, and tissue extending across the midline joining the lower poles (Figs. 8.16–8.18). A Tc^{99m}-DMSA or Tc^{99m} gluco-

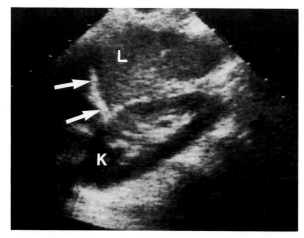

FIG. 8.14. Thoracic kidney. Kidney (*K*) is posterior to right lobe of liver and is herniated through a posterior diaphragmatic hernia. *Arrows* indicate diaphragm anterior to kidney.

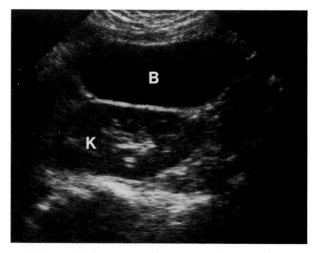

FIG. 8.15. Ectopic kidney. Normal-appearing kidney (*K*) is located in anatomic pelvis posterior to bladder (*B*).

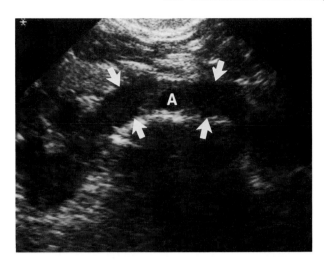

FIG. 8.16. Horseshoe kidney. Transverse scan of fused lower poles of kidneys (*arrows*) that cross anterior to aorta (*A*).

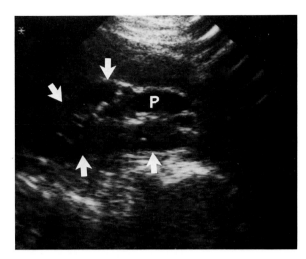

FIG. 8.18. Horseshoe kidney. Kidney (*arrows*) has an abnormal orientation with renal pelvis (*P*) directed anteriorly.

heptonate radioisotope scan is an excellent way to confirm the diagnosis in questionable cases.

Renal Sinus Lipomatosis

There is a variable amount of fat within the renal sinus. When there is subjectively an increase in the renal sinus fat, it is called renal sinus lipomatosis or fibrolipomatosis (Fig. 8.19). This is of no clinical significance and should not be mistaken for renal lipoma, angiomyolipoma, XGP, or replacement lipomatosis of the kidney.

Extrarenal Pelvis

The renal pelvis commonly bulges out of the renal sinus into the perinephric fat (Fig. 8.20). In this situation the pelvis is often large. There is no dilatation of the ureter, infundibula, or calyces. It should not be mistaken for hydronephrosis or UPJ obstruction.

Duplication of the Collecting System

This relatively common anomaly is due to division of the metanephric diverticulum. Incomplete division re-

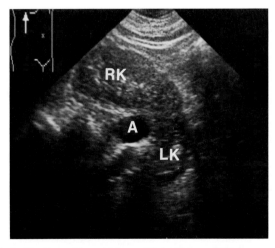

FIG. 8.17. Horseshoe kidney. Right kidney (*RK*) has an abnormal oblique orientation with lower pole crossing anterior to aorta (*A*) where it is fused with left kidney (*LK*).

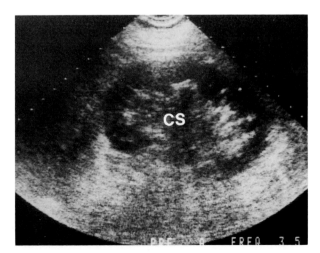

FIG. 8.19. Renal sinus lipomatosis. Excessive fat is present in central sinus (*cs*). This may be relatively hyperechoic or hypoechoic.

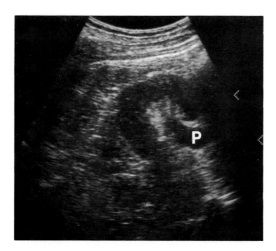

FIG. 8.20. Extrarenal pelvis. Renal pelvis (*P*) extends from central sinus into perinephric fat. There is no evidence of dilatation of calyces or infundibula.

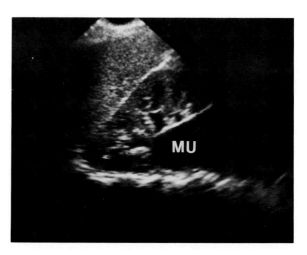

FIG. 8.22. Megaureter. Massively dilated ureter (*MU*) is seen with minimal calyceal dilatation. There was no evidence of obstruction on intravenous urogram or retrograde pyelogram.

sults in a bifid renal pelvis. Complete division results in supranumerary kidney with a bifid ureter or complete duplication of the ureters with a single kidney (14). Ultrasound will show a relatively long kidney with two separate central sinus echo complexes separated by cortical tissue (Fig. 8.21). Further contrast studies would be needed to better define the ureteric anatomy. It should be distinguished from the column of Bertin.

Congenital Megacalyces—Megaureter

This congenital condition consists of nonobstructive enlargement of calyces, which are usually decreased in number. It is often associated with megaureter (Fig. 8.22), in which there is dilatation above a short ady-

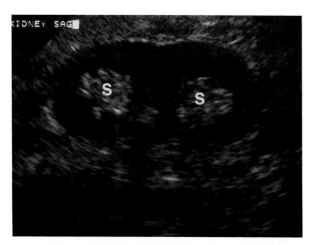

FIG. 8.21. Duplication of collecting system. Two separate central sinus complexes (*s*) are within the kidney. It is not possible to distinguish between a bifid renal pelvis, incomplete ureteric duplication, and complete ureteric duplication.

namic distal ureteric segment (18). The appearances on ultrasound can be identical to obstructive hydronephrosis or dilatation secondary to vesicoureteral reflux. The most common complications are calculus formation and infection secondary to stasis.

8.3 PATHOLOGY

Obstruction of the Collecting System

Hydronephrosis/Hydroureter

Hydronephrosis is dilatation of the pelvicalyceal collecting system caused by incomplete or complete obstruction. Hydroureter is dilatation of the ureter caused by incomplete or complete obstruction. There is usually dilatation proximal to the level of obstruction. Rarely, the collecting system may be obstructed but not significantly dilated.

Congenital conditions are the most common etiology in infants and children. Ureteropelvic junction obstruction is the most common cause of upper tract obstruction, and posterior urethral valves in males are the most common cause of lower tract obstruction. Chronic obstruction that occurs early in life (*in utero* or neonatal) may result in dysplastic changes in the renal parenchyma (Fig. 8.23). Recovery will depend on the extent and severity of the dysplasia. Ureteroceles, ureteric hypoplasia, and ureteric atresia are other causes. Calculi are the commonest cause in adults. Tumors of the kidney, ureter, and bladder are also relatively common in older adults. Miscellaneous causes include edema, stricture, neurogenic bladder, bladder outlet obstruction, and iatrogenesic.

Ultrasound sensitivity for hydronephrosis approaches

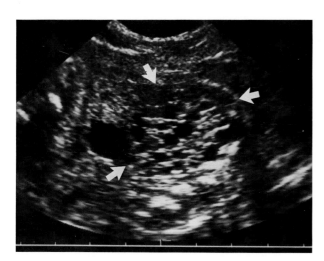

FIG. 8.23. Dysplastic changes in a fetal kidney (*arrows*) caused by bladder outlet obstruction from posterior urethral valves. This may have an identical ultrasound appearance to MCDK depending on severity and duration of obstruction.

100%. However, there are rare situations in which obstruction is present but the collecting system is not distended or the examination is suboptimal. Tables 8.3 and 8.4 list potential pitfalls (18): Ultrasound findings are progressive dilatation of the pelvicalyceal collecting system with separation of the central sinus echoes. Fluid distention of the infundibula is minimal criteria. Fluid within the renal pelvis without infundibular or calyceal dilatation should be regarded as normal. Hydronephrosis may be mild (Fig. 8.24), moderate (Fig. 8.25), or severe (Figs. 8.26 and 8.27).

There is obviously a subjective element in the categorization of severity.

Ultrasound findings of hydroureter are

1. fluid distention of the ureter (Figs. 8.28 and 8.29)
2. tortuosity of the distended ureter (Fig. 8.30)

Doppler ultrasound may be of some value in differentiation of obstructive from nonobstructive dilatation of the collecting system (11). Platt et al. (11) demonstrated an RI of greater than 0.70 in most obstructed kidneys and less than 0.70 in all nonobstructive kidneys.

Intravenous urography and retrograde pyelography may be necessary to better define anatomy and etiology. Quantitative renal function is best assessed by radionuclide techniques. A Whitaker test is the definitive diagnostic test for incomplete obstruction and is usually only necessary in questionable cases.

TABLE 8.4. *False–positive diagnosis of obstruction*

Normal variants
    Distensible collecting system
    Extrarenal renal pelvis
    Full bladder
    Congenital megacalyces or megaureter
    Calyceal diverticulum
Increased urine flow
    Overhydration
    Osmotic diuresis (diuretics, contrast media)
    Diabetes insipidus
    Diuresis in nonoliguric azotemia
Inflammatory disease
    Acute pyelonephritis (generalized dilatation)
    Chronic pyelonephritis (blunted calyces)
    Tuberculosis (cavity formation, papillary necrosis, hydrocalyces)
Renal cystic disease
    Simple cysts (multiple or single)
    Peripelvic cysts
    Adult polycystic kidney disease
    Medullary cystic disease
    Multicystic dyplastic kidney
Other
    Postobstructive or postsurgical dilatation
    Vesicoureteral reflux (past or present)
    Papillary necrosis (noninflammatory)

From Amis et al., ref. 18, with permission.

TABLE 8.3. *False-negative diagnosis of obstruction*

Staghorn calculus—obscured dilated collecting system
Acute obstruction—system not yet dilated
Spontaneous decompression of obstructed system—may see urinoma
Cysts with superimposed hydronephrosis
Hydronephrosis interpreted as cystic disease
Retroperitoneal fibrosis
Calicectasis interpreted as prominent pyramids
Fluid-depleted patient with partial obstruction
Intermittent obstruction
Technical factors—obesity, bowel gas, uncooperative patient

From Amis et al., ref. 18, with permission.

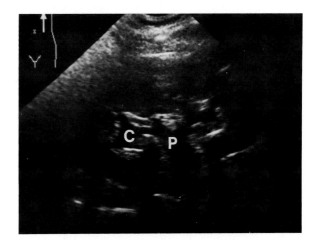

FIG. 8.24. Mild hydronephrosis. There is slight dilatation of the renal pelvis (*P*), calyces (*c*), and connecting infundibula. (Courtesy of Dr. Wayne Tonogai.)

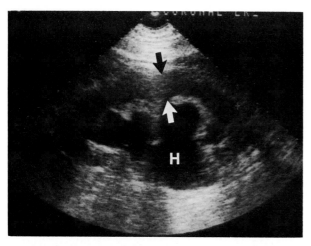

FIG. 8.25. Moderate hydronephrosis. Pelvicalyceal collecting system (*H*) is significantly dilated with preservation of renal parenchymal thickness (*arrows*).

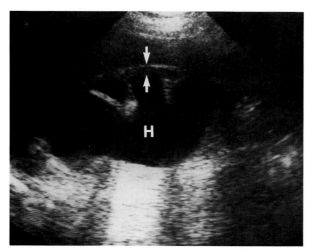

FIG. 8.26. Severe hydronephrosis. There is marked dilatation of pelvicalyceal collecting system (*H*) with thinning of parenchyma (*arrows*).

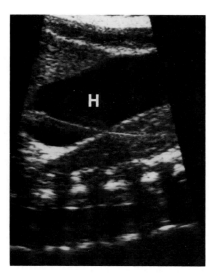

FIG. 8.27. Hydronephrotic sac. Severe long-standing hydronephrosis (*H*) may result in complete atrophy of parenchyma.

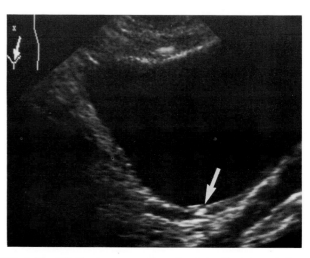

FIG. 8.28. Mild hydroureter. There is slight dilatation of distal ureter caused by a calculus (*arrow*) at uretero-vesicle junction. (Courtesy of Dr. Wayne Tonogai.)

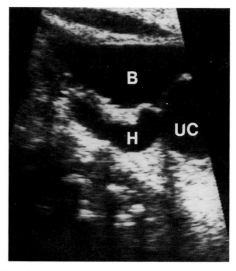

FIG. 8.29. Hydroureter. There is distal hydroureter (*H*) caused by a ureterocele (*UC*) that bulges into bladder (*B*).

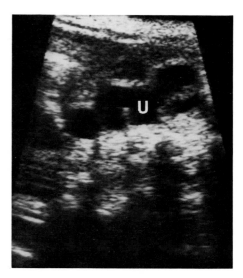

FIG. 8.30. Hydroureter. A tortuous, dilated ureter (*U*) is caused by posterior urethral valves.

Ureteropelvic Junction Obstruction

Ureteropelvic junction obstruction is the most common congenital obstruction of the urinary tract. Current theory suggests that this is due to an adynamic focal segment resulting in stasis and distention (18). Ultrasound findings are moderate to severe hydronephrosis without hydroureter (Fig. 8.31). Fluid challenge may precipitate symptoms of pain.

The differential diagnosis includes an extrarenal renal pelvis. Intravenous urography is the preferred technique for anatomic definition, and radionuclide studies are optimal for quantitative renal function.

Hydronephrosis of Pregnancy

Pregnancy is a physiological state that causes dilatation of the maternal renal collecting systems of the kidneys. Etiology is felt to be caused by hormonal factors and mechanical extrinsic compression. Hydronephrosis increases in degree of severity and incidence throughout gestation. The overall incidence may be as high as 90% on the right and 67% on the left. The degree of dilatation tends to be greater on the right than the left. Associated hydroureter extends to the pelvic brim (19).

Flank pain in the pregnant woman is a relatively common diagnostic dilemma. A coexisting etiology (calculus) should be suspected if there is hydroureter involving the distal third of the ureter below the pelvic brim, left-sided hydronephrosis more severe than the right (especially if it extends below the pelvic brim), and demonstration of a calculus within the pelvicalyceal collecting system or ureter.

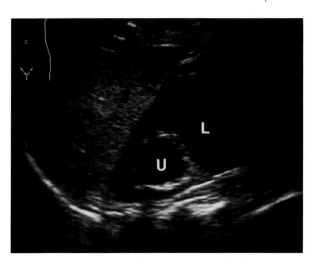

FIG. 8.32. Duplication anomaly with obstruction. There was complete atresia of ureter to lower pole moiety (*L*), causing massive lower pole hydronephrosis. Upper pole moiety (*U*) was hydronephrotic caused by extrinsic compression by lower pole hydronephrotic sac.

Hydronephrosis Associated with Duplication of the Collecting System

Complete duplication of the collecting system has several potential associated disorders. The upper pole moiety is often associated with a ureterocele, which may be nonobstructive or obstructive. The obstructive variant will eventually cause hydronephrosis, hydroureter, and cortical atrophy (Figs. 8.32 and 8.33). The lower pole moiety often refluxes and may have an ectopic insertion outside of the bladder. Reflux may cause cortical atrophy of the mid and lower pole of the kidney. Massive

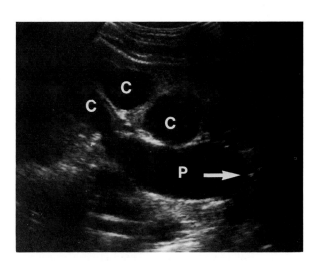

FIG. 8.31. UPJ obstruction. There is moderately severe hydronephrosis with dilatation of calyces (*c*) and pelvis (*P*), which abruptly narrows at level of UPJ (*arrow*).

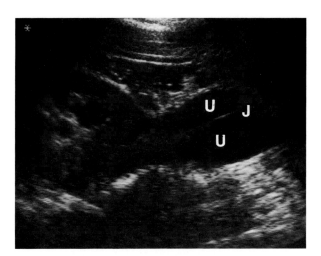

FIG. 8.33. Incomplete ureteric duplication with hydronephrosis caused by a distal ureteric calculus. Dilated proximal ureters (*U*) join in their proximal one third. Only one ureter was seen distal to junction (*J*).

reflux may simulate obstruction with dilatation of the collecting system and dilatation–tortuosity of the ureter.

Intravenous urography is usually recommended for better anatomic detail of the collecting system. Voiding cystourethrogram or radionuclide study may be necessary to assess reflux.

Polar or Segmental Dilatation

Polar dilatation may occur with complete duplication of the collecting system with obstruction of one moiety (Fig. 8.32).

Segmental dilatation may occur as a result of narrowing of an infundibulum because of stricture (e.g., TB, trauma), tumor (transitional cell carcinoma), calculus, or extrinsic compression from a parenchymal mass (e.g., tumor, hematoma, or inflammation).

Pyelocalyceal diverticula communicate with the pelvicalyceal collecting system (20) via a narrow channel. These are usually small and not appreciated on ultrasound. Occasionally, they may be quite large and simulate a renal cyst (Fig. 8.34). The most common complications are stone formation and infection.

Reflux Nephropathy

Reflux is usually due to an ectopic ureteric orifice with an inadequate bladder mural tunnel. Renal parenchyma becomes affected if there is superimposed infection (19).

Ultrasound findings are

1. dilatation of the collecting system and ureter. This may be transient and is nonobstructive (Fig. 8.35).
2. focal cortical scarring (Fig. 8.36). This is due to combination of reflux and infection. Some regard this as the

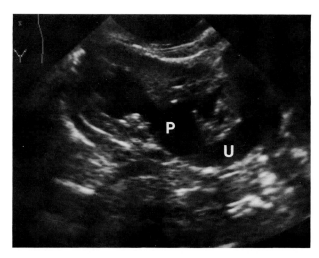

FIG. 8.35. Reflux. This newborn infant had dilatation of the pelvicalyceal collecting system (*P*) and ureter (*U*). Subsequent voiding cystogram demonstrated reflux and no evidence of obstruction.

mechanism of development of chronic atrophic pyelonephritis. The atrophy is usually more prominent in the upper pole but may affect the remainder of the parenchyma in more severe disease. The lower pole and interpolar region may be more severely involved when reflux complicates a complete duplication of the collecting system.

3. diffuse cortical scarring. This may be seen with severe long-standing reflux nephropathy.

In children with infection, voiding cystourethrogram is usually recommended to assess possible reflux. The results will determine whether other tests (e.g., intravenous urogram, radionuclide studies, ultrasound) are necessary (21).

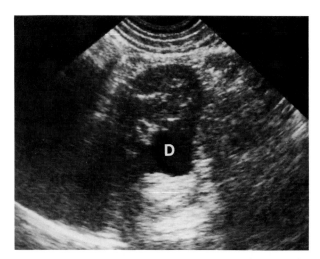

FIG. 8.34. Pyelocalyceal diverticula. Large diverticulum (*D*) was initially thought to be a renal cyst but was subsequently shown to be a large diverticulum arising from renal pelvis on intravenous urogram.

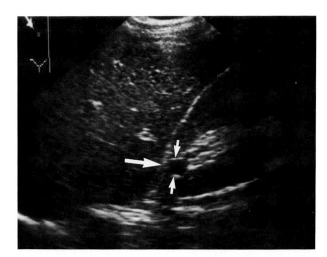

FIG. 8.36. Reflux nephropathy. There is small focal cystic area in upper pole of kidney. It is a dilated calyx (*small arrows*). There is focal cortical thinning (*large arrow*) superficial to dilated calyx. Patient had long-standing reflux.

Renal Papillary Necrosis

Papillary necrosis is most common in renal allografts. It is also seen with analgesic nephropathy, diabetes mellitus, obstructive uropathy, sickle cell disease, pyelonephritis, acute tubular necrosis, renal vein thrombosis, dehydration, and chronic alcoholism (22).

The ultrasound features may simulate hydronephrosis. The sloughed papilla may cause obstruction. In most cases, calycectasis without obstruction is the characteristic feature (Fig. 8.37).

Renal Calculus Disease

Renal calculi are common. Approximately 80% are radio-opaque. Plain radiographs and intravenous urography are the traditional investigations for renal colic. Ultrasound has the advantage of demonstrating non-opaque calculi and hydronephrosis in comparison with the plain radiographs. Ultrasound has the potential of early diagnosis as compared with intravenous urography when there is delayed excretion or nonexcretion.

Ultrasound detected renal calculi in 91% of patients studied by Middleton et al. (23). In another study, renal calculi were diagnosed in 90% of cases by direct visualization of the calculus or unilateral hydronephrosis (24). The major limiting factor is the difficulty in visualizing the middle third of the ureter. Another study regarded ultrasound as inferior to emergency excretory urography in the diagnosis of acute flank pain when a calculus was suspected. In this clinical setting, ultrasound was not as sensitive with mild hydronephrosis or detection of renal or ureteral calculus, or in diagnosing forniceal rupture (25).

Ultrasound features of a calculus are a hyperechoic focus with distal shadowing (Figs. 8.38 and 8.39). Gas

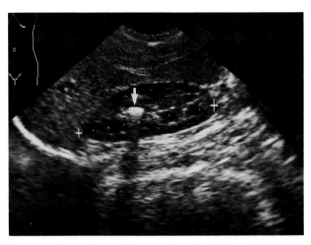

FIG. 8.38. Nephrolithiasis. Calculus (*arrow*) is a well-defined hyperechoic focus with posterior acoustic shadowing.

may cause a similar appearance but may have a "dirty" shadow that is not as sharply defined as would occur with a calculus. There may be associated mucosal edema if the stone is impacted or if there is secondary inflammation or infection. Hydronephrosis and hydroureter may also be present (Fig. 8.28). Tiny calculi may not cause distal shadowing if they are smaller than the focal zone of the transducer. Ultrasound may have false-negative results with small calculi and suboptimal studies (e.g., obesity, uncooperative patient). Ultrasound may have false-positive results with renal parenchymal calcification, vascular calcification, and ureteric catheters. In equivocal cases renal tomography or CT may be necessary to confirm or exclude the diagnosis.

Staghorn calculi may simulate multiple calculi within the collecting system (Fig. 8.40). These can be shown to be connected on real-time scanning. Staghorn calculi often cause hydronephrosis, which is not appreciated be-

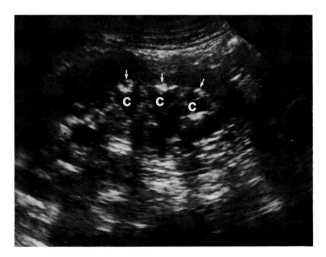

FIG. 8.37. Papillary necrosis. There was mild hydronephrosis. Hyperechoic areas (*arrows*) may be due to mild calcification in papillae peripheral to dilated calyces (*c*).

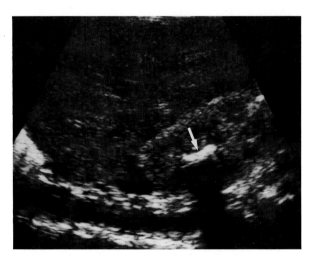

FIG. 8.39. Nephrolithiasis in newborn infant. Large calculus (*arrow*) is due to furosamide therapy.

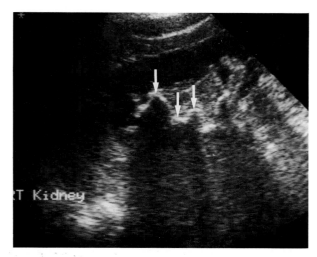

FIG. 8.40. Staghorn calculus. Central focal areas of calcification (*arrows*) can be connected on real-time scanning. There is no obvious hydronephrosis.

cause of the acoustic attenuation by the large stone mass. Careful scanning may show some dilatation of peripheral calyces distal to the calculus. Nevertheless, most staghorn calculi cause some degree of incomplete obstruction (Fig. 8.41). There is also a high incidence of associated infection.

Renal Cystic Disease

Simple Cortical Cyst

Simple uncomplicated cortical cysts are the most common mass in the adult kidney. They are benign, fluid-filled, nonneoplastic cystic masses of unknown eti-

ology. They are usually asymptomatic and require no treatment (26,27).

The ultrasound criteria of a simple uncomplicated cyst are

1. round or oval shape
2. posterior acoustic enhancement
3. absence of internal echoes
4. clear demarcation of the posterior wall

These criteria proved to be 98% accurate for a simple cyst (Figs. 8.42 and 8.43). They may be single or multiple. Each must be individually assessed using the above criteria (26,27).

Simple uncomplicated cortical cysts are uncommon in infants and children (28). In this group, a cortical cyst must be carefully assessed to exclude an obstructed duplication segment or a cystic Wilm's tumor.

Complicated Cortical Cysts

Computed tomography (without and with contrast enhancement) is the next recommended investigation for complicated renal cysts. If there is still concern, percutaneous aspiration biopsy can be performed. However, this should not be a substitute for experience and judgment.

Septations

Thin (<1 mm) delicate septations (Fig. 8.44) are usually of no significance (26). Thick septations (Fig. 8.45) require further evaluation via CT with contrast enhancement. If there is an associated mass, a malignancy must be suspected.

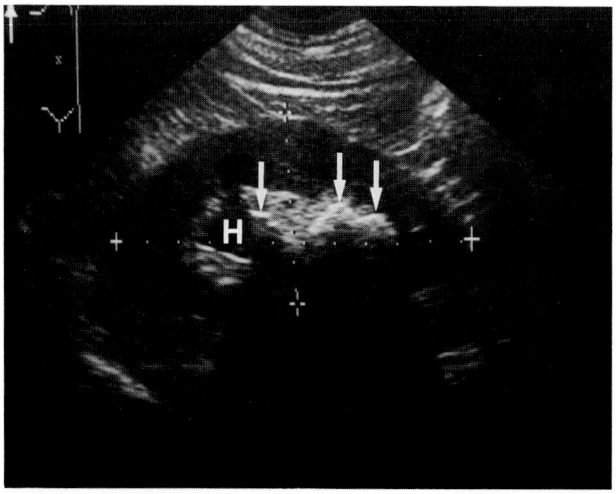

FIG. 8.41. Staghorn calculus with hydronephrosis. Calculus (*arrows*) causes hydronephrosis (*H*) of upper pole collecting system. An element of incomplete obstruction is common.

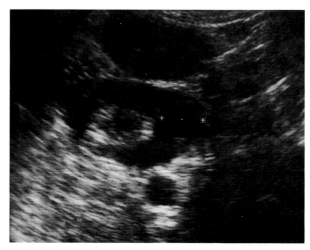

FIG. 8.42. Renal cyst. A small renal cyst may show only slight posterior acoustic enhancement but should demonstrate other criteria.

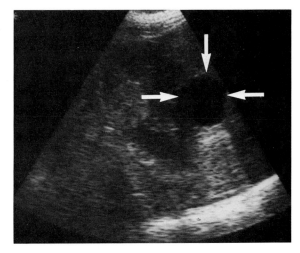

FIG. 8.43. Renal cyst. Acoustic enhancement is obvious posterior to cyst (*arrows*).

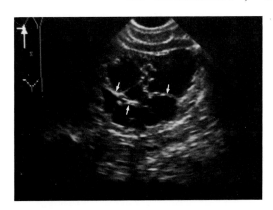

FIG. 8.45. Renal cyst with thick septations. Thick irregular septations (*arrows*) are present in this case of adult polycystic kidney disease.

Abnormal Shape

Septated cysts may be lobulated in contour (Fig. 8.46). This is usually of no significance if the septations are thin and it meets all other criteria of a simple cyst (26).

Calcification

Focal calcification in the wall of a cyst is usually of no significance (Fig. 8.47). It indicates dystrophic calcification from previous infection or hemorrhage (26). If associated with wall thickening or a solid mass, a malignancy must be suspected.

Internal Echoes

Usually internal echoes within a cyst are artifactual, caused by technical factors (e.g., volume averaging,

time-gain curve setting, near or far zone of transducer) (26).

True internal echoes persist after the technical factors have been eliminated. The echoes may be diffuse throughout the cyst, with recent hemorrhage or infection (Figs. 8.48–8.50). There may be layering of echoes in a fluid–debris level (e.g., blood, cellular debris, crystals) (Fig. 8.51). Calcium carbonate crystals in solution will result in a hyperechoic debris–fluid level, with acoustic shadowing (Fig. 8.52) in the far field. This is termed *milk of calcium.*

Focal Thick Wall or Nodule

Focal thick wall or nodule may be due to infection, hemorrhage (retracting clot), or tumor (26) and requires further investigation (Fig. 8.53).

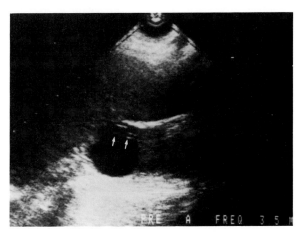

FIG. 8.44. Renal cyst with thin septations (*arrows*).

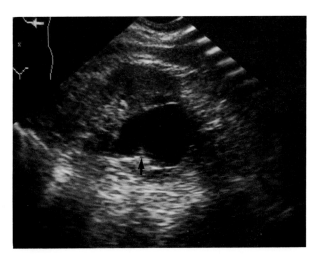

FIG. 8.46. Renal cyst with lobulated contour. Focal indentation (*arrow*) was at the site of a septation (not appreciated on this axis).

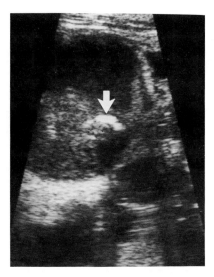

FIG. 8.47. Renal cyst with focal calcification. Focal calcification (*arrow*) is present within a complicated hemorrhagic cyst in a patient with adult polycystic kidney disease.

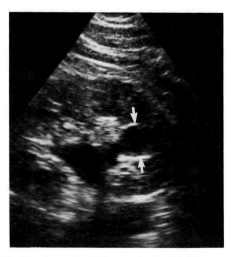

FIG. 8.50. Renal cyst with internal echoes. There were persistent internal echoes around margins of cyst (*arrows*). This simulated a TCC on intravenous urogram and retrograde pyelogram. Pathology demonstrated a hemorrhagic cyst.

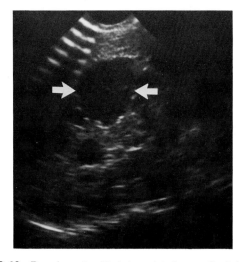

FIG. 8.48. Renal cyst with internal echoes. Cyst (*arrows*) contains diffuse internal echoes caused by a hemorrhagic cyst.

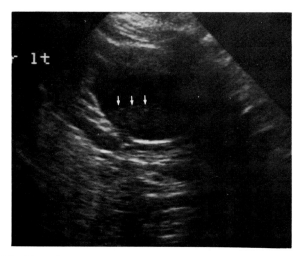

FIG. 8.51. Renal cyst with layering of echoes. Fluid–debris level (*arrows*) is seen within cyst.

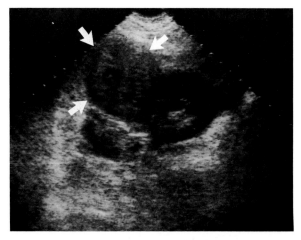

FIG. 8.49. Hemorrhagic renal cyst contains diffuse clot simulating a solid tumor. Earlier scans had shown a simple cyst. Follow-up scans showed resorption of clot.

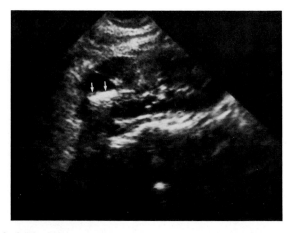

FIG. 8.52. Renal cyst with milk of calcium. Hyperechoic crystals layer out in solution in dependent portion of cyst (*arrows*). There is posterior acoustic shadowing.

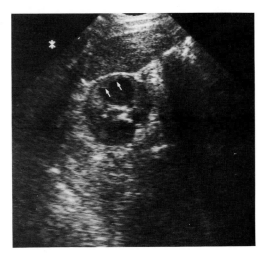

FIG. 8.53. Focal thickening of wall (*arrows*) caused by clot adherent to wall of a cyst.

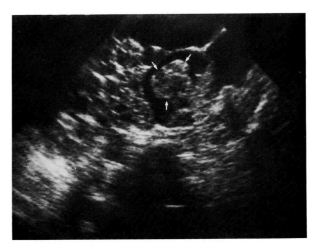

FIG. 8.55. Retracting clot (*arrows*) within a cyst in adult poly-cystic kidney disease.

Solid Component

If the mass is partly solid and partly cystic (Figs. 8.54–8.56), a tumor or retracting clot is most likely (26). Further investigation is mandatory.

Extraparenchymal Cysts

Extraparenchymal cysts are usually not of clinical significance. They may be misinterpreted as renal masses on excretory urography or as hydronephrosis on ultrasound. If they become secondarily infected or complicated by hemorrhage, they may become symptomatic. The uncomplicated cyst has the feature of a simple cyst.

Parapelvic Cysts

Parapelvic cysts are parenchymal cysts that bulge into the central sinus of the kidney (Fig. 8.57). They may cause extrinsic compression on the collecting system or

mass effect on excretory urography. If multiple, they may stimulate hydronephrosis on ultrasound (Fig. 8.58). This error can be avoided by showing that the cystic areas do not communicate with the renal pelvis on real-time ultrasound (29).

Peripelvic Cysts

Peripelvic cysts are lymphatic cysts in the central sinus. These have an identical appearance to parapelvic cysts and cannot be distinguished from parapelvic cysts (29).

Acquired Cystic Disease of the Kidneys

Up to 80% of patients on chronic hemodialysis will develop multiple small cysts within the native kidneys

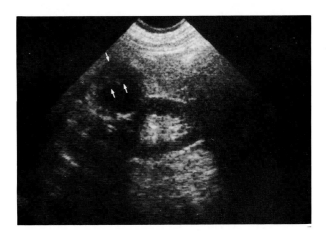

FIG. 8.54. Focal wall thickening (*arrows*) caused by a renal carcinoma involving wall of a cyst.

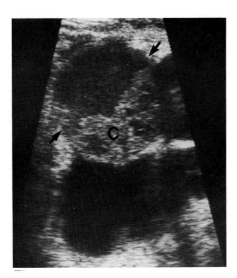

FIG. 8.56. Retracting clot (*C*) within a cyst (*arrows*) that contains internal echoes in fluid caused by blood.

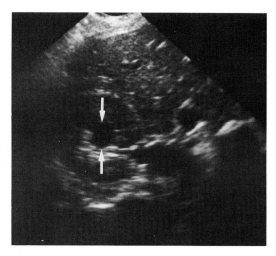

FIG. 8.57. Single parapelvic cyst (*arrows*) extrinsically compresses central sinus complex.

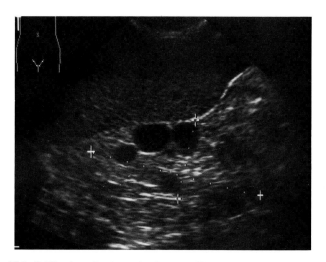

FIG. 8.59. Acquired cystic disease. There are multiple cysts within a kidney, which has increased cortical echogenicity in a patient with chronic renal failure.

(30). Between 8% and 20% of these patients develop renal neoplasms (31,32). The natural history is not well understood. Cysts and tumors usually occur after several years of dialysis. Computed tomography is regarded as more sensitive in detecting small cysts and tumors in comparison with ultrasound (33).

Ultrasound will often show the typical features of cysts (Fig. 8.59). The kidney may be small. The renal cortex is often of increased echogenicity. The kidney may be difficult to identify if the renal cortical echogenicity is similar to the echogenicity of the perinephric fat and central sinus. Ultrasound is valuable as a complementary technique to CT in differentiating between a hemorrhage cyst and a solid mass. Long-term yearly follow-up by CT or ultrasound is recommended.

Unilateral Renal Cystic Disease

This uncommon entity is characterized by multiple cysts involving a portion of one kidney. It is nonfamilial and does not progress, and there is no association with malignancy (34). This has also been described as localized cystic disease of the kidney and unilateral adult polycystic disease of the kidney (35). The latter term is a misnomer, as polycystic kidney disease is hereditary and bilateral. The differential diagnosis includes multilocular cystic renal cell carcinoma, multilocular cystic nephroma, cystic nephroblastoma, mesoblastic nephroma, and segmental MCDK. Each of these usually has thick septations, solid component, or irregular thick wall.

Multicystic Dysplastic Kidney

Multicystic dysplastic kidney is the second most common abdominal mass in neonates. It is due to pyeloinfundibular atresia. Manifestations will depend on the stage at which atresia occurs. Renal artery hypoplasia or agenesis and incomplete or complete ureteric atresia will be present. Contralateral renal abnormalities include UPJ obstruction.

Ultrasound manifestations include (Figs. 8.60 and 8.61) (36)

1. presence of interfaces between cysts
2. nonmedial location of the largest cyst
3. absence of an identifiable renal sinus
4. multiplicity of oval or round cysts that do not communicate
5. absence of parenchymal tissue
6. a single cyst rarely the only manifestation

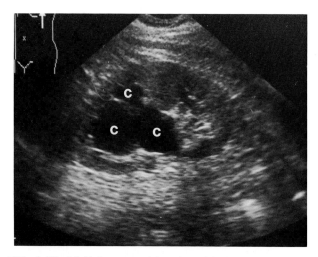

FIG. 8.58. Multiple parapelvic cysts (*c*) simulate hydronephrosis. Intravenous pyelogram showed no evidence of hydronephrosis.

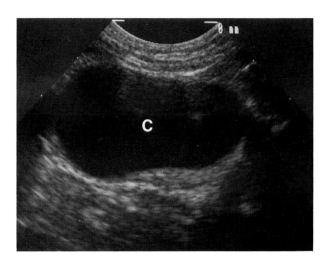

FIG. 8.60. MCDK with a large single cyst (*c*).

The major contribution of ultrasound is to distinguish MCDK from hydronephrosis. If hydronephrosis is still a diagnostic possibility after ultrasound, radionuclide renal scan is recommended. Occasionally, MCDK may be segmental and involve only a part of one kidney. A multiloculated cystic mass in one pole of duplicated collecting system or crossed-fused ectopic kidney should suggest this diagnosis (37). The pathology is the same as MCDK and the differential diagnosis includes multilocular cystic nephroma, cystic nephroblastoma, unilateral renal cystic disease, and cystic renal cell carcinoma. It usually presents as a mass in the newborn period. Ultrasound follow-up is recommended every 6 months for the first 3 years of life. Passive management is recommended unless the MCDK enlarges or becomes complicated by infection or the patient develops hypertension. Multicystic dysplastic kidney disappeared in 9% of patients in one study (38).

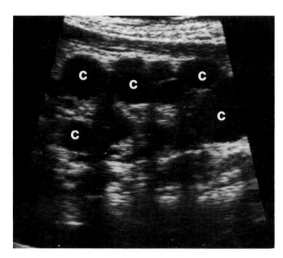

FIG. 8.61. MCDK. There are multiple cysts (*c*) in renal fossa.

Medullary Cystic Disease

Medullary cystic disease is a familial disorder in which autosomal recessive, autosomal dominant, and sporadic cases have been described. It is an uncommon cause of renal failure manifested by salt wasting and anemia. The ultrasound features are multiple small cysts in the central portion of the kidney or at the corticomedullary junction (39). The only significant differential diagnosis is multiple parapelvic cysts.

Infantile Polycystic Kidney

This autosomal recessive disease causes bilateral symmetrical enlarged kidneys. These contain innumerable cystic spaces caused by dilated tubules. Most of the "cysts" are microscopic, although there are rarely macroscopic cysts present. These may present with oligohydramnios *in utero*. These patients often have pulmonary hypoplasia causing respiratory distress, which complicates the early onset of uremia. They usually die in the first few days of life. Some less severely affected individuals may present with bilateral enlargement of the kidneys or abdominal masses with a variable degree of renal failure. Occasionally, because of variable penetrance of the gene, they may present in childhood with hepatosplenomegaly, portal hypertension, and associated complications caused by periportal fibrosis. The underlying renal abnormality is often an incidental finding. However, the renal failure is progressive and will result in uremia eventually (40).

The ultrasound features are (Fig. 8.62) (40)

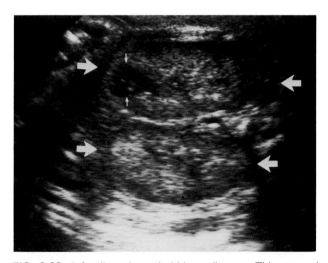

FIG. 8.62. Infantile polycystic kidney disease. This coronal scan shows both kidneys (*large arrows*) to be enlarged and hyperechoic and to have a rim of decreased echogenicity. There is a septated macroscopic cyst (*small arrows*) in one of the kidneys.

1. bilateral symmetrical enlarged kidneys
2. a cortical rim of decreased echogenicity caused by peripherally compressed cortical remnant
3. increased parenchymal echogenicity caused by the multiple tiny cystic spaces
4. macroscopic renal cysts seen rarely
5. findings of hepatosplenomegaly and portal hypertension
6. Liver cysts seen rarely on ultrasound but present in almost all cases on pathology

Adult Polycystic Kidney Disease

This autosomal dominant condition has a high penetrance and affects 0.05% to 0.1% of the population. It may present in infancy or childhood, but it typically presents in the third or fourth decade.

The kidneys contain numerous cysts involving all portions of the nephron and therefore involve the cortex and the medulla. The cysts vary in size from microscopic to macroscopic. They compress functioning nephrons, resulting in progressive deterioration in renal function, eventually resulting in renal failure. Other patients present with hypertension. Bleeding into the cysts may cause pain or hematuria.

Approximately one third of patients have liver cysts, which are usually asymptomatic. Cysts occur less frequently in the spleen, pancreas, and lungs. Between 15% 20% of patients have berry aneurysms of the circle of Willis, resulting in an increased incidence of subarachnoid hemorrhage (41).

In early stages, the kidneys may be enlarged and contain more cysts than expected for the patient's age (Fig. 8.63). In late stages, the kidneys are large and contain numerous cysts with little or any interviewing normal parenchyma (Fig. 8.64). The cysts are frequently complicated by hemorrhage and may contain debris or focal calcification in the wall (Figs. 8.46, 8.54, and 8.55).

Ultrasound is the preferential modality to establish the diagnosis (41). However, ultrasound may miss underlying hydronephrosis. Computed tomography is preferable for the diagnosis of complications such as hemorrhage or infection. Infected cysts can be diagnosed by aspiration for culture and sensitivity. Indium-111-labeled leukocyte scan may help to localize the area of interest, which can then be scanned by ultrasound or CT for diagnostic aspiration.

Neoplasms

Benign Neoplasms

Angiomyolipoma

This common tumor consists of vessels, smooth muscle, and fat. They are important because they may cause pain and hematuria because of hemorrhage and may be confused with other hyperechoic lesions including renal cell carcinoma, liposarcoma, and lipoma (42). They are usually single and unilateral. Approximately 80% of patients with tuberous sclerosis have angiomyolipoma that are usually multiple and bilateral. In most instances, they are incidental findings in asymptomatic patients. Between 85% and 90% of patients are female (43).

Ultrasound is the preferred and most sensitive imaging modality, especially for lesions smaller than 2 cm. Most cases show a well-defined hyperechoic solid mass within the renal cortex (Fig.8.65) (42–43). A few cases show a mixed pattern with hypoechoic areas in a predominantly hyperechoic mass. This is probably due to hemor-

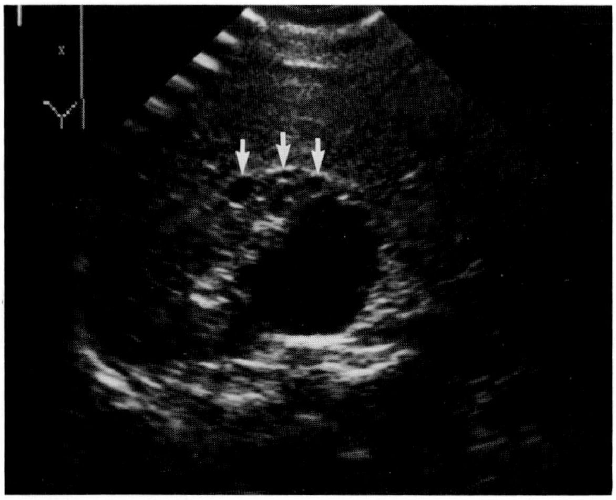

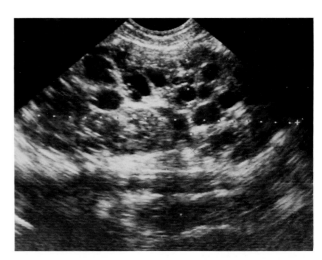

FIG. 8.63. Early adult polycystic kidney disease. *Arrows* indicate a few small cysts as well as a larger cyst. Positive family history of polycystic kidney disease. Significant residual parenchyma is present.

FIG. 8.64. Advanced adult polycystic kidney disease. Kidney is enlarged and contains multiple cysts. As disease process progresses, there is loss of corticomedullary junction and less residual parenchyma.

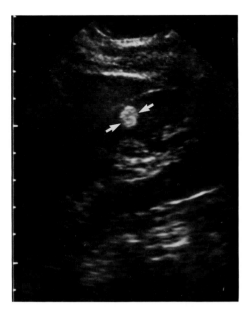

FIG. 8.65. Angiomyolipoma (*arrows*) is seen as a well-defined focal hyperechoic solid mass within parenchyma.

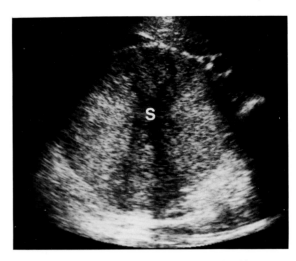

FIG. 8.66. Oncocytoma. Atypical findings in this case are central scar (*S*) with radiating bands extending to periphery. (Courtesy of Dr. Michel Lafortune.)

rhage. It may also present with a subcapsular or perinephric hematoma (43,44). The mass is usually stable over time unless there is an episode of bleeding. However, the ultrasound appearances are not specific.

Computed tomography is a useful complementary technique. If CT demonstrates attenuation numbers in the range of adipose tissue (0–100 Hounsfield units), renal cell carcinoma can be excluded. The only renal masses containing adipose tissue are angiomyolipoma, lipoma, and liposarcoma. The latter two entities are very rare. Computed tomography may fail to identify adipose tissue in small lesions because of partial volume effect. This can be minimized by thin section technique. Computed tomography may show increased attenuation if there has been recent bleeding.

Fine needle aspiration biopsy, angiography, or MRI can occasionally be useful in cases in which the diagnosis is not clear.

Oncocytoma

This rare, benign, solid tumor is usually asymptomatic. The usual ultrasound findings are those of a solid mass. A spoke–wheel pattern of vascularity with a central scar on angiography is suggestive but not diagnostic. Similar features (Fig. 8.66) were described in a single case by ultrasound (45).

Mesoblastic Nephroma

Mesoblastic nephroma has also been called fetal renal hamartoma. It has been diagnosed *in utero*. This uncom-

mon tumor arises from the metanephric blastema and is the most common renal neoplasm in infants. They usually present as a large abdominal mass. Ultrasound features are those of a solid mass. Hemorrhage, necrosis, or cystic degeneration may result in a multiloculated cystic mass (46).

Nephroblastomatosis

This rare congenital condition represents persistent metanephric blastema in the kidney. The most common form is multifocal superficial lesions. Diffuse nephroblastomatosis is less common and may show diffuse renal enlargement or diffuse superficial involvement. It is regarded as a precursor of nephroblastoma (Wilm's tumor) (47).

Ultrasound may show renal enlargement or solid renal mass or masses. In general, the lesions are isoechoic with the normal parenchyma and are difficult or impossible to identify with ultrasound. Therefore, contrast-enhanced CT is the preferred imaging modality (48).

Multilocular Cystic Nephroma

These lesions have many synonyms including benign multilocular cystic nephroma, cystic adenoma, benign cystic differentiated nephroblastoma, cystic partially differentiated nephroblastoma, polycystic nephroblastoma, differentiated nephroblastoma, cystic nephroblastoma, well-differentiated polycystic Wilm's tumor, lymphangioma, and partially polycystic kidney (49). It represents an encapsulated tumor consisting of multiple, noncommunicating cysts separated by multiple septa. It occurs most commonly in males in childhood and females in adulthood. It usually presents as an asymptomatic mass or occasionally with hematuria (49,50). Approximately 3% of patients have one or more microscopic foci of nephroblastoma (Wilm's tumor), and approximately 2% of patients have sarcomatous stroma in multilocular cystic nephroma (49). These cannot be reliably diagnosed by ultrasound or CT. However, change in size or appearance would warrant further investigation. Routine yearly follow-up is recommended.

The ultrasound features are of a well-circumscribed multicystic septated mass (Fig. 8.67). The differential diagnosis includes cystic renal cell carcinoma and cystic nephroblastoma. These entities are usually considered if there is a solid component or the cystic spaces have irregular internal margins (49,50).

Other Benign Tumors

Renal lipoma is rare and consists of fat. It would have features similar to angiomyolipoma on ultrasound, CT, and MRI.

Fibroma and tumor of juxtaglomerular cells (reninoma) are rare and will present as solid masses indistinguishable from the other solid lesions.

Malignant Neoplasms

Renal Cell Carcinoma/Adenoma

These entities are identical pathologically. They are distinguished by size, with 3 cm as the arbitrary criteria. This distinction has recently been questioned (51), and all are currently regarded as malignant. Renal cell carcinoma is relatively common with peak incidence in the fifth and sixth decades and slight male preponderance (52). Patients with *von Hippel-Lindau disease* are at in-

creased risk of renal cell carcinoma. It is a rare familial disease transmitted as an autosomal dominant trait with variable penetrance. Patients may have cerebellar hemangioblastomas, retinal angiomas, renal cysts and renal cell carcinomas, pancreatic cysts and tumors, and pheochromocytomas. Yearly screening by CT or ultrasound is recommended in von Hippel-Lindau disease (52).

Approximately 30% of patients are asymptomatic. Patients may have weight loss, fever, anemia, polycythemia, hematuria, mass, flank pain, hypertension, varicocele, high-output cardiac failure, and hypercalcemia. Many are incidental findings. Approximately 25% of patients have metastasis at the time of diagnosis. The most common metastatic sites in decreasing order of frequency are lungs, bones, lymph nodes, liver, adrenals, and opposite kidney. The latter cannot be distinguished from a synchronous tumor (41). The Robson classification is usually used for clinical staging:

Stage I: Tumor is confined within the renal capsule.
Stage II: Tumor involves perinephric fat but is confined within the pararenal fascia.
Stage III: Tumor invades renal vein, inferior vena cava, or regional lymph nodes.
Stage IV: Tumor invades pararenal fascia, contiguous visceral structures, or distant metastasis.

Ultrasound is an excellent screening modality provided that meticulous technique and strict criteria for distinguishing cysts and solid masses are used. Ultrasound permits a noninvasive method to assess renal vein and inferior vena cava involvement by PW and color Doppler techniques (53). Computed tomography has a higher sensitivity for small tumors of less than 3 cm and is preferred for preoperative staging.

Ultrasound findings include (Figs. 8.68–8.75) (44, 53–56)

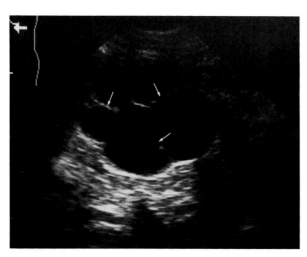

FIG. 8.67. Multilocular cystic nephroma. This multilocular cystic mass contains multiple septa (*arrows*) and is relatively sharply demarcated from contiguous parenchyma.

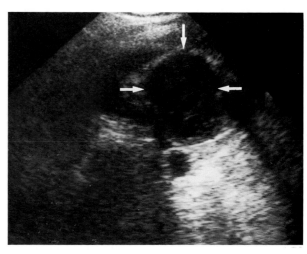

FIG. 8.68. Renal carcinoma. There is a mass (*arrows*) of variable echogenicity caused by tissue necrosis.

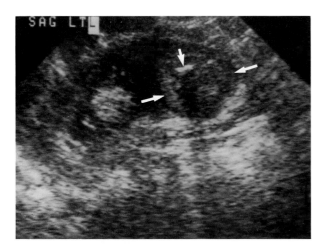

FIG. 8.69. Renal carcinoma with focal calcification. There is a focal area of calcification (*short arrow*) within a solid mass (*long arrows*).

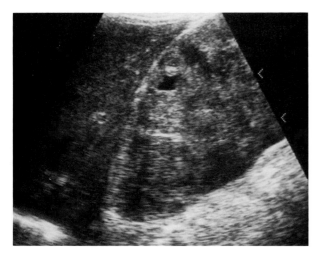

FIG. 8.70. Diffuse renal carcinoma. There is extensive tumor throughout the kidney, causing loss of all normal renal anatomic landmarks.

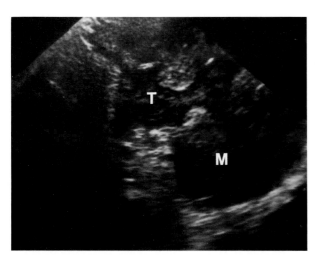

FIG. 8.71. Renal carcinoma invading collecting system. There is a large focal mass (*M*) in lower pole of kidney with tumor (*T*) invasion of pelvicalyceal collecting system.

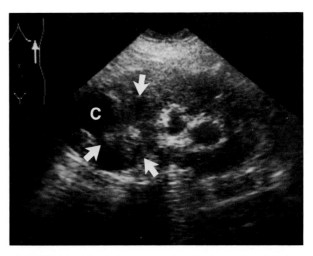

FIG. 8.72. Renal carcinoma causing hydronephrosis. There is a poorly marginated infiltrating mass (*arrows*) that has replaced central sinus complex in the mid to upper polar region causing dilatation and obstruction of upper pole calyx (*c*). Lower pole calyces were slightly dilated but not obstructed on intravenous pyelogram, antegrade pyelogram, and radionuclide study.

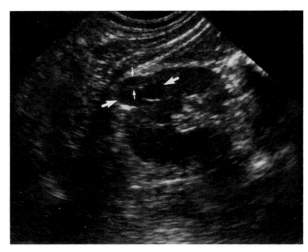

FIG. 8.73. Renal cystic carcinoma. *Arrows* delineate a mass that is predominantly cystic but that has a focal solid component (*small arrows*) that represented tumor.

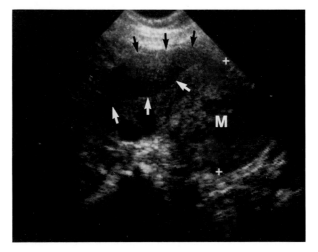

FIG. 8.74. Renal carcinoma with perinephric hematoma. There is a mass (*M*) in lower pole of kidney associated with a perinephric or subcapsular fluid collection (*arrows*) caused by spontaneous hemorrhage.

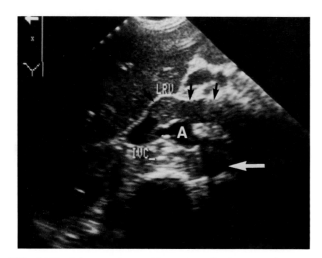

FIG. 8.75. Adenopathy and invasion of left renal vein. Left renal vein (*black arrows*) is enlarged and filled with tumor thrombus. Other views showed extension into inferior vena cava. There is also left paraaortic adenopathy (*white arrow*) contiguous to aorta (*A*).

1. Mass effect distorts the central sinus complex or causes convexity of the renal contour. Occasionally, the tumor will invade the renal pelvis or cause hydronephrosis.
2. Mass is hypoechoic, isoechoic, or hyperechoic relative to the contiguous normal parenchyma.
3. Mass may be sharply or irregularly marginated with the contiguous normal parenchyma.
4. Up to 40% of tumors demonstrate cystic components caused by hemorrhage, necrosis, or tumor vascularity. These may show posterior acoustic enhancement.
5. Calcification within the mass is occasionally demonstrated.
6. Invasion of renal vein and inferior vena cava occurs in 5% to 24% of cases (variously reported) (51).
7. Doppler of the mass may demonstrate a peak-systolic Doppler shift frequency of 2.5 kHz or greater because of tumor vascularity (70% sensitivity). False positive cases involved focal inflammatory masses (56).
8. Metastasis is in the liver, adrenals, and lymph nodes, with direct extension into the retroperitoneum.
9. Rarely, renal tumor may present as a spontaneous perinephric or subcapsular hemorrhage. Renal carcinoma, angiomyolipoma, renal infarction, AVM, hemorrhagic cyst, and abscess should be considered in such case. Renal cell cancer is the commonest cause of spontaneous perinephric or subcapsular hemorrhage (44).

Nephroblastoma (Wilm's Tumor)

Nephroblastoma is the most common abdominal malignancy in children. Most occur before age 5 years. They are bilateral in 5% of cases (41). Fifteen percent are associated with congenital anomalies (e.g., genitourinary, hemihypertrophy, aniridia, neurofibromatosis, Drash's syndrome, Beckwith-Wiedemann syndrome, chromosomal abnormalities) (52). These tumors arise from the metanephric blastema and can consist of different cell types including epithelium, muscle, bone, and cartilage (57). Calcification is present in 15% of cases. Extension into the inferior vena cava is present in 6% of cases. Metastasis is via direct extension, vascular, and lymphatic routes. Therefore metastasis is most common to the lungs, liver, bones, lymph nodes, adrenals, and retroperitoneum. Metastasis is present in 10% of cases at diagnosis (52).

They may have fever, pain, anorexia, hypertension, or hematuria (52). Ultrasound and CT are both regarded as sensitive in detecting the primary lesion. Computed tomography is the preferred method to determine the extent of the lesion and for staging (58,59). Approximately 10% of patients have lung metastasis at the time of diagnosis (52).

Ultrasound findings are (Figs. 8.76–8.78) (46,58,59)

1. solid mass that is usually well circumscribed and of variable echogenicity. The mass may be exophytic or extend into the renal pelvis.
2. focal areas of calcification (15% of cases)
3. cystic areas caused by necrosis. This may appear as a multilocular cystic mass with thick septa and solid foci.
4. liver, adrenal, lymph node, or retroperitoneal metastasis
5. extension into renal vein or inferior vena cava (6% of cases). Duplex Doppler or color Doppler may show mass, narrowing, or complete occlusion of the renal vein or inferior vena cava.

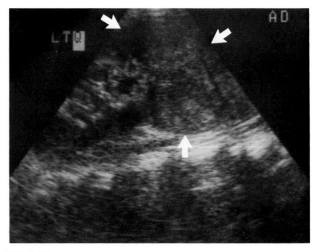

FIG. 8.76. Focal nephroblastoma. There is a large focal solid mass (*arrows*) at lower pole of kidney.

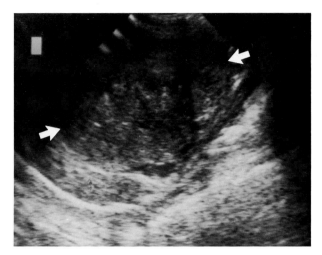

FIG. 8.77. Diffuse nephroblastoma. There is a diffuse mass (*arrows*) in renal fossa with loss of all normal renal anatomic landmarks.

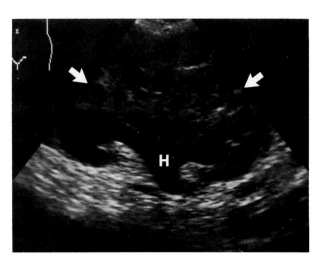

FIG. 8.79. Focal lymphoma. There is a large focal mass (*arrows*) in interpolar region of kidney. There was slight hydronephrosis (*H*) caused by retroperitoneal adenopathy.

Lymphoma

Primary renal lymphoma is rare. Most cases are metastatic. Involvement by non-Hodgkin's lymphoma is more common than Hodgkin's disease. It is estimated that 5% of patients have renal involvement at the time of diagnosis and 33% at autopsy (52,60). Patients are usually asymptomatic but may present with renal failure or ureteric obstruction. In those cases involving the kidney, 50% have a solid solitary mass, 30% have multiple foci, and 20% have diffuse parenchymal infiltration. Most cases show perinephric disease, which may invade the renal sinus (60).

Ultrasound features include (Figs. 8.79–8.82) (60)

1. single or multiple solid hypoechoic masses
2. diffuse renal enlargement
3. perinephric hypoechoic mass
4. mass extending into the central sinus
5. ureteric obstruction by a retroperitoneal mass
6. retroperitoneal or mesenteric lymphadenopathy
7. occasionally, other solid organ involvement

Leukemia

The kidneys are involved in 50% of cases at autopsy of patients with leukemia. Most patients are asymptomatic. There is usually symmetric bilateral enlargement of the kidneys. Focal renal mass or hydronephrosis is occasionally seen (52).

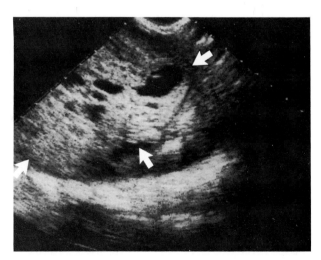

FIG. 8.78. Diffuse nephroblastoma with cystic areas. There is a diffuse mass (*arrows*) that contains focal cystic areas.

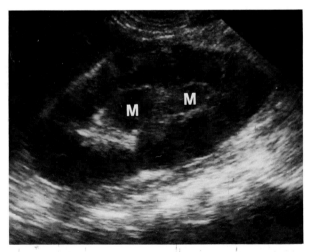

FIG. 8.80. Multifocal renal lymphoma. Renal cortex demonstrates variable echogenicity caused by multiple small masses. There is also focal involvement of central sinus by tumor (*m*).

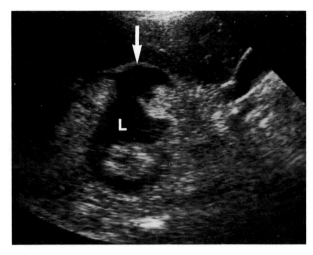

FIG. 8.81. Renal lymphoma with perinephric and pararenal extension. There is focal lymphoma (*L*) involving cortex with extension into perirenal and pararenal space (*arrow*). CT was used to define spaces involved.

Sarcoma

Renal sarcomas are rare. These include liposarcoma, fibrosarcoma, leiomyosarcoma, rhabdomyosarcoma, chondrosarcoma, and malignant fibrous histiocytoma (52). Patients usually present with an abdominal mass and occasionally with hematuria.

Ultrasound features are nonspecific. These include

1. solid mass
2. calcification (most commonly with osteosarcoma)
3. lipomatous component (liposarcoma), which is suggested by a hyperechoic mass. Computed tomography should confirm the lipomatous component.

Transitional Cell Carcinoma of the Renal Pelvis or Ureter

Transitional cell carcinoma accounts for 5% to 10% of all primary renal tumors (41). In 50% of cases there is a concurrent bladder tumor. Forty percent to 80% of patients eventually develop TCC elsewhere in the urinary tract (52). Patients may present with hematuria, ureteral obstruction, or weight loss. Most tumors are small at the time of clinical presentation (52).

Ultrasound is frequently normal (false–negative) because of the small tumor size. However, ultrasound may show a central mass (Figs. 8.83 and 8.84), causing separation of the central sinus echoes (61). A pedunculated mass is rarely seen (Fig. 8.85) (62). A few cases with punctate calcification have been described (63). These may be misinterpreted as a calculus or other cause of calcification. Tumor should be suspected if the calcification is contained within a mass. Hydronephrosis, hydroureter, or mass may be seen with a ureteric TCC (Fig. 8.86).

Metastasis to the Kidney

Metastases to the kidney is common and occurs in 12% of autopsies of patients with cancer. The commonest primary sites are lung, breast, gastrointestinal, lymphoma, and melanoma (52). Patients are usually asymptomatic but sometimes have pain and hematuria. Patients usually have widespread metastatic disease. Ultrasound features include solid mass (Figs. 8.87 and 8.88) or masses in the presence of widespread metastatic disease. They are usually small and multiple. Contrast-enhanced CT is slightly more sensitive than ultrasound in detecting renal metastasis (64).

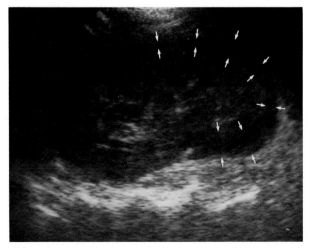

FIG. 8.82. Perinephric lymphoma. There is extensive hypoechoic mass involving perinephric space (*between arrows*). This was initially interpreted as a perinephric hematoma.

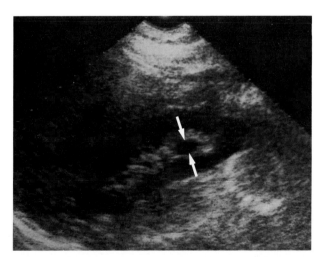

FIG. 8.83. Small TCC. There is a focal mass (*arrows*) that splays the central sinus complex. This would be difficult to distinguish from a parapelvic cyst.

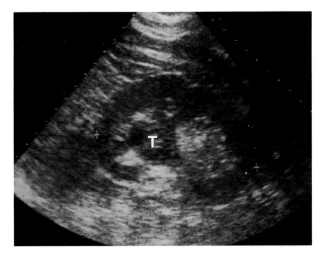

FIG. 8.84. Large TCC. There is a relatively large tumor (*T*) causing splaying of central sinus complex. This would be difficult to distinguish from a large blood clot.

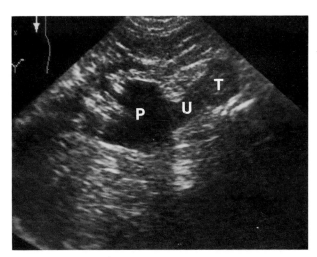

FIG. 8.86. Ureteric TCC. A tumor mass (*T*) causes hydronephrosis with dilatation of ureter (*U*) and renal pelvis (*P*).

Nonneoplastic Parenchymal Disease

Renal Enlargement

Unilateral Renal Enlargement with Smooth Contour

Unilateral renal enlargement may be due to (65)

1. compensatory hypertrophy
2. duplication of the pelvicolyceal system
3. renal vein thrombosis (acute phase)
4. acute arterial infarction
5. obstructive uropathy
6. acute bacterial nephritis

Bilateral Renal Enlargement

Bilateral renal enlargement may be due to (65,66)

1. nephromegaly associated with
   (a) cirrhosis
   (b) hyperalimentation
   (c) diabetes mellitus (commonest cause)
2. proliferative/necrotizing disorders
   (a) acute glomerulonephritis
   (b) polyartheritis nodosa
   (c) systemic lupus erythematosus
   (d) Wegener's granulomatosis
   (e) allergic angiitis

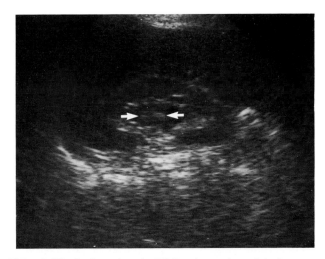

FIG. 8.85. Pedunculated TCC. A pedunculated mass (*arrows*) is seen in renal pelvis. It was mobile but adherent to wall. It was treated via percutaneous endourologic technique. (From Nolan et al., ref. 62, with permission.)

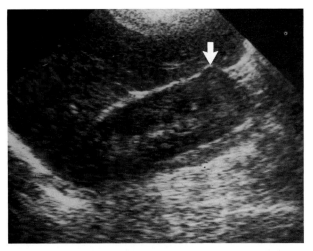

FIG. 8.87. Focal renal metastasis. There is a focal solid mass (*arrow*) in renal parenchyma. There were multiple other sites of metastasis from an unknown primary tumor. Ultrasound features are indistinguishable from a primary tumor.

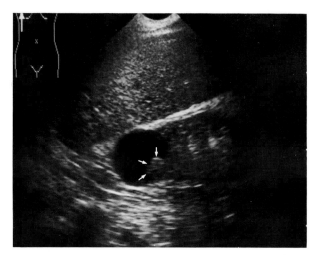

FIG. 8.88. Presumed metastasis to a renal cyst. There is a focal nodule (*arrows*) arising from wall of a cyst. There were multiple other sites of metastasis from an unknown primary tumor.

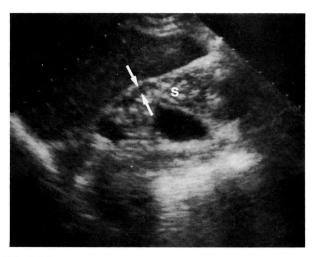

FIG. 8.89. Replacement lipomatosis associated with diffuse renal atrophy. There is diffuse parenchymal thinning (*between arrows*) associated with an increase in renal sinus fat (*S*).

(f) diabetic glomerulosclerosis
(g) Goodpasture's syndrome
(h) Schönlein-Henoch purpura (anaphylactoid purpura)
(i) focal glomerulosclerosis associated with subacute bacterial endocarditis
(j) thrombotic thrombocytopenic purpura
3. amyloidosis
4. multiple myeloma
5. acute tubular necrosis
6. acute cortical necrosis
7. leukemia
8. acute interstitial nephritis
9. acute urate nephropathy
10. acromegaly
11. hemophilia
12. homozygous S disease
13. Fabry's disease
14. physiologic response to contrast material and diuretics

Renal Atrophy

Replacement Lipomatosis of the Kidney

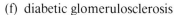

In cases of chronic renal disease with diffuse parenchymal atrophy, there may be an increase in renal sinus fat (Fig. 8.89) (67). Clues to the underlying disease are the presence of cortical atrophy and possibly hydronephrosis or calculus, or both. This should be distinguished from renal sinus lipomatosis, which is of no clinical significance.

Unilateral Diffuse Renal Atrophy

Unilateral renal atrophy (Fig. 8.89) may be due to (65)

1. renal artery stenosis
2. chronic infarction
3. radiation nephritis
4. congenital hypoplasia
5. postobstructive atrophy
6. postinflammatory atrophy
7. reflux nephropathy

Bilateral Diffuse Renal Atrophy

Bilateral renal atrophy may be due to (65)

1. generalized atherosclerosis
2. nephrosclerosis
3. atheroembolic renal disease
4. chronic glomerulonephritis
5. papillary necrosis
6. hereditary nephropathies
   (a) hereditary chronic nephritis (Alport's syndrome)
   (b) medullary cystic disease
7. amyloidosis (late)
8. arterial hypotension

Focal Renal Atrophy

Focal renal atrophy (Fig. 8.90) may be due to (65)

1. reflux nephropathy (chronic atrophic pyelonephritis) (Fig. 8.35)
2. lobar infarction

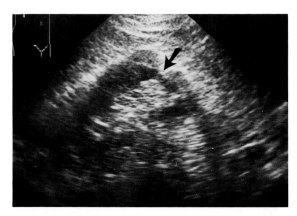

FIG. 8.90. Focal renal atrophy. There is focal atrophy (*arrow*) of renal parenchyma. This to be distinguished from a junctional parenchymal defect.

Increased Renal Parenchymal Echogenicity

Classification of Increased Echogenicity of the Cortex (68)

Grade 0: Normal renal cortical echogenicity is less than that of the liver.

Grade 1: Renal cortical echogenicity equals that of the liver.

Grade 2: Renal cortical echogenicity is greater than that of the liver but less than that of the renal sinus (Fig. 8.91).

Grade 3: Renal cortical echogenicity is equal to that of the renal sinus (Fig. 8.92).

Grade 3 kidneys may be difficult to demonstrate as the perinephric fat will have a similar echogenicity. The kidneys (grade 0–3) may be small, normal, or increased in size. The increase in cortical echogenicity is the result of

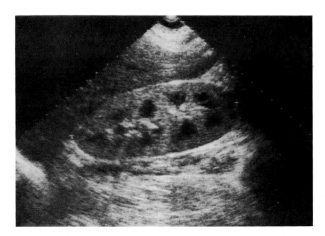

FIG. 8.91. Grade 2 renal parenchyma. There is diffuse increase in renal cortical echogenicity caused by acute tubular necrosis secondary to ingestion of ethylene glycol.

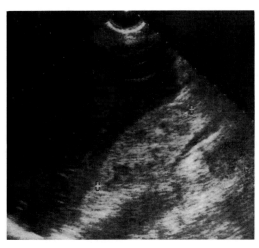

FIG. 8.92. Grade 3 renal parenchyma. There is a diffuse increase in renal parenchymal echogenicity associated with atrophy caused by collagen vascular disease.

changes within the glomeruli, tubules, and interstitium. The changes can be seen in acute and chronic disease processes. However, the appearances are not specific for specific pathologic disease processes. The grade of echogenicity has a positive correlation with the severity of each individual renal disease. However, the degree of overlap in different diseases makes it impossible to distinguish pathologic entities.

Most cases of renal parenchyma disease will be grade 0 on ultrasound examination. Therefore, a normal ultrasound does not exclude medical renal parenchymal disease.

Diseases Associated with Increased Echogenicity of the Cortex

Diseases causing increased cortical echogenicity include (68–70)

1. acute glomerulonephritis
2. chronic glomerulonephritis
3. focal segmental glomerulosclerosis
4. diabetic glomerulosclerosis
5. chronic interstitial nephritis
6. amyloidosis (chronic stage)
7. acute tubular necrosis (occasionally hyperechoic)
8. acute cortical necrosis (chronic stage)
9. leukemia (diffuse infiltration)
10. lymphoma (diffuse infiltration)
11. infantile polycystic kidney disease
12. cortical nephrocalcinosis
    (a) primary hyperoxaluria (oxalosis)
    (b) secondary to acute renal cortical necrosis
    (c) secondary to hypercalcemia
13. end-stage kidney of any etiology

Diseases Associated with Increased Echogenicity of the Medulla

Diseases causing increased echogenicity of the medulla include (71,72)

1. medullary nephrocalcinosis, which may be due to (71)
    (a) skeletal demineralization (primary hyperparathyroidism, primary carcinoma, metastatic tumor to bone)
    (b) increased intestinal absorption of calcium (sarcoidosis, milk-alkali syndrome, hypervitaminosis D)
    (c) miscellaneous (renal tubular acidosis, medullary sponge kidney, hyperoxaluria)
2. hyperuricemia (71)
3. hypokalemia (71)
4. medullary cystic disease (72)
5. Tamm-Horsfall proteinuria (72)

In adults, medullary sponge kidney and renal tubular acidosis are probably the most common causes of nephrocalcinosis. In infants, the most common cause of nephrocalcinosis is furosamide therapy, which causes hypercalciuria. Furosamide therapy may also cause nephrolithiasis in the infant (Fig. 8.38).

This group of disorders is manifested by hyperechoic medullary pyramids (Fig 8.93). If acoustic attenuation is evident, the diagnosis is nephrocalcinosis. If there is no acoustic attenuation (Fig 8.94), the diagnosis is either one of the other medical entities or nephrocalcinosis. Acoustic attenuation will depend on the degree and confluence of calcification and on focal zone characteristics of the transducer.

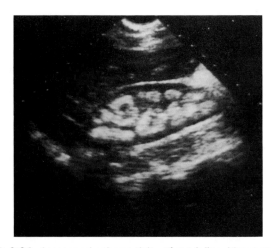

FIG. 8.94. Increased echogenicity of medulla without acoustic shadowing. However, CT showed faint calcification in distribution of medulla, which was not appreciated on ultrasound.

Infection

Most renal infections occur via the ascending route. They are usually caused by contaminants from the intestinal tract. Instrumentation, stasis, calculi, and vesicoureteric reflux are predisposing factors (73). Hematogenous infection also occurs as the result of intravenous drug abuse, endocarditis, cellulitis, and osteomyelitis. *Staphylococcus aureus* is the most common organism (73). Lymphatic spread of infection to the kidney is postulated but not proven (73). Patients with AIDS have an increased incidence of infectious organisms that usually do not infect the genitourinary tract. These include *Pneumocystis carinii, Mycobacterium avium-intracellulare, Mycobacterium tuberculosis,* and cytomegalovirus (74).

Ultrasound is a valuable imaging technique in complicated infection. It is not dependent on renal function. Ultrasound is recommended if there is inadequate clinical response to therapy and in follow-up if a mass is demonstrated.

Plain radiographs of the abdomen can be very useful in XGP if a staghorn calculus is demonstrated. Intravenous urography is normal in 75% of cases with renal infection. It requires the increased cost of contrast media and the small risk of allergic reaction. Radionuclide studies are occasionally a valuable complementary technique. Gallium requires delayed scans (72 hr) and occasionally has false-positive results caused by tumor (lymphoma, metastasis) rather than focal infection. Computed tomography is preferred over ultrasound if the patient is very obese, has a large amount of bowel gas, or is postoperative with multiple incisions or catheters. Computed tomography requires contrast enhancement to be reliable in the diagnosis of renal infection. It is superior in determining the extent of perirenal and par-

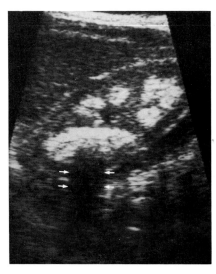

FIG. 8.93. Nephrocalcinosis. There is increased echogenicity in distribution of medulla with a posterior acoustic shadow (*arrows*) at upper pole.

arenal spread of infection. When there is doubt about the diagnosis, percutaneous aspiration for cytology, Gram's stain, and culture can distinguish between tumor and infection.

Pyohydronephrosis–Pyonephrosis

Pyohydronephrosis is the presence of infection superimposed on obstruction. Ultrasound findings are (Figs. 8.95–8.98) (75,76)

1. hydronephrosis–hydroureter
2. echoes throughout the urine
3. fluid–debris level caused by cellular material in the urine
4. gas within the collecting system caused by gas-forming organisms. There will be bright echoes that cast a dirty acoustic shadow.
5. mucosal thickening
6. mass in the collecting system caused by fungus ball. This is most commonly due to infection by *Candida* in an immunocompromised host.

Any combination of the above findings in an appropriate clinical setting is suspicious of pyohydronephrosis. The presence of hydronephrosis and clinical evidence of infection requires drainage via ureteric stent or percutaneous nephrostomy even if the above findings are not evident.

Acute Renal Parenchymal Infection

Acute Pyelonephritis (Acute Bacterial Nephritis)

Acute pyelonephritis will result in diffuse edema of the parenchyma caused by an inflammatory infiltrate. Ultrasound findings are (73,77)

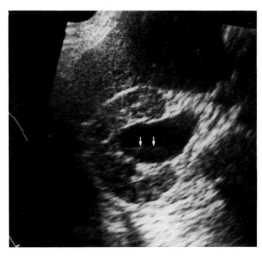

FIG. 8.96. Pyohydronephrosis with fluid–debris level. There is layering of cellular infiltrate (*arrows*) in dependent portion of renal pelvis.

1. usually normal-appearing kidney
2. renal enlargement
3. homogeneous hypoechoic parenchyma
4. compressed echogenic sinus in the early stages caused by edema
5. sinus echoes blending with the parenchyma in more severe infection caused by cellular infiltrate

Acute Focal Bacterial Nephritis (Lobar Nephronia)

Acute focal bacterial nephritis is a focal or multifocal inflammatory process involving the renal parenchyma. There is no liquefaction or necrosis. It is usually due to *Escherichia coli* infection. Ultrasound findings are those

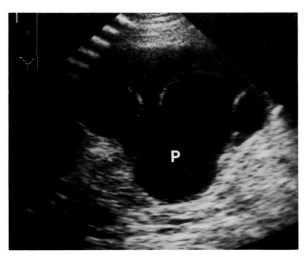

FIG. 8.95. Pyohydronephrosis. There are diffuse echoes throughout hydronephrotic pelvicalyceal collecting system (*P*) with underlying UPJ obstruction.

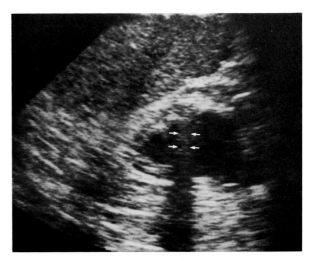

FIG. 8.97. Chronic emphysematous pyohydronephrosis. Kidney is small with a thin renal parenchyma. There is a "dirty" acoustic shadow caused by gas within collecting system.

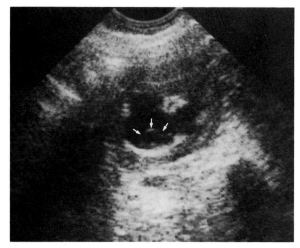

FIG. 8.98. Fungus ball. There is a mass (*arrows*) within dilated collecting system. Patient was an immunocompromised host because of metastatic disease and chemotherapy.

of a focal parenchymal mass (Fig. 8.99), which has the following features (73,77):

1. wedge-shaped
2. poorly demarcated
3. no discernible internal walls
4. hypoechoic, containing low-level echoes
5. disrupts the corticomedullary junction
6. no distal acoustic enhancement

Acute Diffuse Bacterial Nephritis

Acute diffuse bacterial nephritis is a diffuse inflammatory process of the renal parenchyma, which is usually caused by gram-negative organisms including *Klebsiella, Proteus,* and fungi. Ultrasound findings are (Fig. 8.100) (73,77)

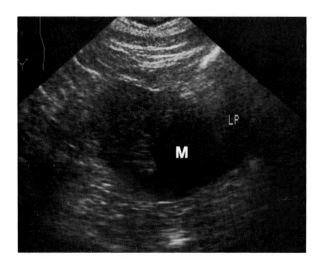

FIG. 8.99. Acute focal bacterial nephritis. There is a focal mass (*M*) in lower pole of kidney. This resolved with antibiotic therapy.

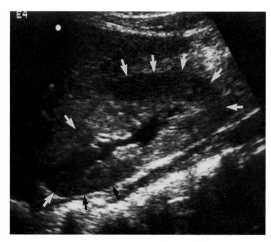

FIG. 8.100. Acute diffuse bacterial nephritis. There are multiple areas (*arrows*) of parenchymal thickening and decreased echogenicity involving upper and lower poles of kidney. These were confirmed by CT and resolved with antibiotic therapy.

1. enlarged kidney
2. patchy disorganized parenchymal pattern with loss of the corticomedullary junction and inhomogeneous echogenicity
3. central sinus blending with the abnormal parenchyma

Acute Renal Abscess

Intrarenal Abscess

Infection that progresses to liquefaction, tissue necrosis, and coalescence of microabscesses results in a parenchymal abscess. It is usually caused by gram-negative organisms including *E. coli, Pseudomonas,* and *Proteus.* Infection may occur via the ascending route or hematogeneously. Occasionally it complicates a pre-existing abnormality such as a cyst or tumor. Up to 25% of cases have negative urinalysis and culture. Ultrasound findings are (Figs. 8.101 and 8.102) (73,77)

1. parenchymal mass that is relatively well defined
2. nearly anechoic mass
3. presence of acoustic enhancement distally
4. irregular internal margins
5. occasionally hyperechoic mass caused by the presence of gas from gas-producing organisms

Perinephric and Pararenal Abscess

Infection that extends through the renal capsule will cause a perinephric abscess. If it extends through the pararenal fascias, it will cause an anterior or posterior pararenal abscess. It may then infect contiguous structures such as the psoas muscle. This usually occurs if there are predisposing factors including urinary tract ob-

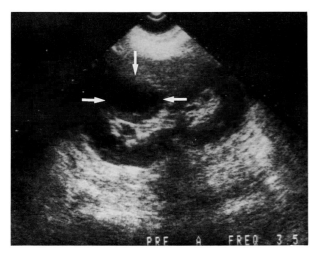

FIG. 8.101. Parenchymal abscess. There is a focal mass (*arrows*) that has a thick wall and is cystic centrally.

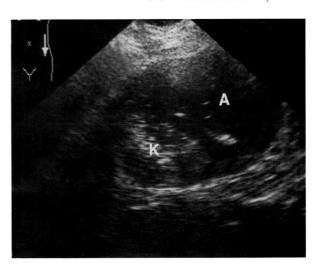

FIG. 8.103. Nephric and perinephric abscess. Kidney (*K*) is extrinsically compressed by an abscess (*A*). Focal echoes within mass are caused by gas. There was loss of tissue plane between kidney and abscess caused by renal–perinephric continuity of inflammatory process. This was drained percutaneously under ultrasound guidance.

struction, immunosuppression, trauma, or intravenous drug abuse in the presence of fulminant infection. Ultrasound findings include (Figs. 8.103 and 8.104) (77)

1. perinephric or pararenal mass
2. hypoechoic zone in the perinephric space
3. mass involving the psoas muscle
4. associated renal parenchymal mass

Chronic Renal Infection

Chronic Atrophic Pyelonephritis

A chronic inflammatory process may result from an initial acute infection. The response will be affected by the virulence of the organism, treatment, and presence of predisposing factors such as reflux. Childhood infections cause diffuse chronic atrophic pyelonephritis more frequently than adult infections. Ultrasound findings include (73,77)

1. focal parenchymal thinning (scar)
2. diffuse cortical thinning, resulting in a small kidney with hyperechoic parenchyma

Xanthogranulomatous Pyelonephritis

Xanthogranulomatous pyelonephritis is an uncommon chronic renal infection that is due to the sequela of

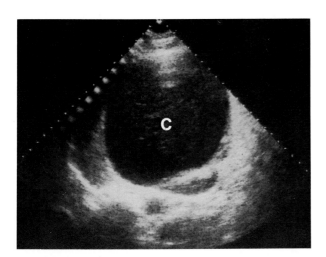

FIG. 8.102. Infected renal cyst. This pregnant patient had a small cyst documented on an earlier scan. She presented with an acute urinary tract infection. There are diffuse echoes throughout a large cystic mass (*C*). It was percutaneously drained of 2 L of pus under ultrasound guidance.

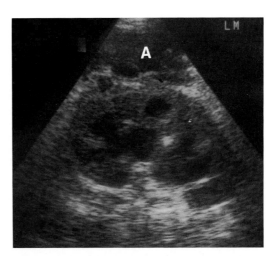

FIG. 8.104. Pararenal abscess. Abscess (*A*) extended from kidney, into perinephric space, and into pararenal space. It was drained percutaneously under ultrasound guidance. It is impossible to appreciate full extent of abscess on this single view.

multiple acute infections or secondary to obstruction from renal calculi. The infection may be focal or diffuse. It is more common in female and diabetic patients. *Proteus mirabilis* is the most common organism. Ultrasound findings are (Figs. 8.105 and 8.106) (77)

1. focal or diffuse renal enlargement with inhomogeneous parenchyma
2. parenchymal masses (abscesses)
3. staghorn calculus
4. possible hydronephrosis

Vascular Disorders

Vascular Calcification

Vascular calcification is a manifestation of atherosclerosis. Calcification of the main renal artery is usually not appreciated. Calcification of intrarenal branches can be appreciated. It is important to recognize the underlying disease process and to avoid misinterpreting vascular calcification as renal calculi (Figs. 8.107 and 8.108). A plain radiograph of the kidneys will usually resolve the potential confusion.

Renal Artery Stenosis

Renal Artery Stenosis in the Native Kidney

Radionuclide studies and arteriography are the preferred techniques in renal artery stenosis of native kidneys. The efficacy of ultrasound is not established for this diagnosis (8). The procedure requires meticulous duplex technique and is tedious at best. The examination may be technically inadequate because of the patient's body habitus. Some ultrasound criteria that have been applied include (8)

1. irregular waveform with spectral broadening
2. rounded or nondistinct peak

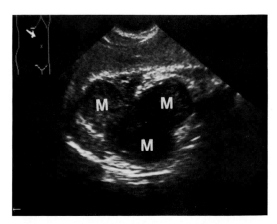

FIG. 8.106. Xanthogranulomatous pyelonephritis. There are focal masses (*M*) containing internal echoes consistent with abscesses.

3. localized increase in peak systolic frequency distal to a focal stenosis
4. peak velocity of 100 cm/sec or more
5. absence of blood flow during diastole
6. absence of blood flow indicating occlusion
7. turbulence
8. ratio of peak renal artery velocity to aortic velocity of greater than 3.5

Although encouraging as a noninvasive screening technique, the ultrasound criteria and techniques need further investigation. Color Doppler has permitted easier visualization of the renal arteries but has low sensitivity and specificity for renal artery stenosis (78).

Renal Artery Stenosis in the Renal Allograph

The position of the renal allograph permits better interrogation of the renal artery. Stenosis or kinking of the main renal artery can occur at the anastomosis site. Mild

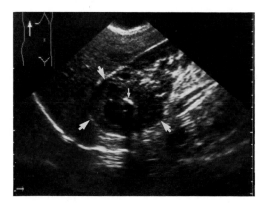

FIG. 8.105. XGP. There is a focal mass (*arrows*) in upper pole of kidney. There is also a focal central calculus (*small arrow*).

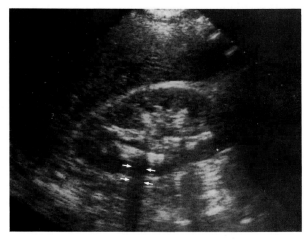

FIG. 8.107. Vascular calcification. Intrarenal vascular calcification with posterior acoustic shadowing (*arrows*) may be misinterpreted as renal calculus.

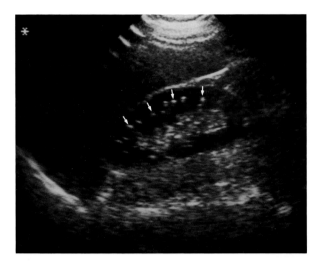

FIG. 8.108. Pseudoxanthoma elasticum. There is extensive calcification of intrarenal vascular structures in distribution of arcuate arteries (*arrows*).

turbulence is a normal finding at the site of surgical anastomosis (8,9). Ultrasound findings of allograph renal artery stenosis are

1. peak frequency shift of greater than 7.5 kHz with a 3-MHz transducer
2. gross turbulence distally

Renal Artery Occlusion

The diagnosis can be made by either PW or color Doppler. Color Doppler has the advantage of ease of identifying the renal artery and flow. The diagnosis is made when flow is absent. False-negative results can occur when flow is detected in collateral vessels. Collaterals can develop with chronic occlusion. A small hyperechoic kidney may also be seen with chronic occlusion (8,9). Acute occlusion may occur with renal artery emboli, atheromatous disease, trauma, and aortic dissection. The kidney may be of normal size or enlarged in this clinical setting. The renal artery is more easily interrogated in the renal allograph. Color Doppler is quicker and easier than duplex technique. The same criteria for diagnosis apply in the renal allograph. The renal allograph may also show segmental occlusion resulting in focal parenchymal infarction. The parenchyma may show a focal hypoechoic area. Arterial flow cannot be demonstrated by duplex or color Doppler techniques. A focal cortical scar may be a late sequela (79,80).

Renal Artery Aneurysm

Aneurysms may be congenital or acquired (e.g., atherosclerosis, infection). An aneurysm of the main renal artery is usually not appreciated on ultrasound. A more peripheral aneurysm may be appreciated. A calcified an-

eurysm may not be appreciated because of the acoustic attenuation. A noncalcified aneurysm may be appreciated by the following ultrasound features (81):

1. mass
2. pulsatile nature
3. arterial Doppler flow (duplex or color)
4. peripheral rim of thrombus (solid rim)

Hemolytic–Uremic Syndrome

The hemolytic–uremic syndrome consists of a clinical triad of hemolytic anemia, thrombocytopenia, and renal failure. It is the most common cause of acute renal failure requiring dialysis in children. This is associated with a renal microangiopathy, which results in abnormal arterial flow. Doppler studies can follow the clinical course of the disease.

Ultrasound features include (82)

1. absent or decreased arterial flow in systole
2. absent or decreased arterial flow in diastole
3. reversed arterial flow in diastole

Arteriovenous Malformation

Arteriovenous malformation (fistula) can be congenital, posttraumatic, or iatrogenic. They may involve the hilar vessels or peripheral vessels within the parenchyma (81). In renal allographs the AVM may be hilar (postsurgical) or peripheral (postbiopsy). A hilar AVM may show (Fig. 8.109) (81)

1. central mass (pseudoaneurysm)
2. peripheral thrombus
3. multiple tubular structures in the central sinus
4. enlarged renal artery

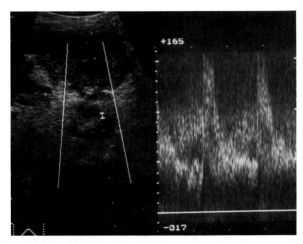

FIG. 8.109. Extrarenal AVM. Cursor is placed on vascular structures near hilum of renal allograph. Spectral display demonstrates turbulence and chaotic, multidirectional flow. Peak velocity is high.

5. large renal vein
6. Doppler flow with turbulence, and arterial-venous signals

Ultrasound features of a peripheral parenchymal AVM are (Figs. 8.110–8.112) (8,9,83)

1. mass (pseudoaneurysm)
2. Doppler flow with turbulence, and arterial-venous signals
3. high-velocity jet
4. decreased RI (0.31–0.50)
5. increased flow velocity (55–180 cm/sec)
6. color Doppler abnormalities:
   (a) arterialization of the venous waveform in the draining vein
   (b) increased color saturation in the artery and draining vein
   (c) perivascular flow artifact caused by localized tissue vibration, resulting in random color assignment in extravascular parenchyma adjacent to the fistula

Renal Vein Thrombosis

Renal vein thrombosis can occur as a result of stasis (extrinsic compression of inferior vena cava or renal vein), with nephrotic syndrome, renal tumors, renal allografts, and trauma. Thrombosis may be complete or incomplete. Ultrasound findings include (Fig. 8.75) (84,85)

1. direct visualization of thrombus within the renal vein or inferior vena cava
2. renal vein dilatation distal to the point of occlusion
3. enlarged kidney—acute phase
4. small kidney—late phase
5. increased parenchymal echoes—late phase

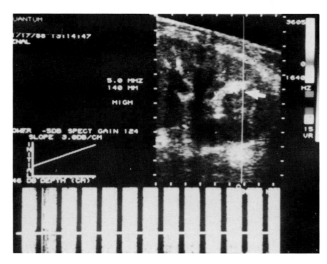

FIG. 8.111. Parenchymal AVM un color Doppler. (*See color image in color plate section B, which follows page 242.*) This is same patient as in Fig. 8.110. *Arrow* indicates area of AVM with a small pseudoaneurysm. There is increased color saturation toward white caused by high velocity. There is also slight perivascular flow artifact in parenchyma caused by tissue vibration.

6. loss of corticomedullary junction—late phase
7. absence of venous flow on PW or color Doppler

Renal Vein Stenosis

Renal vein stenosis is a rare complication of surgery for renal transplantation. Ultrasound demonstrates localized high-velocity shift in the renal vein (9).

Renal Vein Varix

Renal vein varix may rarely occur as a complication of renal vein surgery for renal transplantation. Ultrasound findings are (Fig. 8.113)

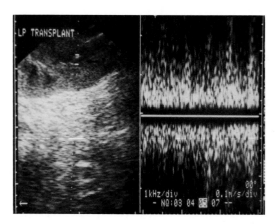

FIG. 8.110. Parenchymal AVM. Cursor is placed on a vessel in lower pole of a renal allograft that has recently had a renal biopsy. Spectral display demonstrates turbulence and chaotic multidirectional flow. Peak velocity is high.

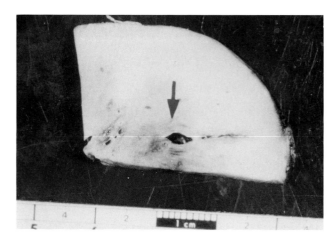

FIG. 8.112. Pseudoaneurysm at site of AVM. (*See color image in color plate section B, which follows page 242.*) Same case as Figs. 8.110 and 8.111.

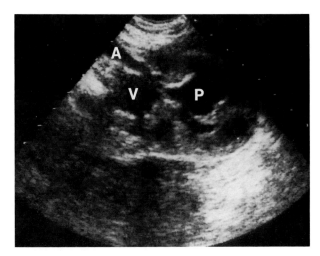

FIG. 8.113. Renal vein varix. A rounded dilated vein (*V*) is located at hilum of a renal allograph. Venous flow was demonstrated on PW Doppler. Renal artery (*A*) and pelvis (*P*) serve as anatomic landmarks.

1. focal dilatation of renal vein
2. venous flow on Doppler
3. no evidence of AVM

Renal Allograph

Normal Renal Allograph

The normal allograph has the same appearance as the normal native kidney. The allograph is usually transplanted in an extraperitoneal location in the patient's contralateral iliac fossa. The renal vessels are anastomosed end-to-side to the patient's external iliac artery and vein. The allograph ureter is anastomosed to the bladder via a ureteroneocystostomy. The hilar structures are the reverse of the native kidney. The most anterior structure is the renal pelvis. The renal vein is the most posterior structure. The renal artery is the middle hilar structure (79).

The allograph lies obliquely in the iliac fossa anterior to the iliacus and psoas muscles. It has an elliptical shape with preservation of the corticomedullary junction. The ratio of the anteroposterior diameter to the length is 0.36–0.54 (79).

Mild dilatation of the intrarenal collecting system is frequent. It is probably due to slight edema at the ureteroneocystostomy, resulting in mild incomplete obstruction.

The normal allograph usually develops hypertrophy and maintains its elliptical shape. The estimated renal volume may increase by 14% to 34%.

Abnormal Renal Allograph

The main indications for ultrasound of the renal allograph are vascular complications, renal failure (e.g., ob-

struction, rejection, acute tubular necrosis, cyclosporine toxicity), and infection. The criteria for infection and vascular disorders as previously described apply to the renal allograph. These will not be repeated in this section.

Peritransplant Fluid Collections

Peritransplant fluid collections are common in the postoperative period. Ultrasound cannot reliably distinguish between the various types of fluid collection (Figs. 8.114–8.116) (86).

Percutaneous needle aspiration will allow accurate diagnosis if the fluid collection is enlarging or if there is clinical suspicion of infection. Both urine and lymph have a similar appearance and require biochemical analysis to distinguish between them. Analysis of the aspirated fluid should include

1. white blood cell count
2. Gram's stain
3. culture and sensitivity
4. hematocrit
5. creatinine
6. total protein

Percutaneous drainage will be of value in abscesses or fluid collections causing obstruction of the collecting system caused by extrinsic compression on the ureter.

Lymphoceles are most common and are also the most common cause of allograph hydronephrosis. Lymphoceles causing hydronephrosis tend to be larger than those without hydronephrosis. They tend to be lobulated, septated, sharply marginated, and contain internal echoes (86).

Abscesses are the second most common. They tend to be lenticular in shape and contain internal echoes (86).

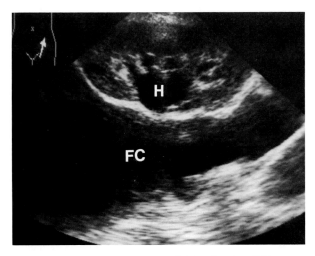

FIG. 8.114. Urinoma. This large fluid collection (*FC*) causes mild hydronephrosis (*H*) in the allograph. It was due to a leak at ureteroneocystostomy.

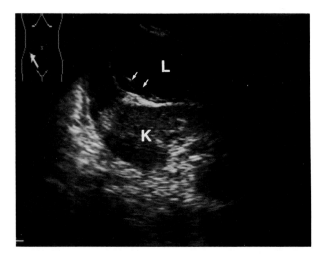

FIG. 8.115. Lymphocele. Lymph collection (*L*) lies anterior and superior to upper pole of kidney (*K*). *Arrows* indicate internal septations.

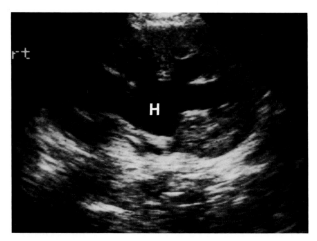

FIG. 8.117. Hydronephrosis of renal allograph. Hydronephrosis (*H*) was due to a stricture at site of ureteric anastomosis. There was also a small leak, which is not shown on this view.

Urinomas are the third most common. They usually occur as a result of a leak from the collecting system caused by ischemia, at the site of the ureteroneocystostomy, or by renal infarction. They tend to occur earlier than other collections. Association with free intraperitoneal fluid should suggest urinary ascites. A radionuclide scan may demonstrate extravasation of radionuclide (86).

Hematomas are the least common of the proven cases. They tend to be lenticular in shape, contain internal echoes, and are sharply marginated (86).

Hydronephrosis of the Allograph

Hydronephrosis (Fig. 8.117) of the renal allograph may be due to extrinsic compression by peritransplant fluid collection (86), leak at the ureteroneocystostomy

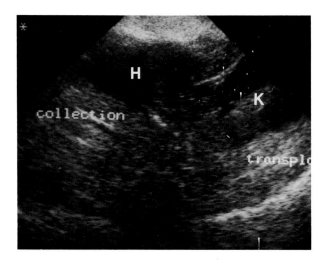

FIG. 8.116. Hematoma. Hematoma (*H*) lies medial to renal allograph (*K*).

site, intrinsic obstruction (e.g., blood clot, calculus, fungus balls), stricture, and leak caused by ischemic necrosis (79). The degree of hydronephrosis does not have a direct correlation with the degree of obstruction (79). Urine production, compliance of the collecting system, and resistance to flow in the ureter are factors that will affect the degree of dilatation. Minimal dilatation caused by edema at the site of ureteroneocystostomy is common in the immediate postoperative period. The ultrasound criteria for hydronephrosis are similar to those applied in native kidneys. Some fluid within the renal pelvis is usually normal. However, dilated infundibula and calyces usually indicate significant hydronephrosis. These findings should be interpreted in the context of clinical and biochemical findings. Doppler studies have shown an elevated RI of greater than 0.70 in obstruction of native kidneys (87). Similar findings were seen in obstruction of the renal allograph (88).

A radionuclide study can provide valuable correlative imaging with some quantitative criteria for the degree of function and obstruction. Occasionally percutaneous antegrade pyelogram is necessary to confirm the diagnosis (complete or incomplete obstruction), to establish the cause (e.g., stricture, calculus, blood clot, fungus ball, extrinsic compression), and to assess complications (urine leak).

Cyclosporine A Toxicity

Cyclosporine A is sometimes used as an immunosuppressive agent. The dosage must be carefully titered with the clinical response, as it is can be nephrotoxic. The diagnosis of nephrotoxicity is complicated by the fact that there are no specific pathologic criteria on biopsy (79). The diagnosis is one of exclusion in the appropriate clinical context. The diagnosis is established when renal function improves as a result of a reduction in the cyclosporine dose (89).

Ultrasound usually appears normal unless there is superimposed rejection. Doppler is normal unless there is superimposed rejection (12,89).

Acute Tubular Necrosis

Renal tubular damage resulting in renal failure is called ATN. The diagnosis is usually suspected when the allograft shows poor function in the early postoperative period. This usually corresponds to the first 3 days. It is more common in cadaver renal transplants and when there is prolonged period between organ harvesting and transplantation (12,79). Recovery is expectant with maintenance of hydration. If recovery does not occur as expected, biopsy is indicated. This often shows superimposed acute rejection (12,79).

Ultrasound usually shows a normal-appearing renal allograph (79). Occasionally, the allograph becomes edematous and swollen and shows some of the signs usually attributed to acute rejection (90). Doppler studies are usually abnormal. Sensitivity is optimized if threshold (top normal values) are used. Therefore, Doppler criteria include (12)

1. PI > 1.8
2. SDR > 4.0
3. DSR < 0.25
4. RI > 0.75

Acute Rejection

Acute rejection occurs as a result of immune response that is modified by histocompatibility matching, and immunosuppression (79). It usually occurs in the first few weeks after transplantation. It may occur acutely at any time remote from the surgery (79). A *clinical* classification of rejection includes the categories (88)

1. *hyperacute*—within the first 24 hr
2. *acute*—usually within the first few weeks
3. *chronic*—indolent, usually late, with fibrosis

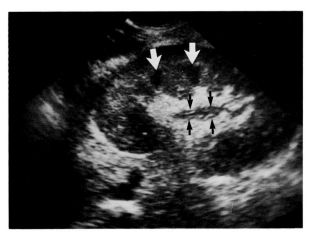

FIG. 8.118. Acute rejection of renal allograph. Kidney appears enlarged. Parenchyma is inhomogeneous. Medullary pyramids (*white arrows*) are prominent. Mucosa (*black arrows*) of renal pelvis is thickened.

The severity can be quantitated by clinical criteria, biochemistry (e.g., BUN, creatinine), and duration.

The histologic classification includes the categories (12)

1. *interstitial* (cellular)—most common
2. *mixed* (interstitial/vascular)
3. *vascular*—least common

Ultrasound is unreliable in excluding mild acute rejection. Moderate and severe acute rejection usually show ultrasound changes on real-time examination (Fig. 8.118). Some of the ultrasound criteria are subjective. There are a multitude of possible criteria (90). The multiple ultrasound criteria will permit a high accuracy of positive prediction for rejection (Table 8.5). Despite these criteria, ultrasound does not permit a specific diagnosis. Similar findings are seen in recurrent glomerulonephritis and ATN.

More recently, interest has been directed at Doppler findings in acute rejection and other diseases affecting renal allographs (Table 8.6). The criteria are not specific to the disease process, thus precluding specific diagnosis. Doppler criteria of acute rejection are (12)

TABLE 8.5. *Ultrasound criteria of acute rejection*

	Normal	Abnormal
Renal sinus fat	hyperechoic	absent or nearly absent
Kidney size	anteroposterior diameter < transverse diameter	anteroposterior ≥ transverse
Corticomedullary ratio	medulla < cortex	medulla ≥ cortex
Corticomedullary sharpness	sharp margin of pyramids	indistinct margin of pyramids
Corticomedullary conspicuity	inconspicuous pyramids	prominent pyramids
Pelvic and infundibular wall thickness	normal inconspicuous	prominent thickened walls
Focal parenchymal abnormality	absent	present

From Hoddick et al., ref. 90, with permission.

TABLE 8.6. *Ultrasound in the diagnosis of allograph dysfunction*

	Anatomy	Doppler
ATN	usually normal	usually abnormal

Acute Rejection	mild-normal or abnormal
	  moderate to severe—usually
	  abnormal
		usually abnormal

Cyclosporine A toxicity	usually normal	usually normal

1. PI > 1.8
2. SDR > 4.0
3. DSR < 0.25
4. RI > 0.75

These criteria are identical to the criteria for ATN. These also have considerable overlap with the lower range of normal (12,89). In the course of acute rejection or ATN, one may see progressive decrease in diastolic flow velocity or reversal of flow (Figs. 8.119–8.122) in diastole. This sequence reflects increase in peripheral vascular resistance caused by worsening of the disease process. There may also be regional variation in blood flow within the parenchyma. Ultrasound has a valuable role in monitoring the progression of the disease process and the result of therapy.

Role of Ultrasound and Other Imaging Modalities

Anatomic and Doppler ultrasound criteria are not specific and cannot make a specific pathologic diagnosis (Table 8.6). These should be interpreted in clinical context. Their greatest value may be in monitoring the progression of the underlying disease process as therapy is modified.

Radionuclide studies cannot reliably differentiate between ATN and acute rejection. Magnetic resonance imaging appearances are nonspecific.

The only way to make a specific diagnosis is via percutaneous biopsy. In the early posttransplantation phase, there may be concurrent ATN and acute rejection. Cyclosporine A toxicity does not have specific pathologic criteria and is a diagnosis made by exclusion.

Unusual Causes of Increased Vascular Impedance in Renal Allographs

Uncommon causes of increased vascular impedance include (88,91)

1. renal vein obstruction (kink)
2. extrarenal compression (hematoma)
3. pyelonephritis
4. hydronephrosis/hydroureter

Chronic Rejection of the Renal Allograph

Little has been written on imaging of chronic rejection. Clinically, there is gradual decline in renal function over a period of months or years (52,88). Histology shows fibrosis of small parenchymal vessels (88). Kidney size correlates poorly with acute versus chronic rejection in children (92). In adults, the kidney is usually small (52).

Doppler criteria are nonspecific. An RI of 0.70 or greater showed a sensitivity of 59% and a specificity of

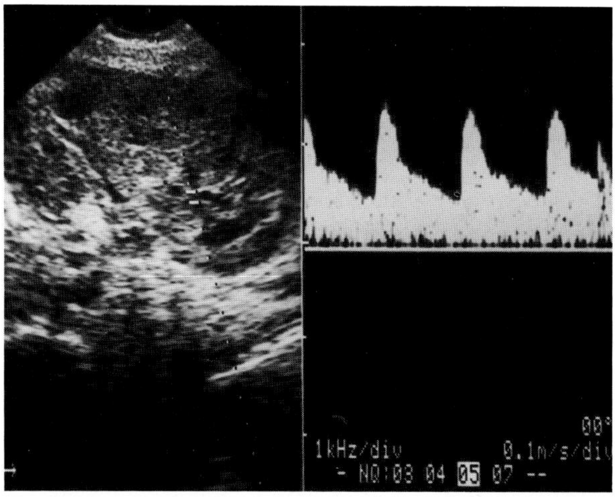

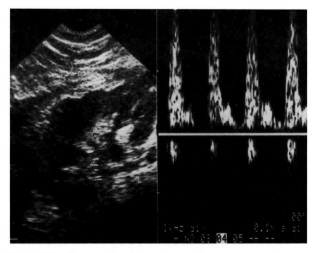

FIG. 8.119. Normal PW Doppler of renal allograph.

FIG. 8.120. Elevated peripheral vascular resistance. There is decreased end diastolic flow velocity.

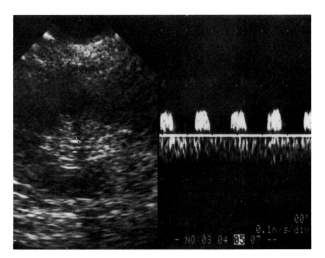

FIG. 8.121. Elevated peripheral vascular resistance. There is absent flow in diastole.

75% in the diagnosis of chronic rejection (86). Doppler should be interpreted in the context of clinical findings.

Trauma

Computed tomography is the preferred imaging modality in major blunt or penetrating abdominal trauma. Ultrasound can be a valuable primary imaging modality if there is contrast media allergy or as a complementary modality to follow the evolution of the injury (93).

Classification

Various classifications of renal trauma exist. A simplified classification is

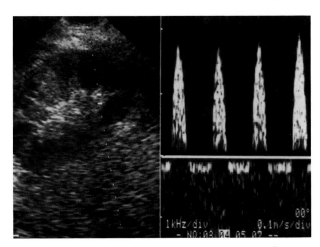

FIG. 8.122. Elevated peripheral vascular resistance. There is reversal of flow in diastole.

Category I: **treated conservatively**
1. contusion
2. focal hematoma caused by a small parenchymal laceration
3. focal parenchymal infarct
4. subcapsular hematoma

Category II: **management is controversial; conservative versus surgical**
1. laceration that enters the collecting system
2. fracture (transection) with two separate fragments
3. perinephric hematoma

Category III: **surgical management**
1. shattered kidney (multiple fragments)
2. vascular pedicle injuries
   (a) venous tear (incomplete)
   (b) venous avulsion (complete)
   (c) arterial tear (incomplete)
   (d) arterial avulsion (complete)
3. laceration of renal pelvis (incomplete tear)
4. Ureteropelvic junction avulsion (complete tear)

Ultrasound Findings in Renal Trauma

Most renal trauma is due to blunt trauma or is iatrogenic. Various combinations of findings are possible because of the spectrum of injuries. Various ultrasound findings are (Figs. 8.123–8.133) (93,94)

1. mass
   (a) usually represents a hematoma (hypoechoic—fresh/recent; hyperechoic—older)
   (b) hilar location suggesting possible vascular pedicle injury or avulsion
   (c) parenchymal location associated with a laceration
   (d) perinephric location usually associated with a parenchymal laceration
   (e) mass within the renal pelvis surrounded by fluid usually representing a clot in the collecting system
2. fluid
   (a) may be urine or blood
   (b) lenticular-shaped collection that compresses the contiguous cortex, usually a subcapsular hematoma
   (c) perinephric fluid possibly blood associated with a laceration or urine associated with a tear of the collecting system
   (d) hilar location suggesting possible laceration of pelvis, UPJ avulsion, or vascular avulsion with fresh blood
3. focal parenchymal abnormality
   (a) focal enlargement—edema or contusion or hematoma
   (b) hypoechoic parenchyma—edema or contusion or hematoma

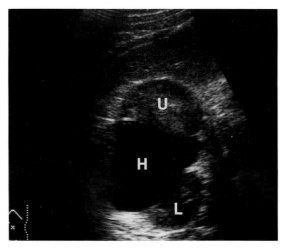

FIG. 8.123. Transection of kidney. Upper (*U*) and lower (*L*) poles of kidney are separated by a large hematoma (*H*). Pelvicalyceal collecting system was intact.

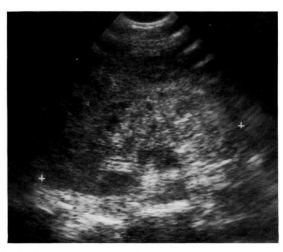

FIG. 8.126. Diffuse contusion. There is enlargement of kidney with loss of normal anatomic landmarks and inhomogeneous echogenicity. This is probably due to a combination of edema and hemorrhage within parenchyma.

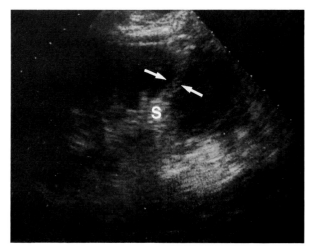

FIG. 8.124. Focal laceration with hematoma. There is a focal band (*arrows*) of increased echogenicity in lower pole of kidney, which extends into central sinus complex (*S*).

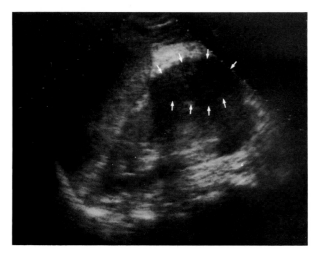

FIG. 8.127. Focal perinephric hematoma. Focal mass (*arrows*) causes slight compression of lower pole parenchyma.

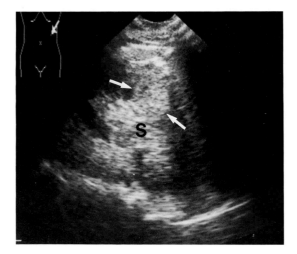

FIG. 8.125. Focal laceration with hematoma. There is a focal hyperechoic mass (*arrows*) involving parenchyma that extends to central sinus complex (*S*).

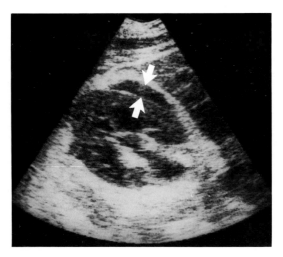

FIG. 8.128. Small subcapsular hematoma. This small lenticular-shaped fluid collection is compatible with a subcapsular hematoma postbiopsy.

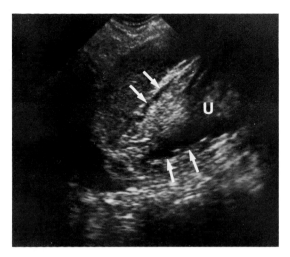

FIG. 8.129. Small urinoma. There is fluid (*arrows*) tracking in perinephric space superior to upper pole of kidney (*U*).

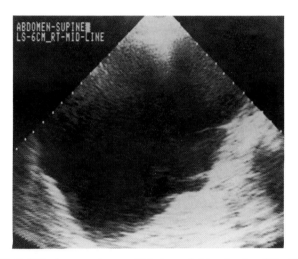

FIG. 8.130. Large urinoma. This large fluid collection (*U*) with septations was due to UPJ avulsion. Kidney was also shattered into multiple fragments. (From Boag et al., ref. 94, with permission.)

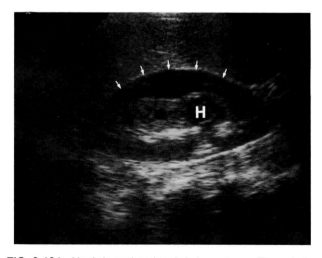

FIG. 8.131. Nephric and perinephric hematoma. There is focal hematoma (*H*) in kidney as well as perinephric fluid collection (*arrows*). This was secondary to renal biopsy.

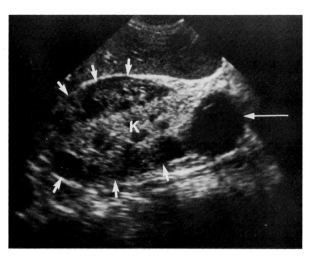

FIG. 8.132. Nephric and perinephric hematomas after renal biopsy. Renal parenchyma is hyperechoic in keeping with medical renal disease. There is a nephric hematoma (*long arrow*) and perinephric hematoma (*short arrows*). Perinephric hematoma caused vascular compression. No signal could be obtained on PW Doppler.

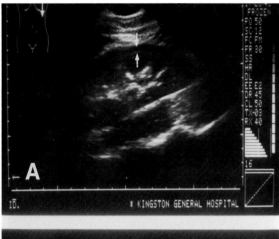

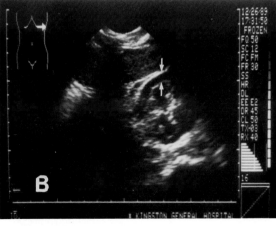

FIG. 8.133. Traumatic renal artery thrombosis. **a:** coronal view; **b:** transverse views. There is fluid (*arrows*) surrounding kidney in keeping with a hematoma. No Doppler signal could be obtained. There was absent flow on radionuclide study and flow to renal hilum on dynamic CT.

191

(c) hyperechoic parenchyma—focal hematoma
(d) disruption of parenchymal contour—laceration
(e) linear hypoechoic defect—laceration
4. enlarged kidney may be caused by
   (a) renal vein thrombosis
   (b) extensive contusion with edema

PW or color Doppler may be useful in evaluating

1. segmental infarction
   (a) parenchyma usually normal-appearing
   (b) segmental absence of flow
2. vascular pedicle injury
   (a) a hilar mass (hematoma)
   (b) a fluid collection (fresh blood)
   (c) mass that may obscure vessels—color Doppler possibly the easiest ultrasound approach to establish presence or absence of flow at the renal hilum and within the parenchyma
   (d) venous thrombosis or avulsion—absence of venous signal in hilum or parenchyma
   (e) arterial thrombosis or avulsion—absence of arterial signal in hilum or parenchyma
   (f) a large perinephric hematoma possibly the cause of vascular compression, resulting in absence of venous or arterial flow

REFERENCES

1. Schlesinger AE, Hedlund GL, Pierson WP, Null M. Normal standards for kidney length in premature infants: determination with US. *Radiology* 1987;164:127–129.
2. Han BK, Babcock DS. Sonographic measurements and appearance of normal kidneys in children. *AJR* 1985;145:611–616.
3. Edell SL, Kartz AB, Rifkin MD. Normal Renal Ultrasound Measurements. In: Goldberg BB, Kurtz AB, eds. *Atlas of Ultrasound Measurements.* Chicago: Year Book Medical Publishers; 1990:146–160.
4. Taylor KJW, Holland S. Doppler US part 1. Basic principles, instrumentation, and pitfalls. *Radiology* 1990;174:297–307.
5. Moore KL. *Clinically oriented anatomy.* 2nd ed. Baltimore: Williams & Wilkins; 1985:252–267.
6. Netter FH. *Atlas of human anatomy.* Summit, New Jersey: CIBA-Geigy; 1989. 319 p.
7. Erwin BC, Carroll BA, Muller H. A sonographic assessment of neonatal renal parameters. *J Ultrasound Med* 1985;4:217–220.
8. Rigsby CM, Burns PN, Taylor KJW. Renal duplex sonography. In: Taylor KJW, Burns PN, Wells PNT, eds. *Clinical applications of Doppler ultrasound.* New York: Raven Press; 1988:201–245.
9. Taylor KJW, Morse SS, Rigsby CM, Bia M, Schiff M. Vascular complications in renal allographs: detection with duplex Doppler US. *Radiology* 1987;162:31–38.
10. Rigsby C, Burns PN, Weltin GG, Chen B, Bia M, Taylor KJW. Doppler signal quantification in renal allographs: comparison in normal and rejecting transplants, with pathologic correlation. *Radiology* 1987;162:39–42.
11. Platt JF, Rubin JM, Ellis JH, Di Pietro MA. Duplex Doppler US of the kidney: differentiation of obstructive from nonobstructive dilatation. *Radiology* 1989;171:515–517.
12. Allen KS, Jorkasky DK, Arger PH, et al. Renal allographs: prospective analysis of Doppler sonography. *Radiology* 1988;169:371–376.
13. Middleton WD, Melson GL. Renal duplication artifact in US imaging. *Radiology* 1989;173:427–429.

14. Moore KL. The urogenital system. In: Moore KL. *The developing human: clinically oriented embryology.* Philadelphia: WB Saunders; 1977:220–258.
15. Patriquin H, Lafaivre JF, Lafortune M, et al. Fetal lobation: an anatomo-ultrasonographic correlation. *J Ultrasound Med* 1990;9:191–197.
16. Carter AR, Horgan JG, Jennings TA, et al. The junctional parenchymal defect: a sonographic variant of renal anatomy. *Radiology* 1985;154:499–502.
17. Lafortune M, Constantin A, Breton G, Vallee C. Sonography of the hypertrophied column of Bertin. *AJR* 1986;146:53–56.
18. Amis ES, Cronan JJ, Pfister RC, et al. Ultrasonic inaccuracies in diagnosing renal obstruction. *Urology* 1982;19:101–105.
19. Peake SL, Roxburgh HB, Langlois SLEP. Ultrasonic assessment of hydronephrosis of pregnancy. *Radiology* 1983;146:167–170.
20. Mellins HZ. Cystic dilatations of the upper urinary tract: a radiologist's developmental model. *Radiology* 1984;153:291–301.
21. Lebowitz RL, Mandell J. Urinary tract infection in children: putting radiology in its place. *Radiology* 1987;165:1–9.
22. Hoffman JC, Schnur MJ, Koenigsberg M. Demonstration of renal papillary necrosis by sonography. *Radiology* 1982;145:785–787.
23. Middleton WD, Dodds WJ, Lawson TL, Foley WD. Renal calculi: sensitivity for detection with US. *Radiology* 1988;167:239–244.
24. Erwin BC, Carroll BA, Sommer FG. Renal colic: the role of ultrasound in initial evaluation. *Radiology* 1984;152:147–150.
25. Laing FC, Jeffrey RB, Wing VW. Ultrasound versus excretory urography in evaluating acute flank pain. *Radiology* 1985;154:613–616.
26. Bosniak MA. The current radiological approach to renal cysts. *Radiology* 1986;158:1–10.
27. Pollack HM, Banner MP, Arger PH, Peters J, Mulhern CB, Coleman BG. The accuracy of gray-scale renal ultrasonography in differentiating cystic neoplasms from benign cysts. *Radiology* 1982;143:741–745.
28. Steinhardt GF, Slovis TL, Perlmutter AD. Simple renal cysts in infants. *Radiology* 1985;155:349–350.
29. Amis ES, Cronan JJ. The renal sinus: an imaging review and proposed nomenclature for sinus cysts. *J Urol* 1988;139:1151–1159.
30. Barbaric ZL. *Principles of genitourinary radiology.* New York: Thieme Medical Publishers; 1991:200–201.
31. Cho C, Friedland GW, Swenson RS. Acquired renal cystic disease and renal neoplasms in hemodialysis patients. *Urol Radiol* 1984;6:153–157.
32. Dunhill MS, Millard PR, Oliver D. Acquired cystic disease of the kidneys: a hazard of long-term intermittent maintenance hemodialysis. *J Clin Pathol* 1977;30:868–877.
33. Taylor AJ, Cohen EP, Erickson SJ, Olson DL, Foley WD. Renal imaging in long term dialysis patients: a comparison of CT and sonography. *AJR* 1989;153:765–767.
34. Levine E, Huntrakoon M. Unilateral renal cystic disease: CT findings. *J Comput Assist Tomogr* 1989;13:273–276.
35. Kutcher R, Sprayregen S, Rosenblatt R, Goldman M. The sonographic appearance of segmental polycystic kidney. *J Ultrasound Med* 1983;2:425–427.
36. Stuck KJ, Koff SA, Silver TM. Ultrasonic features of multicystic dysplastic kidney: expanded diagnostic criteria. *Radiology* 1982;143:217–221.
37. Diard F, Le Dosseur P, Cadler L, Calabet A, Bondonny JM. Multicystic dysplasia in the upper component of the complete duplex kidney. *Pediatr Radiol* 1984;14:310–313.
38. Vinocur L, Slovis TL, Perlmutter AD, Watts FB, Chang CC. Follow-up studies of multicystic dysplastic kidneys. *Radiology* 1988;167:311–315.
39. Rego JD, Laing FC, Jeffrey RB. Ultrasonographic diagnosis of medullary cystic disease. *J Ultrasound Med* 1983;2:433–436.
40. Hayden CK, Swischuk LE, Smith TH, Armstrong EA. Renal cystic disease in childhood. *Radiographics* 1986;6:97–116.
41. Robbins SL, Cotran RS, Kumar V. The kidney. In: Robbins SL, Cotran RS, Kumar V. *Pathologic basis of disease.* Philadelphia: WB Saunders; 1984:991–1061.
42. Hartman DS, Goldman SM, Friedman AC, Davis CJ, Madewell JE, Sherman JL. Angiomyolipoma: ultrasonic–pathologic correlation. *Radiology* 1981;139:451–458.
43. Bret PM, Bretagnolle M, Gaillard D, et al. Small, asymptomatic angiomyolipomas of the kidney. *Radiology* 1985;154:7–10.

44. Belville JS, Morgentaler A, Louglin KR, Tumeh SS. Spontaneous perinephric and subcapsular renal hemorrhage: Evaluation with CT, US and angiography. *Radiology* 1989;172:733–738.
45. Lafortune M, Breton G. Echographic demonstration of an oncocytoma. *J Can Assoc Rad* 1983;34:144–146.
46. Hartman DS, Davis CJ, Sanders RC, Johns TT, Smirniotopoulos J, Goldman SM. The multiloculated renal mass: considerations and differential features. *Radiographics* 1987;7:29–52.
47. Cormier PJ, Donaldson JS, Gonzalez-Crussi F. Nephroblastomatosis: missed diagnosis. *Radiology* 1988;169:737–738.
48. Fernbach SK, Feinstein KA, Donaldson JS, Baum ES. Nephroblastomatosis: comparison of CT with US and urography. *Radiology* 1988;166:153–156.
49. Madewell JE, Goldman SM, Davis CJ, Hartman DS, Feigin DS, Lichtenstein JE. Multilocular cystic nephroma: a radiologic–pathologic correlation of 58 patients. *Radiology* 1983;146:309–321.
50. Banner MP, Pollack HM, Chatten J, Witzleben C. Multilobular renal cysts: radiologic–pathologic correlation. *AJR* 1981;136: 239–247.
51. Curry NS, Schabel SI, Betsill WL. Small renal neoplasms: diagnostic imaging, pathologic features, and clinical course. *Radiology* 1986;158:113–117.
52. Barbaric ZL. *Principles of genitourinary radiology.* New York: Thieme Medical Publishers; 1991:152–187.
53. Schwerk WB, Schwerk WN, Robeck G. Venous renal tumor extension: a prospective US evaluation. *Radiology* 1985;156: 491–495.
54. Coleman BG, Arger PH, Mulhern CB, Pollack HM, Banner MP, Arenson RL. Grey-scale sonographic spectrum of hypernephromas. *Radiology* 1980;137:757–765.
55. Charboneau JW, Hattery RR, Ernest EC III, James EW, Williamson B Jr, Hartman GW. Spectrum of sonographic findings in 125 renal masses other than benign simple cyst. *AJR* 1983;140:87–94.
56. Kier R, Taylor KJW, Feyock AL, Ramos IM. Renal masses: characterization with Doppler US. *Radiology* 1990;176:703–707.
57. Mostofi FK. Tumors of the renal parenchyma. In: *Kidney disease– present status.* IAP Monograph No. 20. Baltimore: Williams & Wilkins, The International Academy of Pathology; 1979:356–412.
58. Jaffe MH, White SJ, Silver TM, Heidelberger KP. Wilms tumor: ultrasonic features, pathologic correlation, and diagnostic pitfalls. *Radiology* 1981;140:147–152.
59. Reiman TA, Siegel MJ, Shackelford GD. Wilms tumor in children: abdominal CT and US evaluation. *Radiology* 1986;160: 501–505.
60. Hartman DS, Davis CJ, Goldman SM, Friedman AC, Fritzsche P. Renal lymphoma: radiologic–pathologic correlation of 21 cases. *Radiology* 1982;144:759–766.
61. Subramanyam BR, Raghavendra BN, Madamba MR. Renal transitional cell carcinoma: sonographic and pathologic correlation. *JCU* 1982;10:203–210.
62. Nolan RL, Nickel JC, Froud PJ. Percutaneous endourologic approach for transitional cell carcinoma of the renal pelvis. *Urol Radiol* 1988;9:217–219.
63. Dinsmore B, Pollack HM, Banner MP. Calcified transitional cell carcinoma of the renal pelvis. *Radiology* 1988;167:401–404.
64. Choyke PL, White EM, Zeman RK, Jaffe MH, Clarke LR. Renal metastasis: clinicopathologic and radiologic correlation. *Radiology* 1987;162:359–363.
65. Davidson AJ. A systematic approach to the radiologic diagnosis of parenchymal disease of the kidney. In: Davidson AJ, ed. *Radiology of the kidney.* Philadelphia: WB Saunders; 1985:118–122.
66. Segel MC, Lecky JW, Slasky BS. Diabetes mellitus: the predominant cause of bilateral renal enlargement. *Radiology* 1984;153: 341–342.
67. Subramanyan BR, Bosniak MA, Horii SC, Megilow J, Balthazar EJ. Replacement lipomatosis of the kidney: diagnosis by computed tomography and ultrasound. *Radiology* 1983;148:791–792.
68. Hricak H, Cruz C, Romanski R, et al. Renal parenchymal disease: sonographic–histologic correlation. *Radiology* 1982;144: 141–147.
69. Kraus RA, Gaisie G, Young LW. Increased renal parenchymal echogenicity: causes in paediatric patients. *Radiographics* 1990;10:1009–1018.
70. Green D, Carroll BA. Ultrasound of renal failure. In: Hricak H, ed. *Genitourinary ultrasound. Clinics in diagnostic ultrasound.* New York: Churchill Livingstone; 1986:55–88.
71. Toyoda K, Miyamoto Y, Ida M, Tada S, Utsunomiya M. Hyperechoic medulla of the kidneys. *Radiology* 1989;173:431–434.
72. Slovis TL. Pediatric renal anomalies and infections. In: Babcock DS, ed. *Neonatal and pediatric ultrasonography. Clinics in diagnostic ultrasound.* New York: Churchill Livingstone; 1989: 157–185.
73. Kuligowska E. Renal infections. In: Hricak H, ed. *Genitourinary ultrasound. Clinics in diagnostic ultrasound.* New York: Churchill Livingstone; 1986:89–112.
74. Kuhlman JE, Browne D, Shermak M, Hamper UM, Zerhouni EA, Fishman EK. Retroperitoneal and pelvic CT of patients with AIDS: primary and secondary involvement of the genitourinary tract. *Radiographics* 1991;11:473–483.
75. Jeffrey RB, Laing FC, Wing VW, et al. Sensitivity of sonography in pyonephrosis: a reevaluation. *AJR* 1985;144:71–73.
76. Stuck KJ, Silver TM, Jaffe MH, Bowerman RA. Sonographic demonstration of renal fungus balls. *Radiology* 1981;142:473–474.
77. Kuligowska E, Newman B, White SJ, Caldarone A. Interventional ultrasound in detection and treatment of renal inflammatory disease. *Radiology* 1983;147:521–526.
78. Berland LL, Koslin DB, Routh WD, Keller FS. Renal artery stenosis: prospective evaluation of diagnosis with color duplex US compared with angiography. *Radiology* 1990;174:421–423.
79. Hricak H, Hoddick WK. Ultrasound in renal transplantation. In: Hricak H, ed. *Genitourinary ultrasound. Clinics in diagnostic ultrasound.* New York: Churchill Livingstone; 1986:161–179.
80. Grenier N, Douws C, Morel D, et al. Detection of vascular complications in renal allografts with color Doppler imaging. *Radiology* 1991;178:217–223.
81. Subramanyam BR, Lefleur RS, Bosniak MA. Renal arteriovenous fistulas and aneurysm: sonographic findings. *Radiology* 1983;149: 261–263.
82. Patriquin H, O'Regan S, Robitaille P, Paltiel H. Hemolytic–uremic syndrome: intrarenal arterial Doppler patterns as a useful guide to therapy. *Radiology* 1989;172:625–628.
83. Middleton WD, Kellman GM, Melson GL, Madrazo BL. Postbiopsy renal transplant arteriovenous fistulas: color Doppler US characteristics. *Radiology* 1989;171:253–257.
84. Braun B, Weilemann LS, Weigand W. Ultrasonographic demonstration of renal vein thrombosis. *Radiology* 1981;138:157–158.
85. Rosenfield AT, Zeman RK, Cronan JJ, Taylor KJW. Ultrasound in experimental and clinical renal vein thrombosis. *Radiology* 1980;137:735–741.
86. Silver TM, Campbell D, Wicks JD, Lorber MI, Surace P, Turcotte J. Peritransplant fluid collections. *Radiology* 1981;138:145–151.
87. Platt JE, Rubin JM, Ellis JH, Di Pietro MA. Duplex Doppler US of the kidney: differentiation of obstructive from nonobstructive dilatation. *Radiology* 1989;171:515–517.
88. Don S, Kopecky KK, Filo RS, et al. Duplex Doppler US of renal allografts: causes of elevated resistive index. *Radiology* 1989;171: 709–712.
89. Buckley AR, Cooperberg PL, Reeve CE, Magil AB. The distinction between acute renal transplant rejection and cyclosporine nephrotoxicity: value of duplex sonography. *AJR* 1987;149: 521–525.
90. Hoddick W, Filly RA, Backman U, et al. Renal allograft rejection: US evaluation. *Radiology* 1986;161:469–473.
91. Warshauer DM, Taylor KJW, Bia MJ, et al. Unusual causes of increased vascular impedance in renal transplants: duplex Doppler evaluation. *Radiology* 1988;169:367–370.
92. Babcock DS, Slovis TL, Han B, McEnery P, McWilliams DR. Renal transplants in children: long-term follow-up using sonography. *Radiology* 1985;156:165–167.
93. Pollack HM, Wein AJ. Imaging of renal trauma. *Radiology* 1989;172:297–308.
94. Boag G, Nolan RL, Nickel JC. Imaging of giant urinomas. *J Med Imaging* 1988;2:36–40.

The Adrenal Glands

INTRODUCTION

The adrenal gland is composed of an outer cortex that secretes steroids (cortisol, aldosterone, androgen, and estrogen) and an inner medulla that secretes catecholamines (dopamine, norepinephrine, and epinephrine). Secretion of the adrenal cortex is regulated by the hypothalamus and pituitary gland, which in turn are under a feedback control exerted by the adrenals. The cortex arises from the mesoderm and predominates in the superior portion of the gland. The medulla arises from the chromaffin ectodermal cells of the primitive sympathetic ganglia and predominates in the inferior portion of the gland.

Identification of the normal adrenal glands in adults by sonography is less accurate and less successful than with CT scanning. This is particularly true for obese patients and for the left gland. However, better visualization is obtained with ultrasound in neonates and infants, in whom the glands are larger and easier to image.

9.1 SCANNING TECHNIQUE

No special patient preparation is required. A high-resolution real-time sector scanner using a 3.5- or 5-MHz transducer is routinely used.

Scanning is usually performed with the patient lying supine for the right gland, with the transducer placed in a right intercostal space in the midaxillary line, using the liver as an acoustic window (Fig. 9.1). The right gland is detected posterior to the IVC in the coronal and transverse scan planes. The left gland is scanned using a more posterior approach, with the patient lying obliquely on the right side and with the transducer placed beneath the ribs in the posterior axillary line, using the spleen as an acoustic window (Fig. 9.1).

9.2 NORMAL ANATOMY

Both adrenal glands, surrounded by areolar fat, are located in the retroperitoneal perirenal space at the level

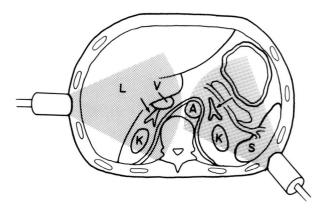

FIG. 9.1. Technique of scanning adrenals. Right adrenal is scanned in right midaxillary line using liver as an acoustic window; left adrenal is scanned in posterior axillary line through spleen. *L,* liver; *V,* vena cava; *A,* aorta; *K,* kidney; *S,* spleen. *Arrows* indicate adrenal glands. (From Yeh, ref. 3, with permission.)

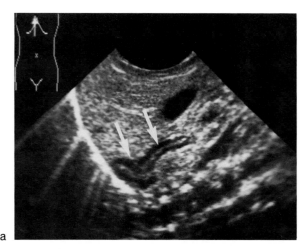
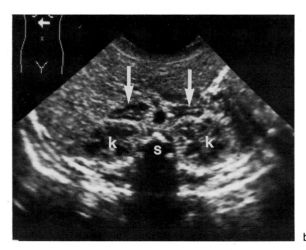

FIG. 9.2. Normal adrenals: sonographic appearance. **a:** sagittal scan; **b:** transverse scan. Gland is outlined by *arrows*. Note hypoechoic cortex surrounding hyperechoic medulla. *k*, kidneys; *S*, spine.

of the eleventh or twelfth rib, lateral to the vertebrae. The right adrenal is related laterally to the posteromedial border of the liver, medially to the right crus of the diaphragm, anteriorly to the IVC, and inferiorly to the upper pole of the right kidney. The location of the left gland is more variable. It may be suprarenal or may be medial to the upper pole and may be as low as the renal hilus. It is lateral to the aorta and crus of the diaphragm and posterior to the pancreatic tail and splenic vein.

Each adrenal gland is composed of three parts: the body or anteromedial ridge and two limbs (the lateral and medial wings). On sonography, the glands are triangular structures (Fig. 9.2a,b).

Normal dimensions of the glands have been determined *in vivo* by CT and ultrasound scanning (Fig. 9.3). Table 9.1 gives the measurements as determined in the fetus (after 30 weeks) (1), in neonates (2), and in adults (3).

The adrenal glands decrease to half their original size in the first 2 days of life, because of involution of the fetal zones that comprise 80% of the thickness of the glands at birth (2). The glands in the adults are more elongated and wider but much thinner than those of infants and children. Adrenal weight is, however, heavier in adults

than in neonates or children. The mean weight is estimated at 5.2 to 6.2 g in neonates, 8.0 to 8.6 g in children, and 13 to 14 g in adults (4).

An adrenal gland that exceeds 1.5 cm in maximal anteroposterior or transverse diameter should be considered suspicious for enlargement either by focal mass or hypertrophy (4). Texture-wise, the normal gland usually shows an echo-poor outer layer, which represents the cortex surrounding an echogenic inner layer, which represents the medulla.

Each gland is supplied by three arteries: (a) the inferior adrenal artery, coming from the renal artery; (b) the middle adrenal artery, arising from the aorta; and (c) the superior adrenal artery, a branch of the inferior phrenic artery. A single central vein emerging from the hilus drains the gland, on the right, into the IVC and, on the left, into the renal vein. These vessels are not detected in routine scanning.

9.3 PATHOLOGY

Congenital Anomalies

Congenital adrenal absence or hypoplasia is rare. Accessory adrenal cortical tissue is more common but only found at autopsies in the kidneys, in the retroperitoneum, and occasionally in the genitalia.

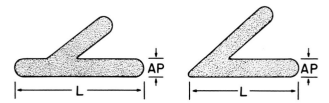

FIG. 9.3. Technique of measuring adrenal. *L*, length; *AP*, anteroposterior diameter. (Modified from Shackelford GD. Adrenal glands, pancreas, and other retroperitoneal structures. In: Siegel MJ, ed. *Pediatric sonography*. New York: Raven Press; 1991:213–256, with permission.)

TABLE 9.1. *Normal adrenal size*

	Transverse (mm)	Anteroposterior (mm)	Length (mm)
Fetus (1)	—	—	14–22
Neonate (2)			
Day 1	17.9 ± 2.7	9.6 ± 2.1	17.3 ± 1.8
Day 2	9.5 ± 1.5	5.7 ± 1.0	7.7 ± 0.9
Adult (3)	20–40	3–6	30–60

The adrenals are present in patients with renal agenesis (5). The ipsilateral gland appears elongated or discoid in shape and may simulate adrenal hypertrophy (6). In renal agenesis or ectopia, the position of the adrenal gland is unaffected.

In CAH, enzymatic deficiencies are inherited as autosomal recessive traits. There is accumulation proximal to the enzyme deficiencies of precursors that act as androgens or minerale-corticoids, leading to ambiguous genitalia, virilism in females, precocious puberty, and salt-losing crisis in males. There is also absence of feedback inhibition of ACTH secretion by the hypothalamus and pituitary, leading to adrenal hyperplasia (7,8). Sivit et al. (8) found a mean adrenal length of 23.7 mm and width of 5.3 mm in symptomatic infants with CAH. The role of ultrasound is (a) to document and monitor adrenal size, (b) to exclude other causes of virilism such as ovarian neoplasms, polycystic ovarian disease, and functional adrenal neoplasms, and (c) to demonstrate pelvic anatomy in patients with ambiguous genitalia.

Morphological Abnormalities

Adrenal Enlargement

An adrenal gland may be considered enlarged when it measures more than 1.5 cm in maximal transverse or anteroposterior diameter (4), either on CT or ultrasound scan.

The enlargement may be due to hemorrhage, tumor, or diffuse hyperplasia (9). Hemorrhagic and neoplastic diseases will be discussed separately in this chapter. Congenital hyperplasia has been previously discussed.

Acquired adrenal hyperplasia is typically bilateral. It may be due to increased secretion of ACTH by a pituitary adenoma (Cushing's disease) or to ectopic ACTH production usually by small cell carcinoma of the lung or bronchial carcinoid (Cushing's syndrome). The enlarged glands retain their normal shape and sonographic architecture, with the echogenic medulla surrounded by a hypoechoic outer cortex (9) (Fig. 9.4).

A confusing situation exists when a focal nodule is detected in a patient with adrenal hyperplasia. Is it an autonomous adenoma (in which case adrenalectomy is indicated), or is it part of macronodular hyperplasia (in which case medical management is the rule)? From the work of Doppman et al. (10), it appears that macronodular hyperplasia occurs more frequently in patients with long-standing Cushing's disease than with Cushing's syndrome. In most instances, diagnosis can only be made by clinical and biochemical findings.

Adrenal Calcifications

Adrenal calcifications are seen in association with many different conditions, including hemorrhage, infec-

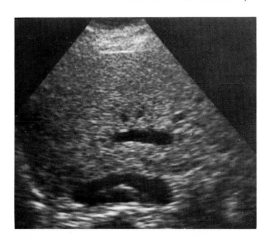

FIG. 9.4. Adrenal hyperplasia. Transverse sonogram shows marked enlargement of right adrenal, which, however, retains its normal configuration and texture (transverse diameter = 5 cm). Left adrenal is also enlarged in this patient with documented Cushing's syndrome.

tions, cysts, and neoplastic diseases. Adrenal hematomas calcify several weeks after the acute hemorrhage (11). When a calcified adrenal mass is seen in a child, appropriate tests should be obtained to rule out a neuroblastoma. Infections that result in adrenal calcification include histoplasmosis, tuberculosis, and neonatal herpes infection. Calcified granulomas are often found in atrophic glands and often are associated with adrenal insufficiency (11,12). Peripheral curvilinear calcification is seen in about 15% of benign adrenal cysts (12). Pheochromocytomas may be cystic but they do not calcify.

About 50% of adrenal neuroblastomas contain granular or psammomatous calcification. About 25% of adrenocortical carcinomas calcify. Calcification is unusual in the other types of adrenal neoplasms (e.g., myelolipoma, pheochromocytoma, and adenoma) (12). An exceptionally rare lipidosis, Wolman's disease, is characterized by dense calcification in enlarged adrenal glands (13).

Ultrasound is much less sensitive than CT in detecting adrenal calcifications, but a knowledge of what adrenal lesions may calcify can be useful in practice. Calcifications when detected are hyperechoic with or without acoustic shadowing.

Hemorrhage

Bleeding into the adrenals is more commonly seen in neonates in whom the glands are normally large. It is typically confined to the subcapsular space. Common causes of NAH are traumatic delivery and fetal hypoxia or asphyxia. In fact, in one study (14), NAH is seen in about one third of cases of neonatal asphyxia in the first few days of life. In adults, predisposing factors are blunt trauma, stress related to sepsis, burns or surgery, bleeding diatheses, and anticoagulant therapy. Eighty-five

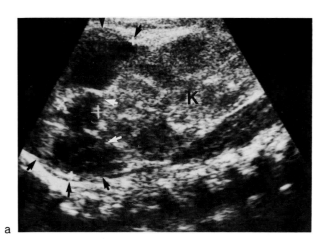
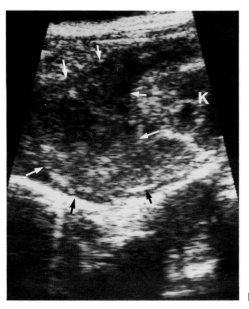

a

b

FIG. 9.5. Acute NAH: parasagittal scan. **a:** sagittal sonogram. Left adrenal (*arrows*) is enlarged (antero-posterior diameter = 4.0 cm) in this female newborn with sepsis and hypoxia. A mass was palpated in left flank 22 hr after birth. Note cystic spaces within enlarged gland. *K*, kidney. **b:** A week later, gland appears smaller and more echogenic. Findings are compatible with resolving hematoma.

percent of adrenal hemorrhage secondary to blunt trauma involves the right gland. Bleeding from anticoagulant therapy occurs most often in the first 3 weeks of treatment (15).

Sonography is the modality of choice in detecting and monitoring adrenal hemorrhage in the neonate. Within the first 24 hr, the hematoma is echogenic (Figs. 9.5a,b and 9.6). Over the next few days, it becomes gradually echo-poor or even echo-free. Eventually, the hematoma may disappear or may calcify in several months (Fig. 9.7). A pseudocyst may persist as a sequela (16,17).

Bilateral adrenal hemorrhage may be complicated by shock, disseminated intravascular coagulation, and adre-

nal insufficiency (15). In children, differential diagnosis with neuroblastoma should always be considered, and appropriate biochemical tests should be obtained whenever in doubt.

Cystic Disease

Adrenal cysts are rare incidental findings in imaging studies.

Sixty percent are true cysts with an epithelial lining and are classified as lymphangiomatous or angiomatous. Thirty percent are pseudocysts, with a fibrous wall, and

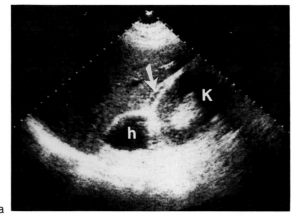
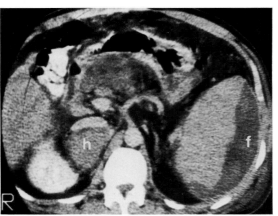

a

b

FIG. 9.6. Posttraumatic adrenal hemorrhage. **a:** sagittal sonogram; **b:** CT scan. Sonogram shows echo-poor mass (*h*) in right adrenal. This corresponds to right adrenal hematoma seen on CT scan. Note small amount of blood in Morison's pouch (*arrow*) and subcapsular splenic hematoma (*f*). Patient was involved in a car accident. *K*, kidney.

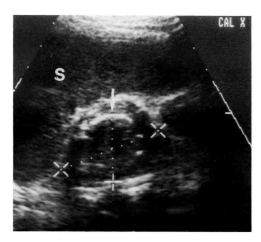

FIG. 9.7. Calcified adrenal hematoma. Curvilinear echo (*arrow*) represents calcification in this left enlarged adrenal gland. Neuroblastoma may have a similar appearance. *S*, spleen.

are considered to be related to previous hemorrhage or infection. Very rare conditions include hydatid cysts and cystic adrenal neoplasms. Typically unilateral, adrenal cysts are bilateral in 15% of cases, and this occurs most often in children. Females are more commonly affected (18,19).

Symptomatic cysts are often large, measuring more than several centimeters in diameter. Typically, they appear as thin smooth-walled spherical echo-free collections with good through transmission (Fig. 9.8a,b). Curvilinear calcification may be detected in the wall either radiographically or sonographically. Occasionally, it may be difficult to distinguish a large left adrenal cyst from a pseudocyst in the tail of the pancreas. If the lesion can be demonstrated to lie anterior to the splenic vein, it is pancreatic in origin. If it lies posterior to the splenic vein, it arises from the adrenal. Symptomatic or atypical

cysts may be aspirated percutaneously under ultrasound or CT guidance for diagnostic and therapeutic purposes (19).

Infection and Abscess

Since the discovery of AIDS, infections of the adrenal glands are more frequently seen in the adult. The common causative agents are histoplasma, *Mycobacterium tuberculosis*, cytomegalovirus, and herpes simplex (20,21). Pyogenic adrenal infection is extremely rare (Fig. 9.9). Adrenal abscesses are more easily detected by ultrasound in the neonates, in whom they are considered to result from infection of adrenal hemorrhages or from maternal infection at the time of delivery (22). Offending organisms include *Escherichia coli*, Group B streptococci, *Staphylococcus aureus*, and *Bacterioides*. Sonographically, a fluid–fluid level may be seen in a hypoechoic adrenal mass (22). Differential diagnosis with NAH, neuroblastoma, and necrotic metastasis is difficult by sonography alone.

Neoplasms

Myelolipoma

This is a rare benign biochemically inactive adrenal neoplasm composed mainly of fat and bone marrow elements. They are usually small and unilateral but may be bilateral and quite large (23).

If the tumor is composed mainly of fat, ultrasound demonstrates a hyperechoic mass (Fig. 9.10a,b). If myeloid elements predominate, the tumor will simulate an adenoma or a metastasis (23). In oncology patients, a fine needle aspiration biopsy is often required (24).

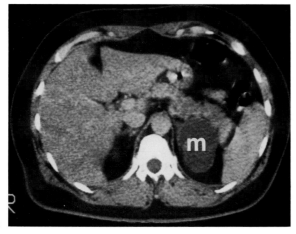

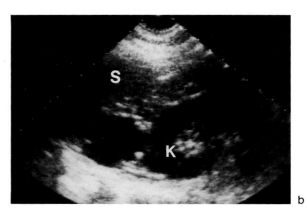

a   b

FIG. 9.8. Adrenal cyst. **a:** CT scan; **b:** parasagittal sonogram. It is difficult to know from CT scan whether left adrenal mass (*C*) is cystic or solid. Sonography demonstrates that mass is cystic. *S*, spleen; *K*, kidney.

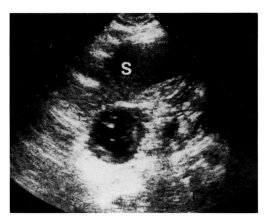

FIG. 9.9. Adrenal abscess. Pus was aspirated from this complex mass in left adrenal. This was seen in a patient with AIDS. *S*, spleen.

Cortical Adenoma

Three types are recognized: nonfunctioning adenoma, adenoma secreting cortisol (one cause of Cushing's syndrome), and adenoma secreting aldosterone (Conn's syndrome).

Nonfunctioning cortical adenomas are commonly found at autopsies and on routine CT and ultrasound scanning. Strict criteria must be met before an adrenal mass can be considered an incidental finding: (a) it should be unilateral; (b) no history of a primary malignancy elsewhere; and (c) no biochemical evidence of adrenal hyperfunction. If the mass is less than 3 cm in diameter, it is wise to perform follow-up scan in 3 to 6 months. Biopsy or surgery should be considered if the mass increases in size or becomes symptomatic (25).

Fifteen percent of Cushing's syndrome is caused by an adrenal cortical adenoma producing excess cortisol. The syndrome is characterized by central obesity, hirsutism, hypertension, edema, impaired glucose tolerance, osteo-penia, and psychological disturbance. Ninety percent of the cortisol-producing adenomas measure less than 5 cm (25). In the typical scintigram with iodomethyl-norcholesterol (NP-59), only the gland containing the neoplasm is visualized as the result of excess cortisol production. The activity of the normal contralateral gland is suppressed because of reduced secretion of ACTH by the pituitary (26).

Excess secretion of aldosterone by the zona glomerulosa of the adrenal cortex results in Conn's syndrome, which is caused, in 80% of cases, by a unilateral cortical adenoma, and in the remaining 20% by bilateral hyperplasia. Ninety percent of Conn adenomas measure less than 3.5 cm in diameter (25). The lesion can be detected by dexamethasone-suppressed, NP-59 cortical scintigraphy or by venous sampling (26).

The sonographic and CT appearance of adrenal adenomas, either nonfunctioning or functioning, is nonspecific, with most appearing as focal homogeneous round solid masses (27). The ability of MRI in distinguishing a benign from a malignant adrenal mass is still under investigation (28).

Diagnosis of functioning adrenal adenoma is usually made clinically and biochemically. The role of imaging techniques (ultrasound, CT, MRI, isotopes) is to establish that hyperfunction is due to focal unilateral neoplasm, which requires adrenalectomy, and not due to bilateral hyperplasia, which should be managed by conservative medical treatment. Ultrasound performs less well than CT or MRI in detecting small adrenal masses (25), but it still is commonly used in assessing children and young adults.

Adrenocortical Carcinoma

Adrenocortical carcinomas are rare. In children, they are more common than adenomas, the ratio being 3:1.

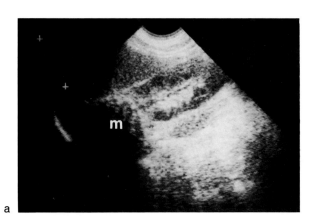

a

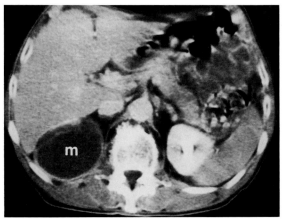

b

FIG. 9.10. Myelolipoma. **a:** sonogram; **b:** CT scan. Myelolipomas are composed of a mixture of myeloid tissue and fat. This myelolipoma (*m*) appears strongly echogenic because of a large amount of fat casting posterior acoustic shadowing. CT scan confirms fatty content of tumor.

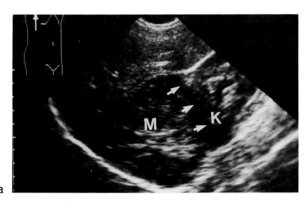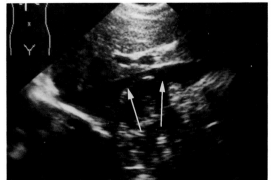

a b

FIG. 9.11. Adrenal carcinoma. **a:** parasagittal scan; **b:** parasagittal scan. Mass (*M*) is large, echogenic, and well demarcated (*short arrows*) from right kidney (*K*). It is posterior to IVC, which is compressed but not invaded (*long arrows*).

They are the most common cause of spontaneous ACTH-independent Cushing's syndrome in the pediatric age group. Females of all ages are more commonly affected than males (29). In the past, before ultrasound and CT, 90% of adrenocortical carcinoma measured more than 6 cm in mean diameter at the time of diagnosis (25). With the high sensitivity of present day imaging equipment, it is expected that carcinomas of much smaller sizes will be detected.

The sonographic appearance is that of a lobulated mass of inhomogeneous echo pattern (Fig. 9.11a,b). Small cystic spaces may be seen representing areas of necrosis. Calcifications are identified in 25% of cases. However, quite a few lesions, especially smaller ones, are homogeneous and indistinguishable from adenomas (29,30). More significant to the diagnosis of malignancy is the sonographic demonstration of vascular invasion (Fig. 9.12a,b) (adrenal or renal vein and IVC) and metastases (lymph nodes and liver). It may be difficult to distinguish large adrenal carcinomas from those arising from the kidneys, liver, or pancreas.

Neuroblastoma

Neuroblastomas are sarcomas arising from the adrenal medulla and in the sympathetic chain. Nearly half of all neuroblastomas originate from the adrenal medulla. The anatomic distribution and percentage of the tumors at each site are given in Table 9.2.

Neuroblastomas account for 7% of all cancers in children, in whom they are the second most common intraabdominal tumor, next to Wilm's nephroblastomas, which account for 12% of all cancers. Eighty percent of all neuroblastomas are found in the first 3 years of life (31). They frequently secrete catecholamines (dopamine and norepinephrine), which are metabolized to HVA and VMA. The urinary levels of these metabolites are used as diagnostic screening tests and as markers for monitoring response to treatment and tumor recurrence. Clinical findings include failure to thrive, hypertension, and abdominal mass.

Neuroblastomas have been diagnosed *in utero* by sonography (32), which is considered the screening modal-

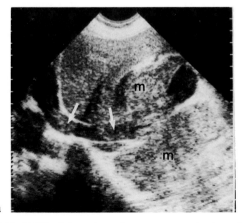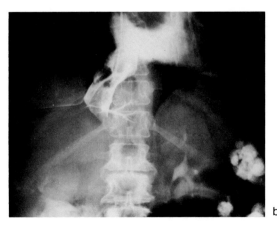

a b

FIG. 9.12. Adrenal carcinoma—vascular invasion. **a:** parasagittal scan; **b:** cavagram. IVC is encased by large solid tumor (*m*). Echogenic masses (*arrows*) representing tumor thrombus are seen in its lumen. Cavagram confirms sonographic findings.

TABLE 9.2. *Primary sites of neuroblastoma*

Location	Percentage
Abdomen	
Adrenal Glands	43–46
Extraadrenal	18
Posterior Mediastinum of Thorax	14
Neck	5
Pelvis	5
Brain	2
Other and unknown	20

Modified from Page D, DeLellis R, Hough A. Tumors of the adrenal. In: *Atlas of tumor pathology*. Washington, DC: Armed Forces Institute of Pathology; 1985, with permission.

ity of choice in the evaluation of abdominal masses in infants and children. Usually, the lesion appears as a solid mass with coarse echoes. It often has ill-defined borders and a tendency to cross the midline (Fig. 9.13a,b). Calcification within the tumor is common, seen in at least 50% of cases. This can be detected by ultrasound as bright echoes with or without acoustic shadowing. Less commonly, the lesion has a complex echo pattern, with cystic components that probably represent areas of hemorrhage or necrosis (25,29,33). This is in contrast to the intrarenal Wilm's tumor, which typically appears evenly echogenic (similar to the texture of normal liver), containing usually small round areas of cystic necrosis but rarely calcification (34). When a neuroblastoma or Wilm's tumor is extensive, differentiation is practically impossible by imaging alone (Fig. 9.14a,b).

Computed tomography and MRI appear to perform better than ultrasound in the staging of the disease, by more accurately detecting lymph node metastases, vascular encasement, and intraspinal extensions (35).

Surgery is the treatment of choice for stage I and II. Prognosis depends on a number of factors including clinical staging at the time of diagnosis, patient's age, and primary site of the tumor. Adrenal neuroblastomas in children older than 2 years of age have the worst prognosis (29,33).

Pheochromocytoma

Pheochromocytoma is a neoplasm arising from chromaffin cells, which secrete catecholamines and which are found in the adrenal medulla, in the organ of Zückerkandl near the aortic bifurcation, or in the paravertebral sympathetic ganglia near the renal hilus. Ten percent of all pheochromocytomas are extra-adrenal; 10% are bilateral; 10% are malignant. About 5% are seen in children. The majority of pheochromocytomas are found as isolated lesions. However, they may constitute a component of the MEN syndromes. They also occur more frequently in the neuro-ectodermal syndromes (von Hippel-Lindau, neurofibromatosis, tuberous sclerosis, and Sturge-Weber) (36).

Symptoms are related to increased secretion of catecholamines. They consist commonly of headache, palpitations, and excessive perspiration and are present in 95% of patients. Diagnosis is made on clinical and biochemical criteria. Imaging tests are used to localize the tumor for surgical removal and for the detection of metastases. They include ultrasound, CT, MRI, and isotope scanning with MIBG.

Adrenal Pheochromocytoma

Ninety percent of all pheochromocytomas are found in the adrenal medulla. When solitary, the right gland is more commonly affected than the left (36).

The size of the tumors varies between 1 to 16 cm, rarely measuring less than 3 cm when found. Sonographically, the appearances reflect the internal architecture of the neoplasms, which are characterized by hypervas-

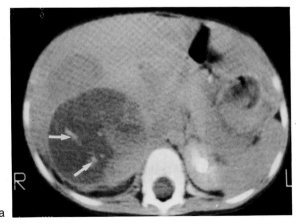
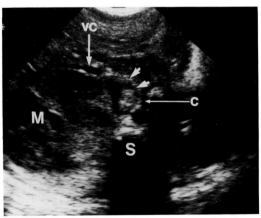

a   b

FIG. 9.13. Neuroblastoma. **a:** CT scan; **b:** transverse sonogram. CT scan shows round mass of inhomogeneous density containing scattered calcifications (*long arrows*). Sonogram demonstrates solid nature of the mass (*M*), which extends across midline (*short arrows*). Note anterior displacement and compression of vena cava (*vc*). Celiac axis (*c*) is stretched. Details are better seen on sonogram. *S*, spine.

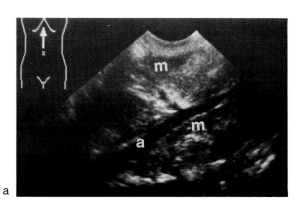

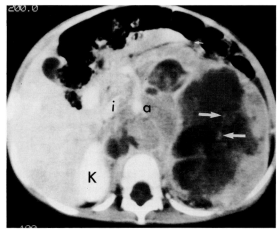

a   b

FIG. 9.14. Enormous neuroblastoma. **a:** parasagittal sonogram; **b:** CT scan. Aorta (*a*) is encased by a large echogenic mass (*m*). CT scan shows calcification (*arrows*) in this huge neuroblastoma, which extends across midline, encasing and displacing vessels. Patient responded well to chemotherapy. *a*, aorta; *i*, IVC; *k*, kidney.

cularity, areas of hemorrhage, necrosis, and cystic degeneration. Consequently, ultrasound usually shows a solid mass with complex or homogeneous echogenicity (Fig. 9.15). Calcification is rare.

Magnetic resonance imaging appears to be the screening modality of choice in the work-up of patients with suspected pheochromocytoma (37). Nevertheless, sonography remains useful in detecting cystic pheochromocytoma and in establishing the cystic or solid nature of a known adrenal mass. Although cystic degeneration is relatively frequent in a pheochromocytoma, purely cystic pheochromocytomas are extremely rare, with only a few cases reported in the literature (Fig. 9.16). Percutaneous aspiration biopsy may be fatal (38).

Extra-Adrenal Pheochromocytomas (Paragangliomas)

Ten percent of all pheochromocytomas are found outside the adrenal medulla. The distribution and percentage of extra adrenal pheochromocytomas are summarized in Table 9.3.

Whereas adrenal pheochromocytomas are usually benign, ectopic pheochromocytomas are often malignant and more commonly seen in MEN syndromes (36). They are better detected by ^{131}I-MIBG scintigraphy and MRI (39). Sonography occasionally can detect tumor in the organ of Zückerkandl and in the wall of the urinary bladder (40).

Adrenal Lymphoma

Isolated primary adrenal lymphoma is a rarity, with only four cases reported in the world literature (41,42). Most often the glands are affected in patients with widespread lymphomatous disease elsewhere or as a site of tumor recurrence after therapy. In one series, adrenal

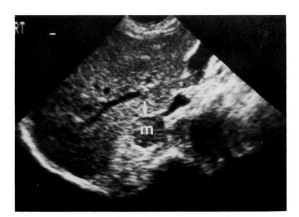

FIG. 9.15. Pheochromocytoma (solid): transverse sonogram. Small echogenic round mass (*m*) is seen posterior to IVC (*arrow*), which is compressed. Diagnosis is established by a positive MIBG scan. An adenoma secreting cortisol or aldosterone or a metastasis may have a similar appearance.

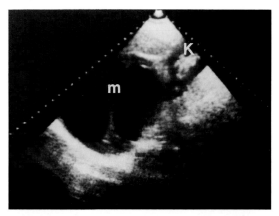

FIG. 9.16. Cystic pheochromocytoma: parasagittal scan. Large lobulated septated mass (*m*) is seen cephalad to upper pole of right kidney (*k*). This patient had a long history of headache and palpitation. He died from cardiovascular collapse during surgery. (Courtesy Dr. H.F.G. Seward, Group Health Centre, Sault Ste. Marie, Ontario, Canada.)

TABLE 9.3. *Distribution of extraadrenal pheochromocytoma*

Location	Percentage
Retroperitoneal sympathetic chain	44
Organ of Zückerkandl	22
Chest	19
Bladder wall	2
Multicentric	10

From Moulton and Moulton, ref. 25, with permission.

involvement was found in 25% of patients with systemic lymphoma (43).

Lymphomatous adrenal masses frequently appear sonographically as echo-poor lesions (Fig. 9.17), although a few may show a septated cystic appearance caused by intratumoral hemorrhage. The masses are bilateral in 50% of cases (43). Diagnosis is suspected in the appropriate clinical settings.

Adrenal Metastases

Metastases to the adrenals are common, detected in 27% of autopsied cancer patients (44). The most common primary sources are lung (33%) and breast carcinoma (30%) and melanoma. Fifteen percent of patients with bronchogenic carcinoma are found to have adrenal metastases on prospective CT studies (25). Virtually any type of malignancy can send secondaries to the adrenals (e.g., melanoma, colon, pancreas, kidney, thyroid).

The sonographic appearance of adrenal metastases is as pleomorphic as that demonstrated on CT scanning. Typically, they are multiple and small (<3 cm in diameter), or they may be single and large, attaining several centimeters diameter. They are bilateral in about 40% of cases (25). Most are hypoechoic, but a few may be hyper-

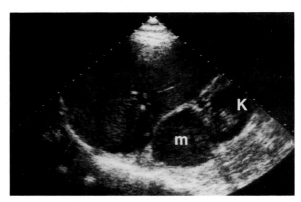

FIG. 9.18. Adrenal metastasis: oblique parasagittal scan. This metastasis (*m*) is seen in patient with bronchogenic carcinoma. Diagnosis was made by percutaneous fine needle aspiration biopsy. *IVC*, inferior vena cava; *K*, kidney.

echoic (Fig. 9.18). Some may show a complex texture caused by internal hemorrhage and calcification (44).

This leads to an interesting problem: the discovery of an adrenal mass in an oncology patient. What to do? It is well established that most adrenal masses found by ultrasound or CT in cancer patients are actually benign (adenoma or cysts) (25). A few recent reports claim that MRI and isotopes (NP-59) may differentiate a benign from a malignant adrenal mass (45). In practice, it is advised to perform a fine needle aspiration biopsy, which is a relatively safe and accurate procedure.

9.4 PITFALLS, ARTIFACTS, AND PRACTICAL TIPS

1. A large fatty neoplasm in the liver or right adrenal (e.g., liver lipoma, adrenal myelolipoma) will cause apparent disruption of the diaphragmatic echo. This is an artifact caused by changes in the propagation speed of the sound beam through the fatty tumor. This is discussed in detail in the section on the diaphragm (Chapter 2).

2. Cytology cannot distinguish a primary adrenocortical carcinoma from direct invasion of the adrenal gland by a renal cell carcinoma. Percutaneous aspiration biopsy is therefore not useful in this situation (46).

3. Metastases to the adrenal glands from bronchogenic carcinoma are missed in 17% of cases screened by CT scanning that show normal size adrenal glands (47).

4. Although a large number of adrenal masses found in oncology patients prove to be benign, such masses should be considered malignant until proven otherwise. A fine needle aspiration biopsy is usually indicated (48).

5. When performing percutaneous adrenal biopsy, one should always take precaution to deal with potentially fatal risk of blood pressure alteration in case of unsuspected pheochromocytoma (49).

6. In practice, CT is the preferred initial imaging mo-

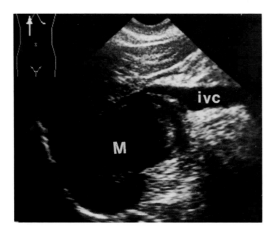

FIG. 9.17. Adrenal lymphoma: parasagittal scan. Note compression of IVC by large lobulated echo-poor mass (*M*). This is seen in a patient with disseminated non-Hodgkin's lymphoma. Lymphomatous masses are often sonolucent but solid. *IVC*, inferior vena cava.

dality for adults or for patients in whom there is strong clinical suspicion of adrenal pathology. Sonography performs better in neonates, children, and thin patients.

REFERENCES

Normal Anatomy

1. Lewis E, Kurtz AB, Dubbins PA, Wapner RJ, Goldberg BB. Real-time ultrasonographic evaluation of normal fetal adrenal glands. *J Ultrasound Med* 1982;1:265–270.
2. Scott EM, Thomas A, McGarrigle HHG, Lachelin GCL. Serial adrenal ultrasonography in normal neonates. *J Ultrasound Med* 1990;9:279–283.
3. Yeh H-C. Ultrasonography of the adrenals. *Semin Roentgenol* 1988;23:150–158.
4. Rifkin MD. Measurements of the normal adrenal gland. In: Goldberg B, Kurtz AB, eds. *Atlas of ultrasound measurements.* Chicago: Yearbook Medical Publishers; 1990:161–164.

Pathology

5. Mitty HA. Embryology, anatomy and anomalies of the adrenal gland. *Semin Roentgenol* 1988;23:271–279.
6. McGahan JP, Myracle MR. Adrenal hypertrophy: possible pitfall in the sonographic diagnosis of renal agenesis. *J Ultrasound Med* 1986;5:265–268.
7. Bryan PJ, Caldamone AA, Morrison SC, Yulish BS, Owens R. Ultrasound findings in the adreno-genital syndrome (congenital adrenal hyperplasia). *J Ultrasound Med* 1988;7:675–679.
8. Sivit CJ, Hung W, Taylor GA, et al. Sonography in neonatal congenital adrenal hyperplasia. *AJR* 1991;156:141–143.
9. Nissenbaum M, Jequier S. Enlargement of adrenal glands preceding adrenal hemorrhage. *J Clin Ultrasound* 1988;16:349–352.
10. Doppman JL, Miller DL, Dwyer AJ, et al. Macronodular adrenal hyperplasia in Cushing disease. *Radiology* 1988;166:347–352.
11. Morrison SC, Comisky E, Fletcher BD. Calcification in the adrenal glands associated with herpes simplex infection. *Pediatr Radiol* 1988;18:240–241.
12. Kenney PS, Stanley RJ. Calcified adrenal masses. *Urol Radiol* 1987;9:9–15.
13. Harrison RB, Franckle P Jr. Radiographic exhibit: radiographic finding in Wolman's disease. *Radiology* 1977;124:188.
14. Banagale RC, Donn SM. Asphyxia neonatorum. *J Family Pract* 1986;22:539–546.
15. Wolverson MK, Kannegiesser H. CT of bilateral adrenal hemorrhage with acute adrenal insufficiency in the adult. *AJR* 1984;142:311–314.
16. Pery M, Kaftori JK, Bar-Maor JA. Sonography for diagnosis and follow-up of neonatal adrenal hemorrhage. *JCU* 1981;9:397–401.
17. Mittlestaedt CA, Volberg FM, Merten DF, Brill PW. The sonographic diagnosis of neonatal adrenal hemorrhage. *Radiology* 1979;131:453–457.
18. Vezina CT, McLaughlin MJ, St. Louis EL, et al. Cystic lesions of the adrenals: diagnosis and management. *J Can Assoc Radiol* 1984;35:107–112.
19. Tung GA, Pfister RC, Papanicolaou N, Yoder IC. Adrenal cysts: imaging and percutaneous aspiration. *Radiology* 1989;173:107–110.
20. Wilson DA, Muchmore HG, Tisdal RG, Fahmy A, Pitha JV. Histoplasmosis of the adrenal glands studied by CT. *Radiology* 1984;150:779–783.
21. Yee ACN, Gopinath N, Ho C-S, Tao L-C. Fine-needle aspiration biopsy of adrenal tuberculosis. *J Can Assoc Radiol* 1986;37:287–289.
22. Atkinson GO Jr, Kodroff MB, Gay BB Jr, Ricketts RR. Adrenal abscesses in the neonate. *Radiology* 1985;155:101–104.
23. Musante F, Derchi LE, Zappasodi F, et al. Myelolipoma of the adrenal gland: sonographic and CT features. *AJR* 1988;151:961–964.
24. Gould JD, Mitty HA, Pertsemlidis D, Szporn AH. Adrenal myelolipoma: diagnosis by fine needle aspiration. *AJR* 1987;148:921–922.
25. Moulton JS, Moulton JS. CT of adrenal glands. *Semin Roentgenol* 1988;23:288–303.
26. Kumar R, David R, Sayle BA, Baniki LM. Adrenal scintigraphy. *Semin Roentgenol* 1988;23:243–249.
27. Davies RP, Lam AH. Adrenocortical neoplasm in children—ultrasound appearance. *J Ultrasound Med* 1987;6:325–328.
28. Chezman JL, Robbins SM, Nelson RC, Steinberg HV, Torres WE, Bernardino ME. Adrenal masses: characterization with T_1-weighted MR imaging. *Radiology* 1988;166:357–359.
29. Daneman A. Adrenal neoplasms in children. *Semin Roentgenol* 1988;23:205–215.
30. Daneman A, Chan HSL, Martin J. Adrenal carcinoma in children: a review of 17 patients. *Pediatr Radiol* 1983;13:11–18.
31. Altman AJ, Schwartz AD. Tumors of the sympathetic nervous system. In: *Malignant diseases of infancy, childhood and adolescence.* Philadelphia: WB Saunders; 1983:368–388.
32. Ferraro EM, Fakhry J, Aruny JE, Bracero LA. Prenatal adrenal neuroblastoma. Case report with review of the literature. *J Ultrasound Med* 1988;7:275–278.
33. Ruppert D, Lamki N, Fan S, Singleton EB. The many faces of neuroblastoma. *Radiographics* 1989;9:859–882.
34. Hartman DS, Sanders RC. Wilm's tumour versus neuroblastoma. Usefulness of ultrasound in differentiation. *J Ultrasound Med* 1982;1:117–122.
35. Saks JB, Bryan PJ, Yulish BS, Gauderer MWL, Haaga JR. Comparison of computed tomography and ultrasound in the evaluation of abdominal neuroblastoma. *JCU* 1985;13:641–645.
36. Johnson CM, Welch TJ, Hattery RR, Sheedy PF II. CT of the adrenal medulla. *Semin Ultrasound CT MR* 1985;6:219–240.
37. van Gils APG, Falke THM, van Erkel AR, et al. MR imaging and MIBG scintigraphy of pheochromocytomas and extra-adrenal functioning paragangliomas. *Radiographics* 1991;11:37–57.
38. Lembke T, Greenberg H. Cystic pheochromocytoma with inadvertent needle biopsy and glucagon administration. *J Can Assoc Radiol* 1987;38:232–233.
39. Quint LE, Glazer GM, Francis IR, Shapiro B, Chenevert TL. Pheochromocytoma and paraganglioma: comparison of MR imaging with CT and I-131 MIBG scintigraphy. *Radiology* 1987;165:89–93.
40. Puvareswary M, Davoren P. Pheochromocytoma of the bladder: ultrasound appearance. *JCU* 1991;19:111–115.
41. Vicks BS, Perusek M, Johnson J, Tio F. Primary adrenal lymphoma: CT and sonographic appearance. *JCU* 1987;15:135–139.
42. Cunningham JJ. Ultrasonic findings in "primary" lymphoma of the adrenal area. *J Ultrasound Med* 1983;2:467–469.
43. Antoniou A, Spetseropoulos J, Vlahos L, et al. The sonographic appearance of adrenal involvement in non-Hodgkin's lymphoma. *J Ultrasound Med* 1983;2:235–236.
44. Gooding GAW. Ultrasonic spectrum of adrenal masses. *Urology* 1979;13:211–214.
45. Francis IR, Smid A, Gross MD, et al. Adrenal masses in oncologic patients: functional and morphologic evaluation. *Radiology* 1988;166:353–356.

Pitfalls, Artifacts, and Practical Tips

46. Koenker RM, Mueller PR, van Sonnenberg E. Interventional radiology of the adrenal glands. *Semin Roentgenol* 1988;23:314–322.
47. Pagari JJ. Normal adrenal glands in small cell lung carcinoma: CT guided biopsy. *AJR* 1983;140:949–951.
48. Glazer HS, Weyman PJ, Sagel SS, Levitt RG, McClennan BL. Nonfunctioning adrenal masses: incidental discovery on computed tomography. *AJR* 1982;139:81–85.
49. Casola G, Nicolet V, van Sonnenberg E, et al. Unsuspected pheochromocytoma: risk of blood pressure alterations during percutaneous adrenal biopsy. *Radiology* 1986;159:733–735.

The Retroperitoneal Blood Vessels

10.1 AORTA

Scanning Techniques

The patient is scanned during quiet respiration in the supine position. The probe is placed on the anterior abdominal wall in the epigastrium, and transverse scan planes are used to localize the aorta. The aorta is traced from the diaphragm to the bifurcation by moving the probe along the abdominal wall. This allows a rapid and accurate initial assessment of the position, size, and morphology of the entire abdominal aorta and surrounding soft-tissue structures (e.g., lymph nodes, IVC, spine, major arterial branches). Sagittal scans are then used to examine the long axis once the course of the aorta has been determined in the transverse scans.

In some cases bowel contents obscure the mid and distal abdominal aorta and iliac arteries. Frequently, graded pressure with the probe will displace the bowel and allow visualization of the aorta. If this does not succeed, coronal scanning with the probe placed in the left or right midaxillary line will demonstrate the aorta. It is usually possible to examine the entire abdominal aorta adequately from one or more of these vantage points. Coronal scans with the patient lying on their right or left side may also be useful.

For PW Doppler interrogation, the aorta is imaged in either sagittal or coronal scan planes. Then the Doppler sample volume is placed in the center of the lumen with the Doppler angle at 60° or less. Color Doppler allows a rapid qualitative assessment of blood flow in the aorta, and the color may be used to guide placement of the PW sample volume in the lumen.

Normal Anatomy

The abdominal aorta is a pulsatile tubular structure, which is round or oval in cross section (Fig. 10.1). The aorta tapers from the diaphragm (mean diameter = 2.3 cm) to the bifurcation (mean diameter = 1.5 cm). The range of normal diameters in the upper abdominal aorta in adults is 1.5 to 2.5 cm (1). The aorta lies anterior to the spine and just to the left of midline. The distance between the posterior aortic wall and ossified vertebral bodies is less than or equal to 0.5 cm (Fig. 10.1) (1). The wall of the aorta is moderately echogenic and thin (1–2-mm thickness). The diameters of the aorta are measured from exterior wall to exterior wall (Fig. 10.1). On real-time ultrasound, one observes symmetric outward expansion of all aortic wall surfaces with ventricular systole.

The first major branch of the abdominal aorta is the celiac artery, which arises from the anterior aspect of the aorta cranial to the pancreatic body, and it gives rise to the common hepatic, left gastric, and splenic arteries (Fig. 10.2). These can be visualized in virtually every patient. One centimeter caudal to the celiac artery, the SMA arises anteriorly at the level of the pancreatic body. The inferior mesenteric artery also arises anteriorly, just cranial to the aortic bifurcation, but this is not routinely visualized in abdominal sonograms (Fig. 10.2).

Abbreviations: **CDU,** color Doppler ultrasound; **IVC,** inferior vena cava; **LLD,** left lateral decubitus; **PW Doppler,** pulse wave Doppler; **RLD,** right lateral decubitus; **SMA,** superior mesenteric artery.

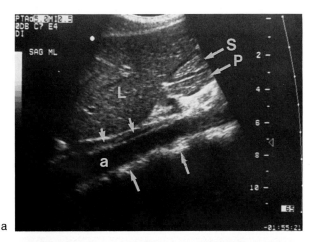

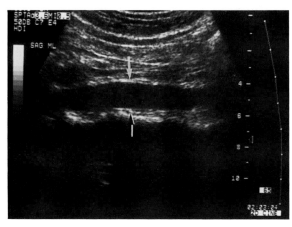

FIG. 10.1. Normal abdominal aorta. **a:** sagittal scan of proximal abdominal aorta (*a*) demonstrates vertebral bodies (*large arrows*) posterior to aorta. Crus of diaphragm (*small arrows*) is anterior to aorta. *L*, liver; *S*, stomach; *P*, pancreas. **b:** sagittal scan of distal abdominal aorta. *Arrows* demarcate exterior margins of aortic wall. **c:** transverse scan of the proximal abdominal aorta. Aorta (*a*) and IVC (*i*) lie anterior to spine (*arrows*). *L*, liver. *Curved arrow*, crus of diaphragm.

The renal arteries are the two lateral aortic branches that can be visualized in many patients. These arise 1 to 2 cm caudal to the SMA origin and are best seen at their origins in transverse scan planes, with the probe on the anterior abdominal wall (Fig. 10.3). The right renal artery courses posterior to the IVC, and it is often visualized on transverse and longitudinal scans of the IVC (Fig. 10.3). Coronal scan planes with the probe placed along the right or left midaxillary line may also demonstrate the origins of the renal arteries (Fig. 10.3).

Normal Doppler

Color Doppler ultrasound and PW Doppler can be used to assess blood flow in virtually all pediatric and adult patients. Color Doppler ultrasound is useful for quick qualitative assessment of blood flow in the aorta and its major branches. Note that the color represents the *average Doppler frequency* and *not peak velocity.* Color Doppler ultrasound may detect blood flow in branches that are not visible by imaging alone, and this serves as a guide for placement of the PW Doppler sample volume.

The PW velocity–time profile changes from the proximal abdominal aorta to the distal aorta. Proximal to the celiac axis, the velocity waveform demonstrates a high systolic velocity peak and low forward diastolic flow. The curve has a clear window below it (Fig. 10.4), and this reflects the "plug" flow in the aorta: the blood flow velocity is almost the same from the center of the lumen out to the vessel walls (2).

Below the renal arteries the velocity in late diastole decreases, and more distally in the aorta there is flow reversal because of the high impedance of blood flow to the muscles of the legs (Fig. 10.4). This rebound of blood helps kidney perfusion. During exercise of the legs, peripheral resistance decreases, and this allows forward flow during diastole in the distal aorta.

Pathology

Atherosclerosis

Atherosclerosis is the most common pathology of the abdominal aorta in ultrasound practice. In milder cases, calcifications are present in the aortic wall (Fig. 10.5), and larger plaques may impinge into the lumen. The aorta is often mildly dilated (i.e., ectatic) and tortuous. Intraluminal thrombus may also be present even with mild dilatation.

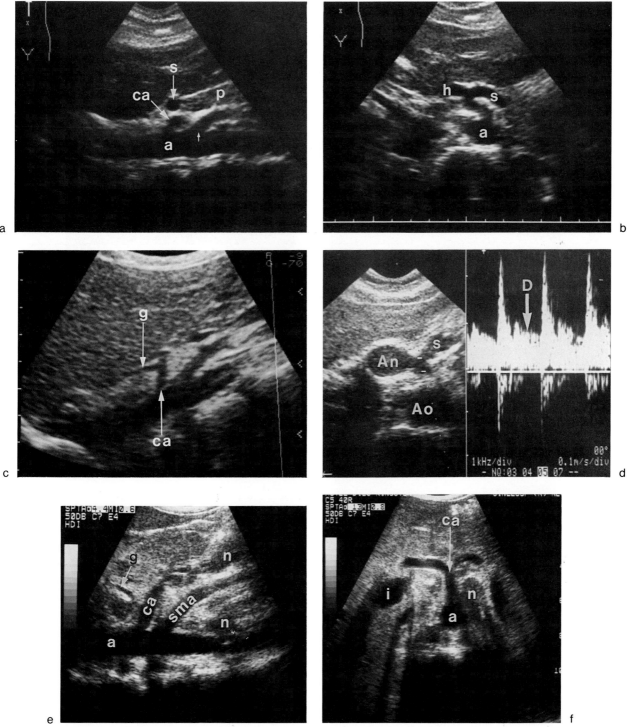

FIG. 10.2. Anterior branches of abdominal aorta. (*See color images of parts **g–l** in color plate section B, which follows page 242.*) **a:** celiac artery and superior mesenteric artery. Sagittal scan demonstrates origin of SMA (*arrow*) and celiac artery (*ca*). *a*, aorta; *p*, pancreas; *s*, splenic artery. **b:** celiac axis. Transverse scan demonstrates tortuous celiac artery (*ca*) arising from aorta (*a*) and branching into common hepatic artery (*h*) and splenic artery (*s*). **c:** left gastric artery. Sagittal scan demonstrates proximal left gastric artery (*g*) arising from celiac artery (*ca*). **d:** aneurysm of common hepatic artery. Transverse scan of celiac axis demonstrates an aneurysm (*An*) of proximal common hepatic artery. Doppler cursor is in celiac artery. Doppler spectrum demonstrates forward flow in systole and diastole (*D*). *s*, splenic artery; *Ao*, aorta. **e:** celiac artery and sma with lymphadenopathy. Multiple enlarged lymph nodes (*n*) surround celiac artery (*ca*) and SMA (*sma*). Note small left gastric artery (*g*). *a*, aorta. (**f**) celiac axis with lymphadenopathy. Transverse scan of same patient as **e** demonstrates enlarged lymph nodes (*n*) stretching celiac artery (*ca*) and its branches. *a*, aorta; *i*, IVC. **g:** color Doppler of celiac axis and SMA: diastole. Sagittal scan during ventricular diastole demonstrates forward blood flow (red) in aorta, celiac artery, and superior mesenteric artery. Note white in center of celiac artery, indicating higher velocity in center of lumen compared with edges of lumen. Note also blue color in left gastric artery, which arises from celiac axis. Blue indicates flow away from probe.

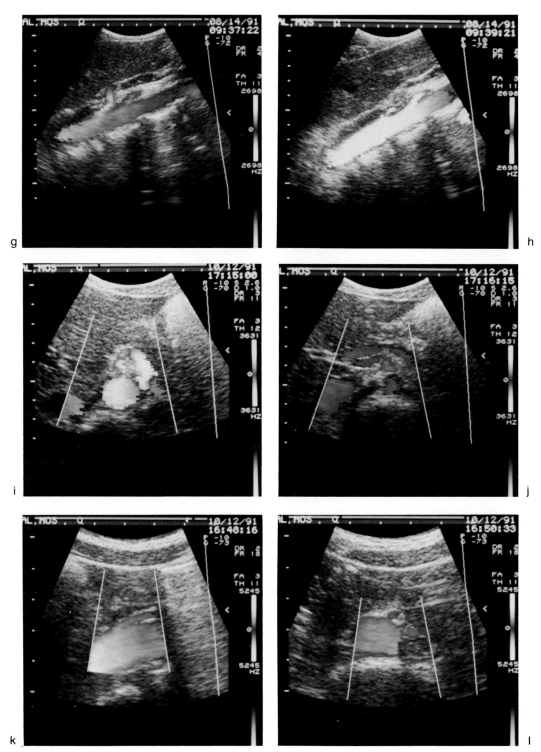

FIG. 10.2. *continued.* **h:** color Doppler of celiac axis and SMA: systole. Sagittal scan during ventricular systole demonstrates higher velocity flow (white versus red) in aorta and superior mesenteric artery. Celiac artery is less well visualized in this scan. **i:** celiac axis—missing hepatic artery (color). Transverse scan demonstrates forward flow in celiac artery (red) and splenic artery (blue because artery courses away from probe). Common hepatic artery is absent (see g). **j:** SMA—replaced common hepatic artery. Transverse scan through proximal SMA demonstrates common hepatic artery arising from right side of SMA and coursing toward porta hepatis (see i). **k:** inferior mesenteric artery: sagittal, color Doppler. Sagittal scan of distal aorta demonstrates origin of IMA at anterior aspect of aorta with forward flow (red) in both vessels. **l:** IMA: transverse, color Doppler. Transverse scan through distal aorta demonstrates IMA along anterior aspect of aorta. Blood flow is toward probe (red) because probe was angled toward head. (Scans c, i, j, k, and l are courtesy of Mr. Tyler Sauerbrei.)

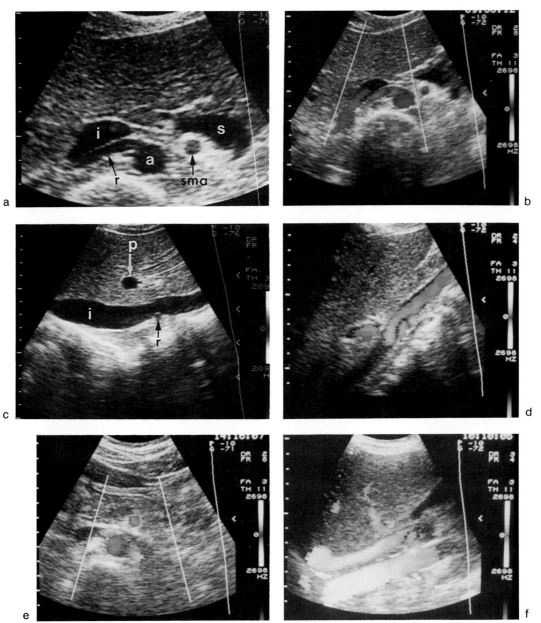

FIG. 10.3. Normal right renal artery. (*See color images of parts **b, d–f** in color plate section B, which follows page 242.*) **a:** transverse scan of upper abdominal aorta (*a*) demonstrates right renal artery (*r*) originating from aorta and coursing posterior to IVC (*i*). There was congenital absence of left kidney and left renal artery in this patient. *s*, splenic vein; *sma*, superior mesenteric artery. **b:** Right renal artery: transverse, color Doppler same patient as a. Flow in proximal right renal artery is coded red because it is toward the probe. Flow in portion of artery behind IVC is blue because it is away from probe. Note red flow (i.e., toward probe, away from right kidney) in right renal vein into IVC. **c:** IVC and right renal artery: sagittal. Sagittal scan of IVC (*i*) demonstrates right renal artery (*r*) posterior to IVC. Right portal vein (*p*) lies anterior to IVC in liver parenchyma. **d:** IVC and right renal artery: sagittal, CDU. Flow in IVC is coded blue because it is away from probe, toward heart. Flow in right renal artery behind IVC is also coded blue because it is away from probe in this case. Red color adjacent to right renal artery represents swirling blood flow in IVC after stream passes over artery. Note also blue coded flow in portal vein anterior to IVC. **e:** Right and left renal arteries: transverse, color Doppler. Origins of right and left renal arteries are visualized and blood flow (blue) is away from probe. Note also flow in SMV (blue) and SMA (red). **f:** Right and left renal arteries: coronal, CDU. Scan through right hepatic lobe demonstrates blood flow in IVC (blue) and aorta (red). Flow in right renal artery (adjacent to IVC) is red (toward probe), whereas flow in origin of left renal artery is a small patch of blue (away from probe). Red flow adjacent to blue is left renal vein (flow toward probe and toward IVC).

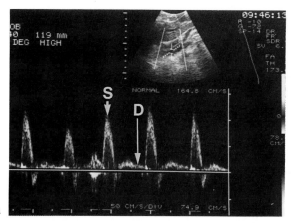 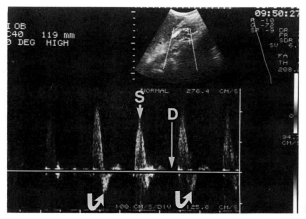

FIG. 10.4. Doppler spectrum of aortic blood flow. **a:** Doppler spectrum of blood flow in proximal abdominal aorta demonstrates continuous antegrade flow in late diastole (*D*). *S*, peak systolic velocity. **b:** Doppler spectrum of blood flow in distal aorta (distal to renal arteries) demonstrates absence of blood flow in late diastole (*D*). *Curved arrows*, reversal of blood flow in early diastole. *S*, systole.

Aortic Aneurysm

Aneurysms of the aorta (i.e., aortic diameter >3 cm) (see Table 10.1) are mainly due to atherosclerosis, although a small number are due to syphilis or trauma. Aneurysms are most common in people older than 50 years of age, and they are more common in men. Aneurysms most commonly involve the mid or distal abdominal aorta (i.e., between the origins of the renal arteries and the aortic bifurcation), but aneurysms may also involve the proximal abdominal aorta (including the origins of the renal arteries, SMA, and celiac artery) or even extend into the thorax (thoracoabdominal aneurysm). Distal aneurysms commonly extend into one or both common iliac arteries and occasionally beyond (into external or internal iliac arteries). Uncommonly, a patient may have iliac aneurysms without an aortic aneurysm.

The main roles of ultrasound in aneurysm assessment are:

1. to determine the proximal and distal extent of the aneurysm
2. to measure the maximum cross-sectional diameter of the aneurysm accurately

The distal extent of the aneurysm is defined with respect to the bifurcation. The aneurysm may end cranial to the bifurcation (Fig. 10.6), end at the bifurcation, or extend into the common iliac arteries, in which case the iliac artery diameters are measured. The proximal extent is defined with respect to the renal artery origins. Because the renal arteries are not routinely visualized, we use the SMA as a landmark and note the distance between the SMA origin and neck of the aneurysm (Fig. 10.6). The SMA origin is usually 1 to 2 cm proximal to

FIG. 10.5. Atheroma of the abdominal aorta. Sagittal scan of aorta. Atheroma cause increased echogenicity and irregularity of aortic walls (*arrows*). No significant stenosis is present.

TABLE 10.1. *Work sheet for aortic aneurysm*

Proximal extent	
Distance between SMA and neck	
of aneurysm	_____cm
Distal extent	
Distance between bifurcation and	
caudal end of aneurysm	_____cm
Aneurysm measurements	
Length	_____cm
Maximum width	_____cm
Maximum anteroposterior diameter	_____cm
Maximum oblique diameter	_____cm
Common iliac arteries	
Right maximum diameter	_____cm
Left maximum diameter	_____cm
Aneurysm thrombus	
Location _____	
Residual lumen diameter	
Anteroposterior	_____cm
Width	_____cm

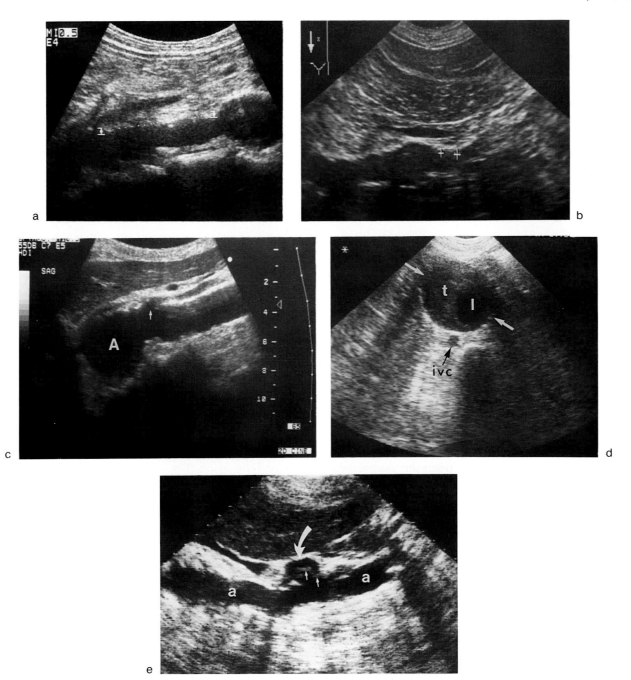

FIG. 10.6. Abdominal aortic aneurysm. **a:** Distance between SMA and aneurysm. Calipers demonstrate distance between origin of SMA and neck of aneurysm. **b:** Distance between aneurysm and bifurcation. Calipers demonstrate distance between distal end of aneurysm and bifurcation into right and left common iliac arteries. **c:** Sagittal scan demonstrates an aortic aneurysm (*A*) proximal to origin of SMA (*arrow*). Aorta distal to SMA is normal in size. **d:** Transverse scan of distal aorta in another patient demonstrates an eccentrically dilated abdominal aorta containing thrombus (*t*). *l*, patent lumen; *ivc*, inferior vena cava. Note that largest diameter lies in an oblique plane and not in anteroposterior nor transverse direction. *Arrows* indicate maximum diameter. **e:** Eccentric saccular aortic aneurysm. Sagittal scan demonstrates an unusual focal aneurysm (*curved arrow*) arising from anterior aspect of abdominal aorta (*a*). Note thrombus (*arrows*) in anterior aspect of aneurysm.

the renal artery origins and thus serves as a marker for renal artery locations (3). In our experience, if the SMA is uninvolved by the aneurysm, a standard repair can be completed with the occasional use of supraceliac clamping (3). When the distance between the SMA origin and the aneurysm neck was less than 3 cm, suprarenal/supraceliac clamping was required in 15% of patients. When the distance was 3 cm or more, suprarenal clamping was necessary in less than 1% of patients.

The diameter of the aneurysm is measured from outer wall to outer wall (Fig. 10.6). This is the same technique as used for CT scans and correlates very well with operative findings (4). A true transverse scan of the aorta (i.e., perpendicular to the long axis of the aorta) at its largest will give an image from which the anteroposterior diameter, the width, and oblique diameters are measured. The maximum diameter may be any of these, but it is often the width. We also measure the maximum anteroposterior diameter in sagittal scans for confirmation.

Other observations made in aortic aneurysms are the presence of intraluminal thrombus and the diameters of the residual patent lumen (Fig. 10.7). Thrombus may be almost echo-free (fresh thrombus) or moderately echogenic (organized clot) (Figs. 10.6 and 10.7) (5). Thrombus often collects anteriorly and laterally. The residual lumen may become very small and rarely may become occluded (Fig. 10.7b,c). The interface between thrombus and fluid blood may form a thin echogenic line that can simulate a dissected aortic intima, but the localized nature of this echo inside the aneurysm and the lack of movement of the echo are signs that favor intraluminal thrombus.

For an aneurysm between 3 and 4.5 cm in diameter, repeat scans are obtained at yearly intervals and the maximum diameter is obtained with the same scan planes and same measurement techniques as the previous scans. The average growth rate for aortic aneurysms between 3- and 5.9-cm diameter is about 0.25 cm/year (6,6A). For aneurysms larger than 5 cm in diameter, expansion rates are estimated to be 0.34 to 0.72 cm/year (6A). In our center, a baseline CT is performed once the aneurysm diameter reaches 4.5 cm, and elective surgery is recommended when the maximum diameter exceeds 5 cm.

Aortic Rupture

For aneurysms less than 5-cm maximum diameter, the rupture rate is less than 1% (7). Rupture of the abdominal aorta most commonly occurs in aneurysms greater than 5 cm in diameter. If the aneurysm is greater than 6 cm in diameter, there is 50% 1-year mortality and if greater than 7 cm, there is 75% 1-year mortality (7). The mortality for elective aneurysm surgery is approximately 5%.

In acute rupture of an aortic aneurysm, ultrasound and CT will demonstrate a retroperitoneal mass or fluid collection along the exterior edge of the aorta, extending into one or both pararenal spaces (Fig. 10.8). A large hematoma may displace one or both kidneys, extend along the psoas muscles, and also extend into the pararenal spaces (8). Computed tomography is significantly better at detecting and delineating retroperitoneal hemorrhage than ultrasound in most patients, but ultrasound may be the first imaging test performed, and some of the hemorrhage is usually visible. With acute aortic rupture and severe abdominal pain, the accompanying ileus impairs ultrasound visualization of the retroperitoneum.

A false aneurysm (or pseudoaneurysm) of the abdominal aorta is an uncommon abnormality that represents a walled-off periaortic hematoma that communicates with the aortic lumen. The pseudoaneurysm may be eccentric, and it may cause pressure erosion on neighboring vertebrae (9,10).

Aortic Dissection

In aortic dissection, intimal lining of the aorta separates from the rest of the wall. The process usually starts in the thoracic aorta and may extend into the abdominal aorta and thus be identified in abdominal sonography. Type A involves the ascending thoracic aorta and type B starts at the origin of the left subclavian artery.

Ultrasound demonstrates an intraluminal thin flap that moves with the aortic pulsations, because fluid blood is in the true lumen and the false lumen (the false lumen is the space between the dissected intima and the aortic wall) (Fig. 10.9) (11). Doppler demonstrates arterial blood flow in both true and false lumens, and it may be impossible to distinguish the two lumens (12). Dynamic CT or angiography are performed to evaluate the extent and location of the dissection with respect to the major aortic branches in the chest and abdomen.

Aortic Grafts

In aortic grafts, the proximal part is a single synthetic tube that is anastomosed to the proximal aorta. The distal portion comprises two sleeves that are anastomosed to the common iliac, external iliac, or femoral arteries. If the proximal anastomosis is end-to-side, the proximal graft lies anterior to the native aorta. If the aneurysm is removed and the proximal anastomosis is end-to-end, the graft lies in the position of the abdominal aorta. If the graft is placed within the native aneurysm and a proximal end-to-end anastomosis is performed, the graft will be surrounded by blood and serous fluid within the native aneurysm (Fig. 10.10).

Ultrasound is useful in assessing graft complications including false aneurysms, hemorrhage, infection,

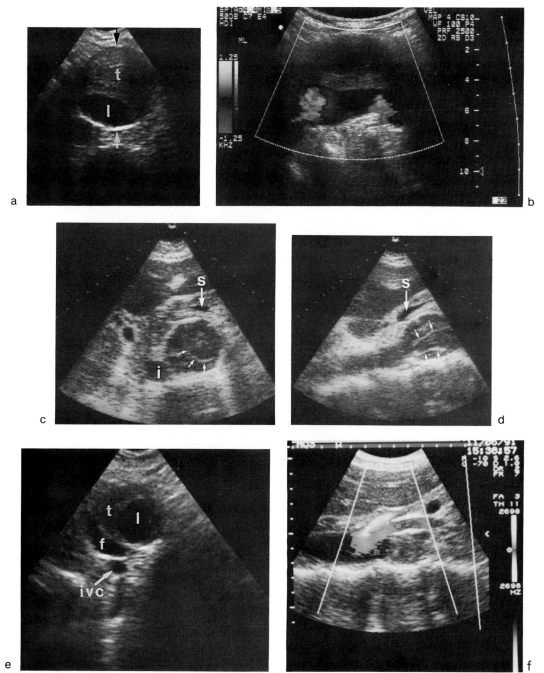

FIG. 10.7. Thrombosis in aortic aneurysms. (*See color images of parts **b** and **f** in color plate section B, which follows page 242.*) **a:** Transverse scan demonstrates thrombus (*t*) in anterior portion of aneurysm. Anterior and posterior walls of aorta are well defined, whereas lateral walls are poorly defined. Therefore width is more difficult to measure accurately than anteroposterior diameter. *l*, patent lumen. **b:** CDU of aortic aneurysm. CDU demonstrates blood flow (red and blue) in residual lumen of aneurysm. Large amount of clot occupies anterior portion of aneurysm. Note lack of color in middle of scan of lumen because ultrasound beam is perpendicular to direction of blood flow. **c and d:** Transverse and sagittal scans of an aortic aneurysm with complete thrombosis of lumen. This patient had poor left ventricular function, and slow blood flow predisposed to thrombosis of aortic lumen. *arrows*, margins of recent thrombus formation within "patent lumen"; *s*, splenic vein; *i*, inferior vena cava. **e:** Recanalization of intraluminal thrombus, mimicking a periaortic fluid collection. Cescent-shaped fluid collection (*f*) represents a blood-filled channel between intraluminal thrombus (*t*) and wall of the aorta. No periaortic fluid collection was found at surgery. *ivc*, inferior vena cava; *l*, patent lumen. **f:** Total occlusion of aorta by thrombus. CDU demonstrates blood flow in proximal aortic lumen (red) and in two major anterior branches (celiac artery and SMA). Just interior to SMA origin, aortic lumen is filled with thrombus. There was no evidence of flow in distal aorta.

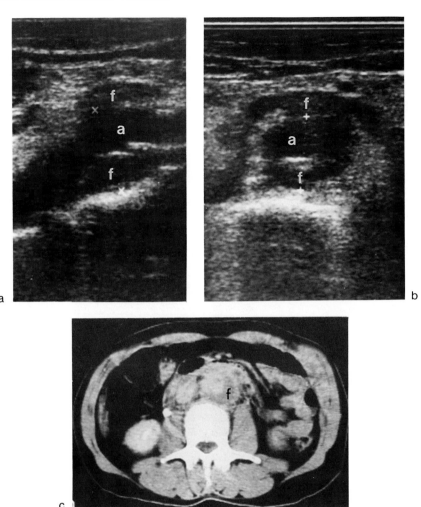

FIG. 10.8. Periaortic fluid collection. **a:** Sagittal scan of midabdominal aorta demonstrates a fluid collection (*f*) anterior and posterior to abdominal aorta. *a*, aortic lumen. **b:** Transverse scan of abdominal aorta. *f*, periaortic fluid collection; *a*, aortic lumen. **c:** CT scan of abdominal aorta demonstrates a low-density fluid collection (*f*) around abdominal aorta. At surgery a periaortic abscess (streptococcus) was found. In ultrasound and CT imaging in this patient, it is impossible to distinguish between a periaortic hematoma and an abscess.

occlusion, and graft failure. A false aneurysm (or pseudo aneurysm) represents a walled-off blood-filled space that communicates with the arterial lumen, usually at the site of anastomosis. These most commonly occur at the femoral artery anastomosis and not in the aorta or iliac arteries. Real-time ultrasound will demonstrate synchronous pulsatility of the arterial and pseudoaneurysm walls. Doppler interrogation reveals blood flow within the pseudoaneurysm. Graft failure (rare) will manifest as focal or diffuse enlargement of the graft itself.

The development of a new fluid collection around or adjacent to a graft may be due to hematoma, seroma, or abscess. Needle aspiration may be required to differentiate. If bubbles of gas are present around the graft, this suggests abscess, although gas may be present in the week after graft placement and not represent infection.

Graft occlusion may be diagnosed with CDU or PW Doppler. Present ultrasound systems can reliably demonstrate normal arterial blood flow within the deep and superficial components of the graft system. The absence of observable blood flow indicates an occlusion or a high-grade stenosis. Angiography may be required to distinguish between occlusion and a tight stenosis.

Pitfalls, Artifacts, and Practical Tips

Measuring Aortic Aneurysms

The width of the aneurysm is less accurate than the anteroposterior diameter because the beam is parallel to the lateral aortic walls, and thus the lateral walls are often poorly defined (Fig. 10.7a). Unfortunately, the aneurysm width is often the maximum diameter, and there-

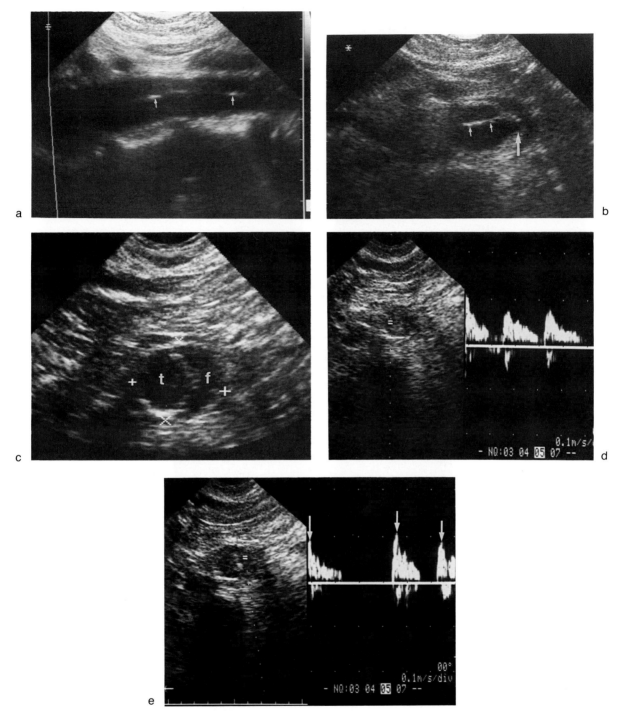

FIG. 10.9. Aortic dissection. **a:** Sagittal scan demonstrates a thin membrane (*arrows*) in anterior half of aorta. **b:** Transverse scan of same patient demonstrates membrane (*arrows*) anterior to origin of left renal artery (*arrow*). True lumen lies posterior to membrane, and therefore blood flow into the left renal artery is unaffected. **c:** Transverse scan of another patient with aortic dissection. Dissected intima lies in a sagittal plane separating true lumen (*t*) from false lumen (*f*). **d:** Duplex Doppler scan of the same patient as c demonstrates a normal velocity spectrum in true lumen of aorta. **e:** Duplex Doppler of false lumen also demonstrates pulsatile blood flow within this space. This implies that blood is flowing from true lumen through intima, into false lumen, and then out through another hole in intima more distally, back into true lumen. *Arrows*, systolic velocities.

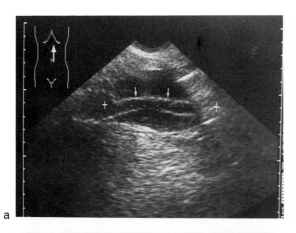

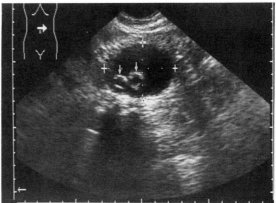

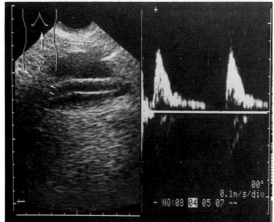

FIG. 10.10. Aortic graft within native aneurysm. **a:** Sagittal scan of aortic aneurysm demonstrates graft material (*arrows*) lying within the aneurysm. **b:** Transverse scan of same patient demonstrates two limbs of aortic grafts (*arrows*) lying within the aortic aneurysm, which is outlined by cursors (+). **c:** Sagittal duplex Doppler scan of same patient demonstrates an arterial spectrum within the lumen of the graft.

fore there is an inherent inaccuracy in measuring maximum diameter in these cases.

If the transverse scan is obliqued in any fashion, the width or anteroposterior measurements will be falsely high. It is therefore useful to also measure the maximum anteroposterior diameter in sagittal scans. Sagittal scans allow a better appreciation of the location of the maximum anteroposterior diameter in the length of the aneurysm (Fig. 10.6).

The measured aortic diameter can be incorrect because the calipers are not placed at the outer edge of the aortic wall. The anterior and posterior walls are usually well defined, and the exterior margins are usually visible even if the walls are thickened because of atheroma (Fig. 10.5). Therefore, accurate anteroposterior diameter measurements are possible in most patients.

The biggest problem for aortic ultrasound is to measure aneurysm size in sequential scans in a consistent and accurate fashion. With CT, sequential measurements are consistent and accurate because scan planes are reproducible. Real-time ultrasound scan planes are more difficult to reproduce and there is a tendency to measure the aneurysm in different places on sequential scans (*especially* if different technologists and different radiologists are involved). To minimize these deficien-

cies, it is important to perform sequential scans utilizing the same scan techniques, to measure the outer wall diameter and to measure the aneurysm in the same location in sequential scans. To this end, the sonographer should obtain two or three sets of transverse and sagittal scans through the largest portion of the aneurysm and label these appropriately. Electronic calipers can be used to measure the anteroposterior diameters, widths, and oblique diameters, but the reporting radiologist will make the final decision regarding diameter measurements by assessing these scan results, by using hand-held calipers if necessary and by comparing with previous scans.

Dissection Versus Intraluminal Thrombus

The interface between fluid blood and a hypoechoic intraluminal thrombus is a thin line on ultrasound that may mimic a dissection. If the thin line represents a dissection membrane however, real-time ultrasound will demonstrate a mobile membrane, and Doppler will demonstrate blood flow on both sides of the thin line. If the false lumen becomes thrombosed, distinction may be impossible.

Retroaortic Fat

When copious retroperitoneal fat is present, there may be more than 0.5 cm of fat interposed between the posterior aortic wall and the lumbar spine. One must then distinguish between fat and other material such as lymphadenopathy and fluid collections (Fig. 10.11). In some circumstances, a CT scan may be required (Fig. 10.11).

Aortic Position

The aorta may lie in midline or slightly to the right of midline instead of slightly to the left of midline. This is especially true when the aorta is atheromatous and tortuous.

Pseudo Double Aorta

Occasionally, transverse scans of the abdomen with the probe placed on the midline will produce a duplicated aorta because of beam refractions at the interface between the rectus abdominis muscles and the collection of fat deep to the linea alba (Fig. 10.12). This is the same phenomenon that causes duplication artifacts in pelvic sonography (13).

Proximal Extent of Aortic Aneurysm

If the aortic dilatation involves the aorta proximal to the SMA, one must assess the aorta up to the level of the diaphragm. If the dilatation extends to the diaphragm, a CT of the chest is required to assess the proximal extent.

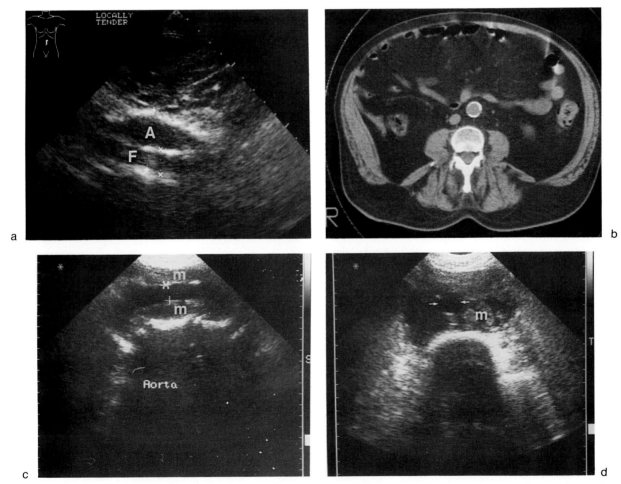

FIG. 10.11. Retroaortic fat. **a:** sagittal scan of abdominal aorta demonstrates excess soft tissue (*F*) between abdominal aorta (*A*) and spine posteriorly. **b:** CT scan of same patient as a demonstrates that soft tissue between aorta and spine is retroperitoneal fat and not a tumor. **c** and **d:** sagittal and transverse scan of another (d) patient demonstrating excess soft tissue (*m*) between aorta and spine. This soft tissue was periaortic lymphadenopathy caused by lymphoma. Note also soft tissue (*m*) anterior to aorta. *Arrows*, lateral margins of aorta.

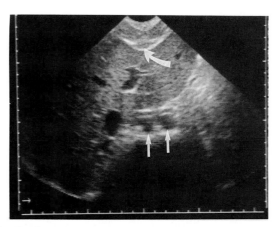

FIG. 10.12. Split image artifact. Transverse scan of upper abdominal aorta apparently demonstrates two aortas (*arrows*); however, scans performed just to right of midline confirm that only one aorta was present. Apparent double aorta is due to a refraction artifact from collection of fat (*curved arrow*) deep to rectus abdominis muscles.

Retroaortic Renal Vein

Occasionally renal anomalies are present in association with an aneurysm. If the left renal vein or branch thereof passes posterior to the aorta, this will affect the surgical approach for aneurysm repair. This information must be conveyed to the surgeon in a timely manner.

10.2 INFERIOR VENA CAVA

Scanning Techniques

The intrahepatic portion of the IVC can be visualized with real-time ultrasound in virtually all adults and children in the supine position during quiet respiration. Re-spiratory expiration will distend the IVC and make it more obvious. Sagittal scans are obtained with the probe on the right anterior abdominal wall and coronal scans with the probe in an intercostal space in the right mid-axillary line. For transverse scans of the IVC, the probe is placed on the anterior abdominal wall and swept caudally to the common iliac veins.

The infrahepatic portion of the IVC may be more difficult to visualize because of overlying bowel gas and the smaller caliber of the IVC distally. Coronal views through the right kidney are often useful in these cases.

Doppler scans are obtained in sagittal or coronal scan planes with the PW sample volume in the center of the IVC lumen and the Doppler angle at 60° or less. Color Doppler ultrasound assessment may be performed in longitudinal and transverse scans. The color flow is often best elicited in transverse scan planes, with the scan plane tilted toward the patient's head or feet. This maneuver will decrease the Doppler angle and accentuate Doppler shifts in the sound frequency.

Normal Anatomy

The IVC is formed by the merging of the right and left common iliac veins along the anterior aspect of vertebral body L_5, just to the right of midline. From this position, the IVC courses cranially just to the right of midline along the lumbar vertebral column. At the L_2 level it passes behind the pancreatic head and then posterior to the portal vein before entering the liver. The IVC courses slightly anteriorly before passing through the diaphragm to enter the right atrium (Fig. 10.13).

The major tributaries visible on ultrasound and CT are the common iliac veins, the renal veins, and the main

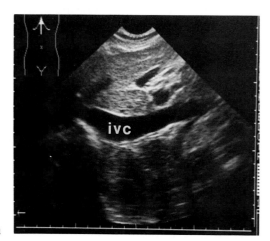

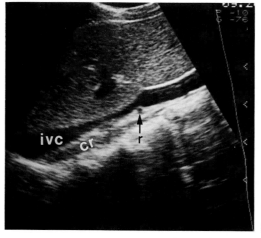

FIG. 10.13. Normal IVC during active expiration. **a:** inferior vena cava (*ivc*) is prominent but normal. Relative enlargement is a normal finding during active expiration. Note course of IVC as it approaches the diaphragm. IVC courses anteriorly as it approaches the right atrium. **b:** normal IVC during active inspiration. IVC is almost collapsed during normal active inspiration. Note right renal artery (*r*) posterior to IVC and hypoechoic band of tissue posterior to right renal artery corresponding to crus of the diaphragm (*cr*).

hepatic veins. The renal veins lie anterior to the renal arteries and enter the IVC at the L_2–L_3 level. The main hepatic veins enter the intrahepatic IVC just beneath the diaphragm, before the IVC enters the right atrium.

The size of the IVC changes with the respiratory and cardiac cycles, with valsalva, and with patient position (14,15). The size of the IVC is decreased with inspiration and valsalva and increased with expiration and suspended respiration after maximum inspiration. Inspiration creates a negative pressure in the chest and draws blood out of the IVC into the right atrium and thus decreases the IVC size. Valsalva is the contraction of abdominal wall muscles (after full inspiration) that increases intra-abdominal pressure, which, in turn, forces blood out of the IVC into the chest (Fig. 10.13).

Nakao et al. (16) examined the anteroposterior diameter of the IVC in RLD, supine, and LLD positions in adults. The IVC was measured 5 cm caudal to the diaphragm during the expiratory phase of respiration. The mean diameter (±SD) in these positions was

RLD 22 (±3.0) mm
Supine 15 (±5.0) mm
LLD 7.0 (±3.0) mm

In the LLD position, an IVC diameter of more than 10 mm was associated with raised right atrial pressure (i.e., >8 mm Hg) (predictive accuracy 95%, sensitivity 84%, specificity 96%).

Normal Doppler

Color Doppler ultrasound is sensitive in detecting the presence of flow in the IVC and the direction. Pulse wave Doppler is performed in a long-axis scan (sagittal or coronal) through the IVC with the Doppler angle less than 60° if possible. The velocity profile is the same as that of the main hepatic veins. There is a triphasic curve wherein the first downward peak represents blood flow toward the heart caused by right atrial diastole, the second downward peak is due to right ventricular diastole, and the third upward peak represents flow away from the heart caused by right atrial contraction (Fig. 10.14) (2).

Congenital Anomalies

Congenital anomalies are not commonly seen in ultrasound practice, but they are important for two reasons:

1. If surgery is performed, preoperative knowledge of the anomaly is very useful.
2. A knowledge of possible venous anomalies will avoid false-positive diagnoses (i.e., diagnosing a venous structure as some other abnormal structure).

Formation of IVC

The right-sided IVC is formed from the development of three pairs of cardinal veins in the embryo and selective regression of various components of these cardinal veins (see Table 10.2) (17,18).

The three pairs of cardinal veins (right and left) are

1. posterior cardinal veins (appear at 4 weeks embryonic life)
2. subcardinal veins (appear at 5 weeks embryonic life)
3. supracardinal veins (appear at 6 weeks embryonic life)

The more common venous congenital anomalies are

1. interrupted IVC with azygous or hemiazygous continuation
2. circumaortic left renal vein
3. retroaortic left renal vein
4. transposition of the IVC
5. duplication of the IVC

Interrupted IVC with Azygous/Hemiazygous Continuation

In this anomaly, the suprarenal segment of the IVC (formed from the right subcardinal vein) fails to develop (i.e., the segment of IVC between the hepatic veins and renal veins is missing). Venous drainage from below the diaphragm is shunted to the azygous/hemiazygous veins, which lie posterior to the crus of the diaphragm in the abdomen. The azygous vein courses into the chest and empties into the superior vena cava. The hepatic vein confluence drains directly into the right atrium.

Ultrasound demonstrates the absence of the suprarenal IVC segment deep to the right hepatic lobe (Fig. 10.15) and the presence of an enlarged hemiazygous vein between the right diaphragmatic crus and the spine. This anomaly is usually an isolated finding, but it may be associated with the asplenia or polysplenia syndromes or cardiac anomalies.

Circumaortic Left Renal Vein

The normal left renal vein passes anterior to the aorta and posterior to the SMA. In circumaortic left renal vein, a second left renal vein passes posterior to the aorta, 2 to 4 cm caudal to the preaortic renal vein.

Retroaortic Left Renal Vein

The entire left renal drainage is via a vein that passes posterior to the aorta at the expected level of the left renal vein or caudal to this level. If ultrasound or CT fails to demonstrate a normal left renal vein, one should

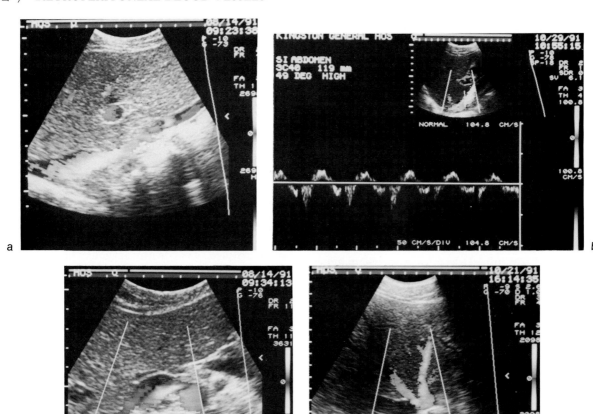

FIG. 10.14. Doppler of normal IVC and branches. (*See color images of parts a–d in color plate section B, which follows page 242.*) **a:** CDU demonstrates net flow (blue) toward chest. Red color in distal IVC represents local turbulence with net flow toward ultrasound probe. Note blood flow in right portal vein and smaller adjacent right hepatic artery (red color). **b:** Normal Doppler spectrum from IVC. Doppler cursor lies in middle of IVC lumen (blue represents flow away from probe at the point in time). Doppler spectrum demonstrates two peaks directed below baseline and one above baseline in opposite direction. First negative peak represents right atrial diastole, and second negative peak represents right ventricular diastole. Positive peak (flow away from chest) represents right atrial contraction. **c:** CDU of right renal vein. Blood flow in right renal vein is coded red (toward probe), as it flows into IVC. Right renal artery (blue) passes posterior to IVC. **d:** CDU of hepatic vein. Transverse scan demonstrates flow toward IVC (blue) in middle and left hepatic veins. (Scans b and d are courtesy of Dr. Patrick Llewellyn, Resident in Radiology, Queen's University, Kingston, Canada.)

TABLE 10.2. *Formation of the inferior vena cava*

Adult anatomy	Embryonic derivative
Below the diaphragm	
Hepatic segment of IVC	Formed by confluence of main hepatic veins
Suprarenal segment of IVC	Right *subcardinal* vein
Renal segment of IVC and renal veins	Anastomosis between *subcardinal* and *supracardinal* veins
Infrarenal segment of IVC	Right *supracardinal* vein
Above the diaphragm	
Azygous vein (right-sided)	Right *supracardinal* vein
Hemiazygous vein (left-sided)	Left *supracardinal* vein

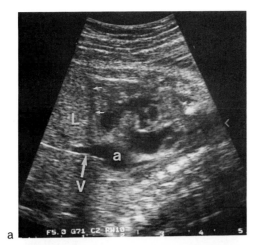

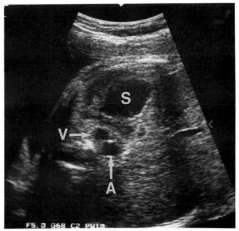

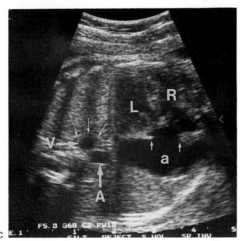

FIG. 10.15. Azygous continuation of IVC. **a:** Sagittal scan of a 36-week fetus demonstrates a very short segment of inferior vena cava (v) coursing from dome of the liver (L) into right atrium. The rest of the IVC was absent. A, atrium; *arrows*, diaphragm. **b:** Transverse scan of same fetus through upper abdomen. Abdominal aorta (A) lies anterior to spine, and blood vessel to left of aorta (v) is a left-sided IVC or hemiazygous vein. s, stomach. **c:** Transverse scan of fetal heart of same patient. Note common atrium (a) and AV canal detect at level of mitral and tricuspid valves (*short arrows*). L, left ventricle; R, right ventricle; A, aorta; V, left-sided IVC or hemiazygous vein; *longer arrows*, crus of diaphragm.

search for a retroaortic vein. This knowledge is important for surgical procedures such as aortic aneurysm repair and renal surgery.

Transposition of the IVC

The infrarenal segment of the IVC (derived from the right *supracardinal* vein) fails to develop. Instead the *left supracardinal* vein remains patent. Ultrasound demonstrates the lower IVC (infrarenal component) to the left of the aorta. The IVC crosses the midline (either anterior or posterior to the aorta) at the level of the renal veins and assumes a normal course cranial to the renal veins.

Duplication of the IVC

A left IVC is present, coursing from the left common iliac vein up to the left renal vein. This is caused by failure of regression of the *left supracardinal vein.* The right-sided IVC is also present. The right of left infrarenal IVC may be larger.

Pathology

IVC Thrombosis

Benign thrombus inside the IVC is usually due to extension of thrombus from the common iliac veins, pelvic veins, or renal veins. In neonates and infants, causes include in-dwelling catheters (umbilical vein catheters), dehydration, and sepsis.

Ultrasound can evaluate the IVC from the right atrium to the renal veins in most adults and children and is useful in the detection of IVC thrombosis. In the infrarenal segment, evaluation is more difficult because of overlying bowel, but careful, persistent scanning with graded compression will be successful in most patients. The thrombus may partially fill the lumen or completely fill and distend the IVC. The thrombus usually has low- to mid-level internal echoes. Occasionally, a long-standing thrombus becomes calcified (19). After recanalization of a clot, residual plaques may persist for some time along the walls of the IVC. CDU is an excellent method to visualize blood flow in the IVC and to highlight the presence of intraluminal clot. It also allows detection of small channels of blood flow around and through the thrombus. With imaging only, it is very difficult to distinguish between benign thrombus and tumor thrombus, although Doppler assessment makes distinction possible in some cases (see below). The goal of the ultrasound examination is to document the presence of IVC thrombus, the cranial and caudal extent, and major branch involvement (hepatic, renal, and common iliac veins).

IVC Dilatation

The IVC may enlarge because of proximal obstruction from many causes including right heart failure (commonly caused by atherosclerotic heart disease), chronic pulmonary disease, pulmonary hypertension, pericardial effusion with tamponade, constrictive pericarditis, atrial tumor, and tricuspid valve disease. With proximal obstruction, the normal respiratory variation of IVC caliber will be lost, and blood flow will slow. The blood may become echogenic (Fig. 10.16), and thus flow becomes

visible with real-time scanning. Doppler will also demonstrate loss of respiratory variation of blood flow. In adults the anteroposterior diameter of the IVC (supine position) is usually less than 20 mm (16). In the left-side-down decubitus position, the diameter should be 10 mm or less (16).

IVC Tumor

Tumors may involve the IVC in several ways

1. extrinsic compression
2. direct invasion from adjacent neoplasm
3. venous extension of tumor from a vein draining into the IVC
4. primary tumor of the IVC wall

The most common tumor involvement is by extrinsic compression by a neighboring tumor without invasion through the wall. Common examples are liver tumors, adrenal tumors, tumors arising in the pancreatic head, and retroperitoneal lymphadenopathy (Fig. 10.17). Extrinsic tumors may obliterate the lumen, but respiratory

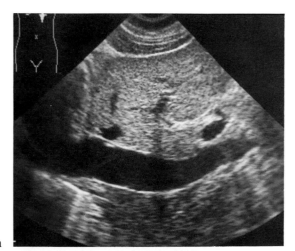

a

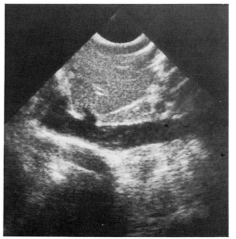

b

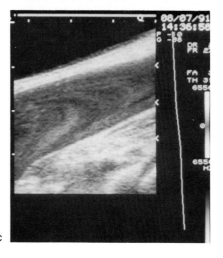

c

FIG. 10.16. IVC dilatation and echogenic blood. (*See color image of part c in color section B, which follows page 242.*) **a:** Sagittal scan demonstrates dilatation of IVC (anteroposterior diameter is 2.8 cm in supine position). There was very little variation in size with respiration. This patient had right heart failure. **b:** Sagittal scan of IVC demonstrates multiple low-level echoes within lumen of IVC. These are due to aggregates of red blood cells (Rouleaux formation). **c:** Scan of a partially obstructed internal jugular vein demonstrates a similar phenomenon. Real-time scanning demonstrated very slow blood flow within jugular vein. Slow flow and enlarged vein both predispose to clumping of red blood cells and thus to visible echogenic blood.

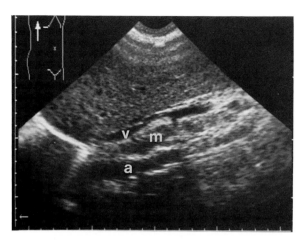

FIG. 10.17. Lymphadenopathy between IVC and aorta. Coronal scan from right side demonstrates multiple masses (*m*) between inferior vena cava (*v*) and abdominal aorta (*a*). Lymphadenopathy was due to lymphoma.

efforts often cause some blood to be visible in the lumen. Color Doppler ultrasound and PW Doppler are useful in demonstrating blood flow in compressed lumens.

Direct invasion of the IVC wall is very uncommon but can be seen with retroperitoneal sarcomas, renal cell carcinoma, and hepatocellular carcinoma.

Intravenous extension of tumor into the IVC is most commonly seen with hepatomas and renal cell carcinomas. A hepatoma can invade into hepatic veins and thence into the IVC and right atrium. Primary renal tumors extend via the renal veins into the IVC (Fig. 10.18). In adults, renal cell carcinoma will have venous extension in 9% to 30% of cases (20), and in children, Wilm's tumor has venous extension in 5% of cases (21).

Rarely a primary malignant tumor (leiomyosarcoma) may arise in the IVC wall (Fig. 10.19) (22), and this may be very difficult to distinguish from venous tumor extension or tumor invasion from surrounding tissue.

IVC Filters

If anticoagulation therapy fails to prevent pulmonary emboli from venous thrombosis in the pelvic veins or leg veins, a mechanical filter may be placed in the IVC to prevent blood clot from traveling to the heart and then to the pulmonary arteries (e.g., Kimray-Greenfield filter, Mobin-Udin filter). The optimal location of the filter is between the renal veins and IVC bifurcation (23).

Radiography can be used to check the level of the filter with respect to the lumbar spine, but ultrasound will give the exact location of the filter with respect to the renal

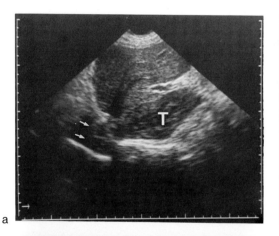

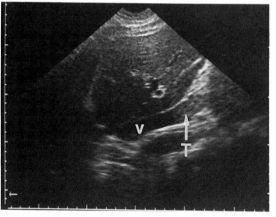

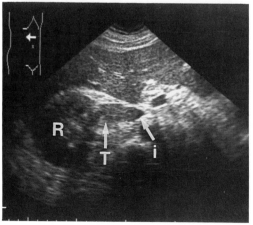

FIG. 10.18. Tumor thrombus in IVC. **a:** Sagittal scan of IVC demonstrates intraluminal tumor thrombus (*T*) distending IVC. Tumor extends into right atrium (*arrows*). **b:** Sagittal scan of IVC of another patient demonstrates tumor thrombus (*T*) within lumen of IVC. Most of visible inferior vena cava (*v*), however, is free of tumor. **c:** Transverse scan of same patient as b demonstrates tumor thrombus distending right renal vein (*T*) and extending into inferior vena cava (*i*). *R*, right kidney.

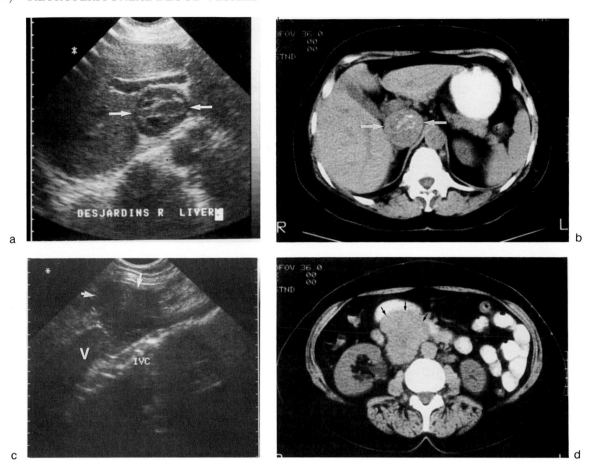

FIG. 10.19. Leiomyosarcoma arising from IVC. **a:** Transverse scan demonstrates enlargement of IVC (*arrows*). Echogenic material fills lumen of IVC. **b:** CT scan at same level demonstrates material filling and extending IVC (*arrows*). A small amount of intraluminal contrast material is seen as white material within the lumen. **c:** Sagittal scan of lower IVC demonstrates a tumor (*arrows*) extending anterior to IVC. Note echogenic material in lumen (*v*) proximal to this mass. **d:** CT scan at same level demonstrates soft tissue mass (*arrows*) extending anterior to IVC. At surgery a malignant tumor arising in wall of IVC was found. This was a leiomyosarcoma. (All scans are courtesy of Dr. Ian Hammond, Chief of Radiology, Ottawa General Hospital, Ottawa, Ontario, Canada.)

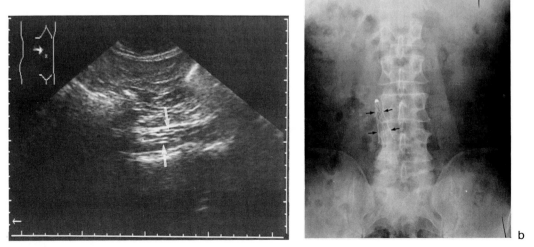

FIG. 10.20. IVC filter. **a:** Sagittal scan of IVC demonstrates multiple linear echoes (*arrows*) within lumen. **b:** Plain radiograph demonstrates Greenfield filter (*arrows*) at level L3-4.

veins (Fig. 10.20) (24) and allow detection of various complications such as thrombosis around the filter and perforation through the IVC wall, which may be associated with a retroperitoneal hematoma. Color Doppler ultrasound or PW Doppler provides a sensitive method for detecting blood flow adjacent to the filter. In the absence of demonstrable blood flow, an inferior vena cavagram should be performed to confirm occlusion.

Pitfalls, Artifacts, and Practical Tips

Visualizing Distal IVC

The upper third of the IVC (segment in posterior aspect of liver) is visualized in virtually all patients. The middle third (posterior to the pancreas) and distal third (posterior to bowel loops) are more difficult to visualize. Graded compression with the ultrasound probe will help displace loops of bowel and thus improve visualization. Maneuvers to distend the IVC will also help (i.e., expiration, RLD position). Sensitive CDU may also demonstrate flow when the IVC lumen itself is difficult to see on real-time imaging.

Distinguishing Aorta and IVC on Sagittal Scans

In hard-copy sagittal images of the aorta and IVC, one distinguishes between aorta and IVC by noting the following: The IVC curves anteriorly as it enters the right atrium, and the aorta courses posteriorly as it passes into the thoracic cavity, along the thoracic spine (Figs. 10.2a and 10.13a).

Echogenic Blood in IVC

Occasionally real-time imaging demonstrates visible echogenic blood flowing in the IVC of normal people (Fig. 10.16). This is usually seen in people with larger IVCs and slow blood flow. The echoes are thought to arise from red cell aggregates whose formation is favored in blood flow that is slow and in larger vessels where the shearing forces are reduced.

Reverberation Artifact in IVC

We have noted a reverberation artifact in sagittal scans of the upper IVC, related to the porta hepatis structures

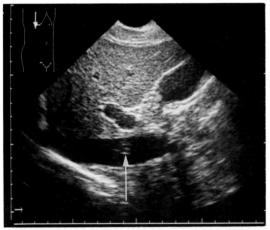

a

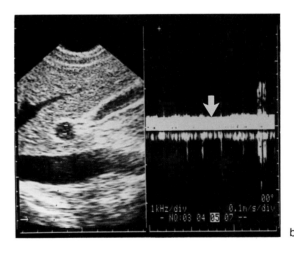

b

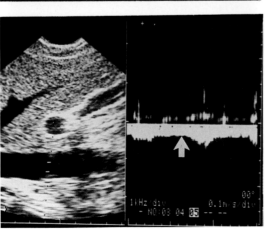

c

FIG. 10.21. Artifact in IVC. **a:** Sagittal scan of IVC demonstrates multiple linear echoes (*arrows*) within lumen of IVC. **b:** PW Doppler scan at same time demonstrates a normal velocity spectrum (*arrow*) in portal vein. **c:** PW Doppler scan at same time within echoes of IVC lumen demonstrates portal vein blood flow (*arrow*) within this structure which represents a duplication artifact of portal vein within IVC.

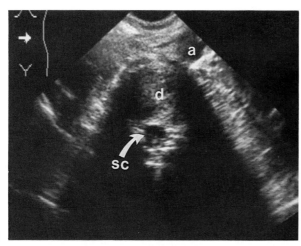 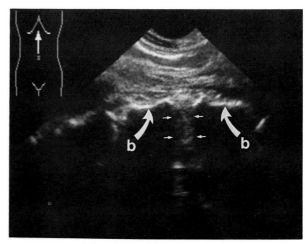

a   b

FIG. 10.22. Intervertebral disc mimicking a retroperitoneal tumor. **a:** Transverse scan of mid abdomen demonstrates a soft tissue structure (*d*) in midline. Note round fluid-filled structure (*sc*) posterior to it. *a*, abdominal aorta; *d*, intervertebral disc; *sc*, spinal cord. **b:** Sagittal scan of same patient confirms that soft tissue structure (*d*) is intervertebral disc (*arrows*). *b*, anterior aspect of vertebral bodies.

anterior to the IVC (Fig. 10.21). This can be very confusing and mimic IVC thrombosis, tumor, intraluminal membrane, or an intraluminal filter. By placing a PW Doppler sample within the intraluminal echoes, one can demonstrate portal venous blood flow and thus prove that the echoes inside the IVC are due to reverberation echoes from the portal vein.

Intervertebral Disc Mimicking a Retroperitoneal Tumor

Transverse scans through an intervertebral disc will demonstrate a soft tissue mass posterior to the IVC and aorta (Fig. 10.22). This can be mistaken for a pathological lesion. Sagittal scans will verify that the tissue corresponds to the lumbar spine disc and neural canal (Fig. 10.22).

REFERENCES

Aorta

1. Dahnert WF, Dubbins PA. Vascular ultrasound measurements. In: Goldberg BB, Kurtz AB, eds. *Atlas of ultrasound measurements.* New York: Raven Press; 1990:72–96.
2. Taylor KJW, Burns PN, Woodcock JP, Wells PNT. Blood flow in deep abdominal and pelvic vessels: ultrasonic pulsed-Doppler analysis. *Radiology* 1985;154:487–493.
3. Brown PM, Westerberg B, Nolan R, Bourgeois D, Sauerbrei E, Nguyen K. Computed tomography of the superior mesenteric artery origin in the preoperative assessment of abdominal aortic aneurysms. *Journal of Vascular Surgery.* (*submitted*)
4. Papanicolau N, Wittenberg J, Ferrucci JT Jr, et al. Preoperative evaluation of abdominal aortic aneurysms by computed tomography. *AJR* 1986;146:711–715.
5. Gooding GAW. Aneurysms of the abdominal aorta, iliac and femoral arteries. In: Raymond HW, Zwiebel WJ, eds. *Seminars in ultrasound. Vol. 3.* New York: Grune and Stratton; 1982:170–179.

6. Gomes MN. Clinical and surgical aspects of abdominal aortic aneurysms. In: Raymond HW, Zwiebel WJ, eds. *Seminars in Ultrasound. Vol. 3.* New York: Grune and Stratton; 1982:156–169.
6a. Canadian Task Force on the Periodic Health Examination. Periodic health examination, 1991 update: 5. Screening for abdominal aortic aneurysm. *Can Med Assoc J* 1991;145:783–789.
7. Wheeler WE, Beachly MC, Ranniger K. Angiography and ultrasonography: a comparative study of abdominal aortic aneurysms. *AJR* 1976;126:95–100.
8. Clayton MJ, Walsh JW, Brewer WH. Contained rupture of abdominal aortic aneurysms: sonographic and CT diagnosis. *AJR* 1982;138:154–156.
9. Brown P, Sauerbrei EE. Chronic sealed rupture of the abdominal aorta. *J Thorac Vasc Surg* 1986;4:529–532.
10. Atlas SW, Vogelzang RL, Bressler EL, Gore RM, Bergan JJ. CT diagnosis of a mycotic aneurysm of the thoracoabdominal aorta. *J Comput Assist Tomogr* 1984;8:1211–1212.
11. Conrad MR, Davis GM, Green CE, Curry TS III. Real-time ultrasound in the diagnosis of acute dissecting aneurysms of the abdominal aorta. *AJR* 1979;132:115–116.
12. Giyanani VL, Krebs CA, Nall LA, Eisenberg RL, Parvey HR. Diagnosis of abdominal aortic dissection by image-directed Doppler sonography. *JCU* 1989;17:445–448.
13. Sauerbrei EE. The split image artifact in pelvic ultrasound: the anatomy and physics. *J Ultrasound Med* 1985;4:29–34.

Inferior Vena Cava

14. Dahnert WF, Dubbins PA. Vascular ultrasound measurements. In: Goldberg BB, Kurtz AB, eds. *Atlas of ultrasound measurements.* New York: Raven Press; 1990:88–90.
15. Grant E, Rendano F, Sevnic E, Gammelgaard J, Holm HH, Grønvall S. Normal inferior vena cava: caliber changes observed by dynamic ultrasound. *AJR* 1980;135:335–338.
16. Nakao S, Come PC, McKay RG, Ransil BJ. Effects of positional changes on inferior vena cava size and dynamics and correlations with right-sided cardiac pressure. *Am J Cardiol* 1987;59:125–132.
17. Moore KL. *The developing human: clinically oriented embryology.* 4th ed. Philadelphia: WB Saunders; 1988:287–291.
18. Garris JB, Kangarloo H, Sample WF. Ultrasonic diagnosis of infrahepatic interruption of the inferior vena cava with azygous (hemiazygous) continuation. *Radiology* 1980;134:179–183.
19. Kassner EG, Baumstark A, Kinkhabwala MN, Ablow RC, Haller

JO. Calcified thrombus in the inferior vena cava in infants and children. *Pediatr Radiol* 1976;4:167–171.

20. Hill MC, Sanders RC. Sonography of the upper abdominal venous system. In: Hill MC, Sanders RC, eds. *Ultrasound annual 1983.* New York: Raven Press; 1983:271.

21. Slovis TL, Philippart AI, Chusing B, et al. Evaluation of the inferior vena cava by sonography and venography in children with renal and hepatic tumors. *Radiology* 1981;140:767–772.

22. Fong KW, Zalev AH. Sonographic diagnosis of leiomyosarcoma

of the inferior vena cava: a correlation with computed tomography and angiography. *J Can Assoc Radiol* 1987;38:229–231.

23. Dunne MG, Goldstein WZ. Computed tomographic and ultrasound appearance of Kim-Ray Greenfield vena caval filters and potential for non-invasive localization. *J Comput Tomogr* 1983;7:375–380.

24. Pasto ME, Kurtz AB, Jarrell BE, et al. The Kimray-Greenfield filter: evaluation by duplex real-time/pulsed Doppler ultrasound. *Radiology* 1983;148:223–226.

CHAPTER 11

Other Retroperitoneal Structures

INTRODUCTION

One must have a good anatomic knowledge of the retroperitoneal spaces to appreciate the pathology located in each space. The retrofascial space is anatomically separate from the retroperitoneal spaces but is usually discussed with the former by convention and clinical practice. These spaces are usually better defined by CT than US. Despite this, the anatomic principles and knowledge of pathology in each space are equally applicable to the practice of US.

An understanding of the anatomic spaces and the structures contained in each space gives insight into the potential types of pathology that may occur in each space.

11.1 NORMAL ANATOMY

The *retroperitoneal space* is bounded anteriorly by the posterior parietal peritoneum and posteriorly by the muscle fascias. The *lumbar fossa* extends from the diaphragm superiorly to the iliac crest inferiorly. It is subdivided into three spaces: the *anterior pararenal space*, the *perirenal space*, and the *posterior pararenal space* (Fig. 11.1). These spaces are fused superiorly and loosely joined inferiorly at the iliac crest. The *lumbar fossa* is

continuous inferiorly with the *iliac fossa* (Fig. 11.2) (or "false pelvis"), which extends from the iliac crest to the ileopectineal line (bony margin extending from the ileum superiorly to the pubic bone inferiorly) of the pelvic brim. The retroperitoneum of the iliac fossa is continuous with the retroperitoneum of the true pelvis inferior to the ileopectineal line (1,2).

The *retrofascial space* is bounded anteriorly by the *iliac fascia* and *anterior thoracolumbar fascia* (Fig. 11.3). These are continuous inferiorly with the *iliac fascia*, which is continuous inferior to the ileopectineal line as the *pelvic fascia*. These muscle fascias are continuous laterally with the *transversalis fascia* of the abdominal wall (2–5). The transversalis fascia (or *enteroabdominal fascia*) blends superiorly with the deep fascial planes of the chest (endothoracic fascia) and inferiorly with the deep fascial planes of the thigh (fascia lata) (4,5).

Retroperitoneum of the Lumbar Fossa

Anterior Pararenal Space

The anterior pararenal space is bounded anteriorly by the *posterior parietal peritoneum*, posteriorly by the *anterior pararenal fascia*, and laterally by the *lateroconal fascia* (Fig. 11.1). The latter is formed by the fusion of the lateral margins of the anterior and posterior pararenal fascias (1,2). The space is continuous across the midline. Inferiorly, a weak fusion of the layers of the anterior and posterior pararenal fascias results in a potential communication of these spaces at the level of the iliac crest (Figs.

Abbreviations: **AIDS**, acquired immune deficiency syndrome; **CT**, computed tomography; **HIV**, human immunovirus; **IV**, intravenous; **IVC**, inferior vena cava; **MIBG**, metaiodobenzylguanidine; **Tc**, technetium; **US**, ultrasound.

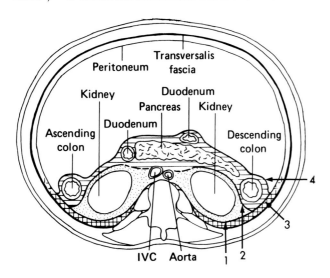

FIG. 11.1. Retroperitoneal compartments. *Striped areas,* anterior pararenal space; *stippled areas,* perirenal space; *crosshatched areas,* posterior pararenal space; *1,* posterior pararenal fascia; *2,* anterior pararenal fascia; *3,* lateroconal fascia; *4,* peritoneum. (From Meyers, ref. 1, with permission.)

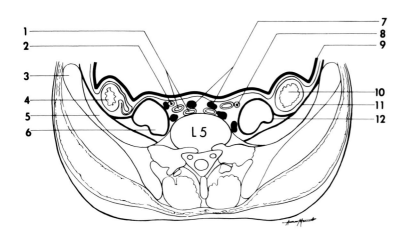

FIG. 11.2. Iliac fossa of retroperitoneum. This transverse diagram is approximately at L5 lumbar vertebral level. Iliac fossa is a potential space lying between the peritoneum (*9*) and the iliacus fascia (*11, 12*), which invests the iliacus (*5*) and psoas (*6*) muscles. *1,* iliac vessels; *2,* right ureter; *3,* ileum; *4,* ascending colon; *7,* lymph nodes; *8,* left ureter; *10,* descending colon. (From Koenigsberg et al., ref. 2, with permission.)

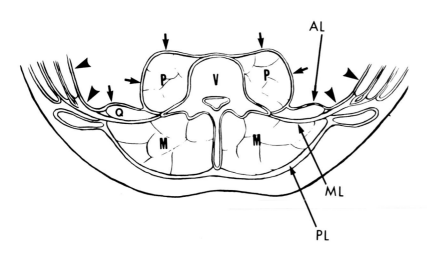

FIG. 11.3. Retrofascial space. Iliac fascia (*small arrows*) covers psoas (*P*) and iliacus muscles. Anterior layer (*AL*) of thoracolumbar fascia (*larger arrows*) covers quadratus lumborum muscles (*Q*). Middle layer (*ML*) is between quadratus lumborum muscles and deep muscles of back. Posterior layer (*PL*) is posterior to deep muscles of the back. Three layers of thoracolumbar fascia are continuous laterally with transversalis fascia (*arrowheads*) of abdominal wall. V; vertebra. (From Van Dyke et al., ref. 3, with permission.)

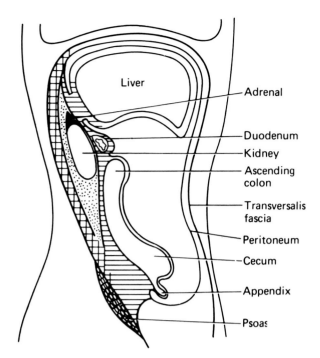

FIG. 11.4. Sagittal diagram of right retroperitoneal spaces. *Striped areas,* anterior pararenal space; *stippled areas,* perirenal space; *cross-hatched areas,* posterior pararenal space. (From Meyers, ref. 1, with permission.)

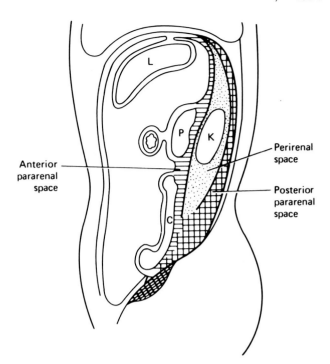

FIG. 11.5. Sagittal diagram of left retroperitoneal spaces. *Striped areas,* anterior pararenal space; *stippled areas,* perirenal space; *cross-hatched areas,* posterior pararenal space. (From Meyers, ref. 1, with permission.)

11.4 and 11.5). Similarly, the lateroconal fascia disappears at the level of the iliac crest, permitting communication between the anterior pararenal space with the properitoneal fat (between the parietal peritoneum and the transversalis fascia) of the flank (1,2).

The anterior pararenal space contains the ascending colon, descending colon, duodenal loop, pancreas, arteries, veins, lymphatics, lymph nodes, nerves, and fat.

Perirenal Space

The perirenal space is bounded anteriorly by the *anterior pararenal fascia,* posteriorly by the *posterior pararenal fascia,* and laterally by the *lateroconal fascia,* which is formed by the fusion of the anterior and posterior pararenal fascias (Fig. 11.1).

There is no continuity across the midline. The anterior pararenal fascia blends into the connective tissue of the great vessels. The posterior pararenal fascia fuses with the muscle fascias overlying the psoas or quadratus lumborum muscles. Inferiorly, the anterior and posterior pararenal fascias are weakly fused, permitting a potential communication of the perirenal space with the anterior and posterior pararenal spaces and with the iliac fossa. Superiorly, the anterior and posterior renal fascias are firmly fused to the diaphragmatic fascia (Figs. 11.4 and 11.5).

The perirenal space contains the kidneys, adrenal glands, ureters, arteries, veins, lymphatics, lymph nodes, nerves, and fat. The fat may be hypoechoic or hyperechoic (relative to the kidney) depending on the number of acoustic reflectors (presumably fibrous strands) within the fat (Fig. 11.6).

Posterior Pararenal Space

The posterior pararenal space is bounded anteriorly by the *posterior pararenal fascia* and posteriorly by the *psoas fascia* and *quadratus lumborum fascia* (Fig. 11.1). It is continuous laterally with the properitoneal fat of the abdominal wall (1) and inferiorly with the iliac fossa (1,2). There are potential communications inferiorly with the anterior pararenal space and perirenal space (Figs. 11.4 and 11.5).

The posterior pararenal space contains fat, arteries, veins, lymphatics, and lymph nodes (2).

Retroperitoneum of the Iliac Fossa

The iliac fossa is bounded anteriorly by the *posterior parietal peritoneum* and posteriorly by the *iliac fascia* (Fig. 11.2). It is continuous with the lumbar fossa superior to the iliac crest and with the pelvic fossa inferior to the ileopectineal line (1,2).

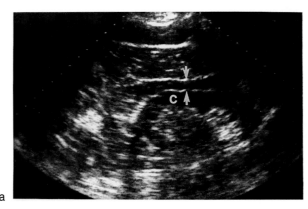
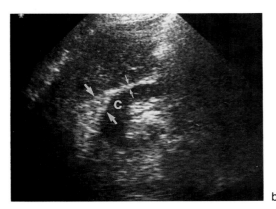

FIG. 11.6. Perinephric fat (*between arrows*) may be hypoechoic (**a**) or hyperechoic (**b**). *C*, renal cortex.

The iliac fossa contains the ureters, arteries, veins, lymphatics, lymph nodes, nerves, and fat.

Retrofascial Space

The posterior boundary of the retroperitoneum is the muscle fascias that enclose the muscles of the posterior abdominal wall. The retrofascial space has intimate anatomic relationships with the posterior pararenal space anteriorly, the erector spinae muscles posteriorly, the spine medially, and the transversalis fascia laterally. Therefore pathology in any of the contiguous anatomic structures may spread to and simulate primary disease of the retrofascial space. Similarly, disease of the retrofascial space may involve contiguous structures simulating primary disease of the contiguous space or structure.

The *iliac fascia* covers the psoas and iliacus muscles (Figs. 11.1–11.3).

The *psoas minor* is absent in 40% of individuals. It originates from the vertebral bodies of T12 and L1 and inserts on the ileopectineal line of the innominate bone and the iliac fascia (3). It runs along the anterolateral aspect of the psoas major and is usually not visualized on scanning.

The *psoas major* arises from (a) the transverse processes of L1 to L5; (b) the sides of the intervertebral discs and adjacent margins of the vertebral bodies T12 to L5; (c) the tendinous arches that bridge over the lumbar arteries adjacent to the vertebral bodies. It inserts on the lesser trochanter via the psoas tendon (3,5). It is visualized as a paraspinal tubular structure medial to the kidneys on longitudinal scans. It is seen as a rounded or oval structure on transverse scans (2).

The *iliacus muscle* arises from the iliac wing and inserts into the psoas tendon and lesser trochanter of the femur (2,5). It appears as a hypoechoic elliptiform structure anterior to the iliac crest (2).

The *thoracolumbar fascia* splits into three layers (Fig. 11.3). The anterior layer is anterior to the quadratus lumborum muscles. The middle layer is between the quadratus lumborum muscles and the deep muscles of the back. The posterior layer is posterior to the deep muscles of the back.

The quadratus lumborum originates from the twelfth rib and inserts on the iliac crest. It is lateral to the psoas muscles and posterior to the kidney. On longitudinal scans it is a fusiform structure that is thickened inferiorly. On transverse scans, it appears as a lenticular structure (2,5).

The deep muscles of the back are located lateral to the lumbosacral spinous processes and posterior to the transverse processes. They include the interspinalis, intertransversarius lateralis and medialis, multifidus, longissimus, and iliocostalis muscles.

The iliac fascia and the thoracolumbar fascia are continuous laterally with the transversalis fascia of the abdominal wall.

Anatomic Groups of Lymph Nodes

In general, lymph node groups parallel vascular structures and often have a similar name (e.g., common iliac nodes). Other node groups are related to organs and are named according to the related organ (e.g., splenic, hepatic). All organs have lymphatic drainage so nodes may be seen related to any organ. There are usually multiple communicating lymphatic channels between node groups. A detailed knowledge of lymphatic drainage patterns can be of assistance in oncologic staging of tumors. The reader is referred to definitive texts (5,6) for more detailed anatomic classification of lymph node groups and drainage pathways.

A simplified classification of lymph node groups based on clinical experience (6,7) and classical anatomy (4,5) is presented in Table 11.1 and Fig. 11.7. The most commonly visualized groups include the right lumbar chain (consisting of pericaval and interaortocaval groups), the left lumbar chain (left periaortic group), and preaortic nodes (consisting of celiac, superior mesenteric, and inferior mesenteric groups) (4,8). The right and left lumbar

TABLE 11.1. *Simplified classification of lymph node groups*

Simplified group	Classical anatomic node groups	Organs drained
Periaortic	Right lumbar-pericaval, interaortocaval	Retroperitoneal organs, pelvic organs, bowel
	Left lumbar	
Kidney hilum	Right lumbar	Genitourinary—adrenal, kidney, testis, ovary, ureter
	Left lumbar	
Epigastric	Coeliac, cardiac, left gastric, gastroepiploic, pyloric, pancreaticoduodenal, and superior pancreatic	Stomach, duodenum, bowel, pancreas
Liver hilum	Cystic, hepatic	Liver, bile ducts
Spleen hilum	Splenic	Spleen
Mesenteric	Mesenteric, paracolic, ileocolic, appendicular, cecal, right colic, middle colic, sigmoid	Bowel
Pelvic	Common iliac, internal iliac, external iliac, sacral	Bladder, prostate, seminal vesicles, uterus, cervix
	Superior rectal, middle rectal	Rectum

chains have multiple cross-connecting channels. The *intestinal trunk* is formed via lymphatics from mesenteric, spleen, liver, and epigastric groups. The intestinal trunk and lumbar chains fuse to form the *cisterna chyli*, which is located posterior to the crura of the diaphragm at L1–2 levels. The *thoracic duct* arises from the cisterna chyli at approximately T12 level and passes posterior to the right crus through the aortic hiatus into the mediastinum. The thoracic duct empties into the left subclavian vein.

Although discrete nodes may be visualized, lymphatic channels, intestinal trunk, cisterna chyli, and thoracic duct are not visualized by US.

11.2 SCANNING TECHNIQUES

Depending on body habitus, and the degree of superimposed bowel gas, the retroperitoneal and retrofascial

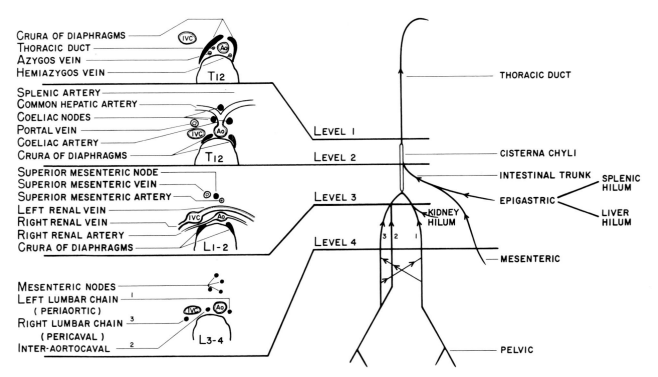

FIG. 11.7. Lymph node groups. This line drawing incorporates a simplifed classification of lymph node groups. *Arrows* indicate normal direction of flow and simplified communications between groups of nodes. *1*, periaortic group; *2*, interaortocaval group; *3*, pericaval chain.

spaces are usually scanned with a 3- or 5-MHz transducer. Routine scans are performed in longitudinal and transverse planes. Oblique and coronal scan planes are used to identify specific structures that are not adequately visualized by routine scan planes. Because the tissue planes separating the various spaces are not readily visualized on US, the involved space may be inferred by position, depth, shape, and involvement of specific organs (e.g., kidney in perirenal space).

Ultrasound does not normally identify masses or lymph nodes of less than 1 cm. Computed tomography is more sensitive in assessing the retroperitoneum for masses and adenopathy and has the advantage of characterizing some masses accurately by the demonstration of fat or gas. Computed tomography can accurately define the various retroperitoneal compartments in most patients. Ultrasound does not normally identify the fascial planes but infers location by correlation with contiguous structures. Nuclear medicine studies have limited efficacy in anatomic localization but may have significant pathophysiologic value in iodine[131] MIBG scans for functioning paragangliomas, and gallium or Tc[99M] white blood cell studies for inflammatory or neoplastic diseases. These will focus the direction of other imaging modalities (US, CT), which will permit more accurate anatomic localization.

11.3 PATHOLOGY

There are several categories of diseases involving the retroperitoneal and retrofascial spaces. These include inflammation, tumor, and hemorrhage. Pathology related to specific organs or structures (e.g., kidney, adrenal gland, vascular structures) previously discussed will not be repeated.

Adenopathy

There is *not* total concurrence on the definition of adenopathy. Most proposed criteria are based on largest short-axis diameter of nodes on CT rather than US. The following recommendations are a consensus of several reports (9–14):

Retroperitoneal ≥1.5 cm—abnormal
Retroperitoneal multiple 1.0–1.5 cm—abnormal
Retroperitoneal single 1.0–1.5 cm—indeterminate
Retroperitoneal ≤1.0 cm—normal
Retrocrural >0.6 cm—abnormal

Some authors (9,10) use 2 cm, whereas others (11–14) use 1.5 cm as the critical diameter for abnormality. Approximately 10% of patients with lymphoma will have normal size lymph nodes (15). Therefore, normal size nodes do not exclude pathology. Similarly, enlarged

nodes do not have a specific pathologic diagnosis. Enlarged nodes may be due to tumor, infection, or inflammatory processes.

Ultrasound normally does not demonstrate retroperitoneal lymph nodes of less than 1 cm (2). Of all nodes demonstrated by US, only 3% were 1 cm or less in largest diameter on a study by Smeets et al. (7). Brascho et al. (16) reported a 98% accuracy in detecting retroperitoneal lymph nodes larger than 2 cm in patients with lymphoma.

Lymph nodes usually present as hypoechoic structures (Figs. 11.8–11.11). The degree of echogenicity is dependent on many variables including size, depth, histologic uniformity, frequency and focal zone of transducer, and time gain curve. The shape is variable and may be spindle-shaped (elongated), oval, or round. Small nodes must be distinguished from vascular structures by imaging in two planes perpendicular to each other. If there is still doubt, Doppler US should clarify the situation. Larger nodal masses may have mass effect by displacing contiguous structures. Larger nodal masses may have a lobulated contour. Secondary infection or therapy may cause central necrosis. Occasionally necrosis occurs spontaneously. This presents as a complex mass with poorly marginated central cystic areas.

Periaortic nodal masses may obscure the tissue planes with contiguous vascular structures resulting in encasement of the great vessels (aorta, IVC) (Fig. 11.10). A tissue plane around the vascular structures is usually preserved with mesenteric adenopathy (Fig. 11.11).

The differential diagnosis of retroperitoneal adenopathy includes retroperitoneal fibrosis, retroperitoneal hematoma, inflammatory mass or abscess, retroperitoneal sarcoma, and extramedullary hematopoiesis. Clinical history, physical findings, and ancillary laboratory data will usually narrow the potential differential diagnosis.

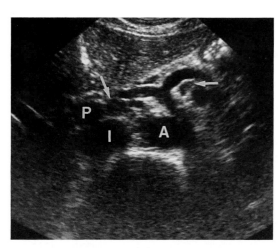

FIG. 11.8. Minimal adenopathy. Transverse scan at level of celiac axis shows small lymph nodes (*arrows*). Portal vein (*P*), inferior vena cava (*I*), and aorta (*A*).

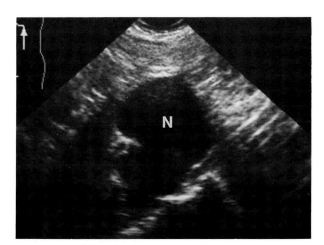

FIG. 11.9. Retroperitoneal adenopathy. Coronal scan of left retroperitoneum demonstrates a lobulated, hypoechoic mass caused by lymph nodes (N).

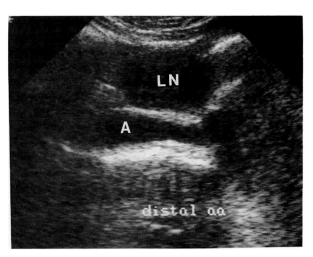

FIG. 11.11. Mesenteric adenopathy. Sagittal scan shows preservation of tissue plane between aorta (A) and mesenteric lymph node mass (LN).

Benign Etiology

Although not a definitive sign, benign lymph nodes tend to be more elongated (7). Echogenic fat in the node hilum (hilar fat sign) may be rarely seen and is regarded as a sign of benignancy (7). The distribution of nodes in this group is similar to the distribution with malignant disease (7). Nodes were less numerous and smaller with benign diseases. Because there is considerable overlap in size of nodes with benign and malignant diseases, this cannot be used as a reliable discriminator. Central necrosis is uncommon.

Diseases that may cause reactive hyperplasia of lymph nodes include tuberculosis, sarcoidosis, Crohn's disease, chronic liver diseases, and immune-mediated diseases (e.g., celiac disease, mastocytosis, rheumatic diseases, AIDS). Immunocompromised patients (positive HIV serology, transplantation, IV drug abusers) may develop

adenopathy as an immune response to repeated antigen stimulation (7). Some patients (e.g., transplantation, AIDS) have increased risk of infection and malignancy.

Castleman's disease (Figs. 11.12 and 11.13) is a rare disease that rarely involves the retroperitoneum, mesentery, and pelvis. It is manifest as lymphadenopathy, which may be focal and discrete, or diffuse and massive. It is usually regarded as a benign disease but may have a malignant clinical course if multifocal in nature (17,18).

Malignant Etiology

There are no characteristic features to distinguish benign from malignant adenopathy. Malignant lymph nodes tend to be more rounded in shape, larger in size,

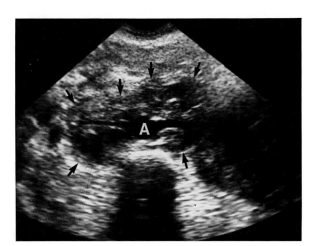

FIG. 11.10. Periaortic adenopathy. Transverse scan shows massive retroperitoneal adenopathy (arrows) encasing aorta and renal arteries. Tissue planes around aorta are lost.

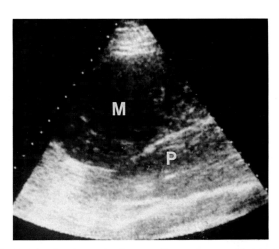

FIG. 11.12. Castleman's disease. Coronal scan of left kidney demonstrates a nodal mass (M) in central sinus of the kidney. Psoas muscle (P) is posteromedially. (From Nolan et al., ref. 17, with permission.)

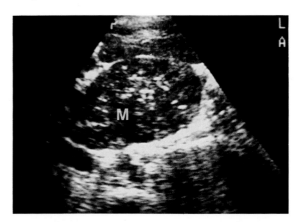

FIG. 11.13. Castleman's disease. A large nodal mass (*M*) contains focal hyperechoic specular echoes caused by small foci of calcification within nodes.

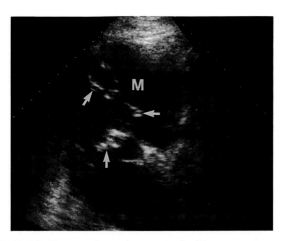

FIG. 11.14. Retroperitoneal metastasis. Transverse scan in area of right iliac fossa demonstrates a large hypoechoic mass (*M*) caused by a metastatic tumor involving right ilium and iliacus muscle. Hyperechoic areas (*arrows*) represent focal areas of calcification within mass related to lytic expansile lesion. Disruption of iliac cortex indicates underlying lytic process.

and more numerous than with benign etiologies. They are more commonly demonstrated in epigastric, periaortic, and liver hilum locations than in other locations (7).

The etiology of malignant adenopathy includes a wide spectrum of primary and secondary tumors. The commonest group is primary gastrointestinal tract malignancies including stomach, esophagus, and other locations (e.g., colon, small bowel) in decreasing frequency. The second most common group is hematologic malignancies including non-Hodgkin's lymphoma, leukemia, and Hodgkin's disease in decreasing frequency. The third group is the genitourinary tract malignancies (7). One cannot reliably differentiate between these entities based on the US or CT appearance alone.

Pitfalls in the Diagnosis of Adenopathy

Lymph nodes may appear anechoic and simulate a cyst (19). This is usually not a problem if technique is optimized.

Other structures may simulate adenopathy. Normal veins, varices, aneurysms, localized hematoma, extramedullary hematopoiesis, and bowel may simulate adenopathy (20). The crus of the diaphragms may be prominent and lobulated, simulating adenopathy (21). This can be excluded by scanning in several planes with real-time visualization. An accessory spleen may simulate a splenic hilar node. Most of these can be correctly categorized by optimal technique, Doppler, and awareness of the pitfalls.

Other Neoplasms

Most tumors involving the retroperitoneal and retrofascial spaces are metastatic (Fig. 11.14). They may invade contiguous spaces by direct extension (e.g., bowel, peritoneum, axial skeleton), by seeding to contiguous

surfaces (peritoneum), and by lymphatic metastasis. The latter is probably the cause of apparent muscle involvement by metastatic tumor and lymphoma (3,22). The US findings are focal or diffuse enlargement of the muscle or group of muscles. There may also be loss of tissue planes and occasionally calcification within the mass. These may invade a contiguous space.

Most primary tumors of the retrofascial space are sarcomas of the muscles and tumors of the nervous system (3). These are relatively rare. The US findings are similar to those of metastatic tumor to muscles. These may invade a contiguous space.

Primary tumors of the retroperitoneum may be be-

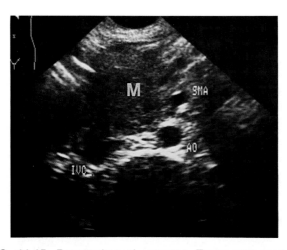

FIG. 11.15. Retroperitoneal sarcoma. Transverse scan in upper abdomen demonstrates a large mass (*M*) anterior to inferior vena cava (*IVC*) and aorta (*A*), which caused displacement of superior mesenteric artery (*SMA*) to left. It was indistinguishable from head of pancreas but did not cause biliary or pancreatic obstruction.

nign or malignant (23–26). They are relatively rare. The commonest benign tumors are lipoma, teratoma, neurofibroma, and paraganglioma. *Lipomas* tend to be hyperechoic masses of varying size (26). *Teratomas* may be a complex mass with cystic and solid components. They may contain a focus of calcification or a fluid–debris level (27). *Neurofibromas* present as a hypoechoic mass. A *paraganglioma* is usually solid but may have an area of central necrosis or focal areas of calcification. These have been described with adrenal pheochromocytomas.

Primary malignant retroperitoneal tumors (Fig. 11.15) are relatively rare. Liposarcoma (Fig. 11.16) is usually regarded as the most common (6,22). Malignant fibrous histiocytoma, leiomyosarcoma, and fibrosarcoma are variably reported as the most common or next most common (6,24,25).

Depending on the pathologic characteristics, liposarcomas contain a variable amount of fat, myxomatous tissue, stellate cells, spindle cells, round cells, and primitive mesenchymal cells. Lipogenic liposarcomas tend to be hyperechoic on US (26). Other pathologic variants may have varying degrees of echogenicity.

Most other primary malignant retroperitoneal masses will appear as a solid hypoechoic mass. Leiomyosarcomas have a tendency to undergo central necrosis, which will appear as a mass with echogenic rim and central cystic component (28).

There are no characteristic US features that permit specific pathologic diagnosis of the various secondary and primary tumors of the retroperitoneal and retrofascial spaces. The differential diagnosis should include tumor, infection, and hemorrhage in most cases. Clinical clues, percutaneous biopsy, or open surgical biopsy are necessary in many cases (3).

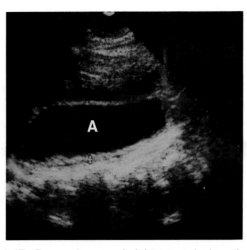

FIG. 11.17. Psoas abscess. A right paraspinal cystic mass (*A*) is located in right psoas and is due to a paraspinal tuberculous abscess.

Infection

Infection usually spreads from contiguous organs (e.g., kidney, pancreas, bowel, appendix, spine, uterus, adrenal). It may also be a complication of surgery. Uncommonly, it may be the result of septic emboli (3).

Extraperitoneal infection may not present as acutely or severely as intraperitoneal infection (29). Immunosuppressed patients may not show the usual clinical or laboratory findings.

The US spectrum is wide. There may be a focal or diffuse textural abnormality with loss of tissue planes or mass effect. The mass may be cystic (Fig. 11.17), solid, or complex (cystic and solid components). Cystic collec-

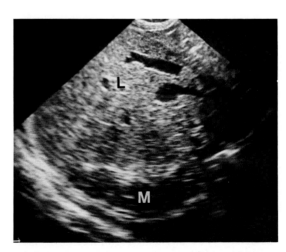

FIG. 11.16. Retroperitoneal liposarcoma. A mass (*M*) is seen posterior to liver (*L*). It also caused poor tissue planes in subhepatic space. It was clinically thought to be a retroperitoneal hemorrhage but was a liposarcoma at time of surgical biopsy.

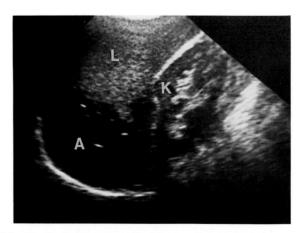

FIG. 11.18. Retroperitoneal abscess. This patient had a recurrent retroperitoneal abscess from a previous duodenal perforation. Abscess (*A*) contains small focal specular echoes from small foci of gas. Abscess involved anterior pararenal space between upper pole of kidney (*K*) and liver (*L*). It extended superiorly posterior to the liver.

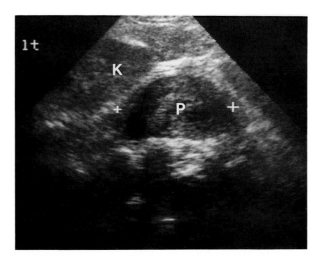

FIG. 11.19. Psoas hematoma. Coronal scan shows an enlarged psoas muscle (P), which is of variable echogenicity. The study was done after an episode of trauma. Kidney (K) is seen adjacent to psoas (P) and serves as an anatomic landmark.

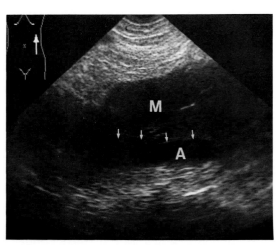

FIG. 11.21. Periaortic hematoma caused by aortic rupture. Large periaortic retroperitoneal mass (M) has poor definition of tissue plane with wall (arrows) of aorta (A). Loss of tissue plane confirms periaortic location.

tions may contain internal echoes, septations, or fluid–debris level. Gas is seen in approximately 25% of abscesses and may appear as a bright echo (Fig. 11.18) with or without a "dirty" acoustic shadow. If there is a large amount of gas, the collection may be mistaken for bowel. The collection may be contiguous to a retroperitoneal structure or spine, which may give a clue to the source of infection.

The differential diagnosis includes tumor and hemorrhage. The clinical and laboratory findings are often very suggestive, whereas percutaneous aspiration for Gram's stain, culture, and sensitivity are usually diagnostic.

Hemorrhage

Hemorrhage may be due to coagulopathy, anticoagulant therapy, ruptured aortic aneurysm, postsurgical complication, and trauma (3). One should look for an underlying cause such as aneurysm or mass in a contiguous organ.

Ultrasound may demonstrate focal or diffuse enlargement of one of the retrofascial muscles (Figs. 11.19 and 11.20). A focal muscle mass is usually hypoechoic. The tissue planes of the retroperitoneal and retrofascial spaces may be obliterated (Figs. 11.21) or may cause dis-

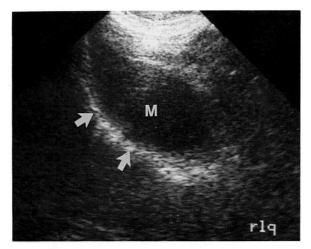

FIG. 11.20. Iliacus hematoma. Hematoma causes a mass (M) involving right iliacus muscle. Ilium (arrows) is intact and serves as an anatomic landmark.

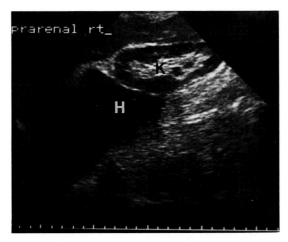

FIG. 11.22. Upper pole of kidney (K) is displaced anteriorly by a large hematoma (H) that is located in posterior pararenal space.

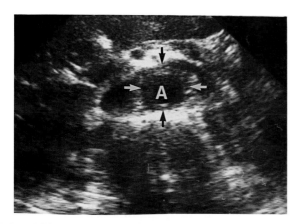

FIG. 11.23. Retroperitoneal fibrosis. Transverse scan demonstrates rim of tissue (*arrows*) surrounding aorta (*A*). At this level, aorta appears to have a "thick" wall.

placement of retroperitoneal structures (Fig. 11.22). The mass may be well defined or poorly defined. It may be cystic, solid, or complex (cystic and solid components). Cystic areas may contain internal echoes or a fluid–debris level.

The history is the most important clue to the diagnosis. The differential diagnosis includes tumor and infection.

Miscellaneous Pathology

Retroperitoneal fibrosis is a rare disease consisting of fibrotic plaque (30). It is usually confined to the retroperitoneum but may be in other locations occasionally. Approximately two thirds of all cases are idiopathic. Twelve percent are due to ingestion of methysergide, which is an ergot derivative that was formerly prescribed for migraine headaches. Eight percent to 10% of cases are

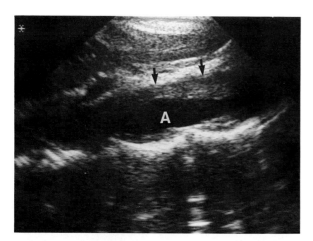

FIG. 11.24. Retroperitoneal fibrosis. Sagittal scan demonstrates tissue anterior to distal abdominal aorta (*A*) with loss of tissue plane between mass and aorta. Loss of tissue plane confirms periaortic location.

due to metastatic tumor with desmoplastic response. Five percent to 10% are due to perianeurysmal fibrosis. Other possible causes include infection, vasculitis, systemic collagen disease, and autoimmune disease process. It usually results in encasement and entrapment of ureters and vascular structures. The commonest presentation is related to ureteric obstruction with hydroureter and hydronephrosis proximal to the level of obstruction. Less commonly it causes arterial, venous, or lymphatic compromise, resulting in claudication, ischemia, edema, or thrombophlebitis. It usually presents as a hypoechoic mass anterior to the lower lumbar or sacral region (Figs. 11.23 and 11.24). Because the mass may be very small, CT is the preferred imaging modality (30). The differential diagnosis includes adenopathy, primary or secondary retroperitoneal tumor, extramedullary hematopoiesis, hematoma, and amyloidosis.

Lymphoceles are usually a complication of lymph node dissection or renal transplant surgery. It appears as a cystic mass with internal septations. Those containing substantial internal echoes and debris are more likely to be infected (31).

Occasionally pelvic vein thrombosis may cause diffuse swelling of the iliopsoas muscles (3), simulating primary disease. Various neuromuscular disorders including scoliosis may cause asymmetry of the retrofascial muscles (3), which may simulate a mass.

Pancreatic pseudocysts and urinomas may involve the retroperitoneal and retrofascial spaces, but these have been discussed elsewhere.

REFERENCES

1. Meyers M. The extraperitoneal spaces: normal and pathologic anatomy. In: Meyers M, ed. *Dynamic radiology of the abdomen: normal and pathologic anatomy,* 2nd ed. New York: Springer-Verlag; 1982:105–185.
2. Koenigsberg M, Hoffman JC, Schnur MJ. Sonographic evaluation of the retroperitoneum. *Semin Ultrasound* 1982;3:79–96.
3. Van Dyke JA, Holley HC, Anderson SD. Review of iliopsoas anatomy and pathology. *Radiographics* 1987;7:53–84.
4. Netter FH. *Atlas of human anatomy.* Summit, New Jersey: CIBA-GEIGY Corporation, 1989.
5. Moores KL. *Clinically oriented anatomy,* 2nd ed. Baltimore: Williams & Wilkins, 1985.
6. Bragg DG, Rubin P, Yonker JE, eds. *Oncologic imaging.* New York: Permagon Press; 1985.
7. Smeets AJ, Zonderland HM, van der Voorde F, Laméris JS. Evaluation of abdominal lymph nodes by ultrasound. *J Ultrasound Med* 1990;9:325–331.
8. Lee JKT. Retroperitoneum. In: Lee JKT, Sagel SS, Stanley RJ, eds. *Computed body tomography with MRI correlation.* New York: Raven Press; 1989:707–754.
9. Glazer GM, Goldberg HI, Moss AA, Axel L. Computed tomographic detection of retroperitoneal adenopathy. *Radiology* 1982;143:147–149.
10. Lee JKT, Balfe DM. Computed tomography evaluation of lymphoma patients. *CRC Crit Rev Diagn Imaging* 1982;18:1–28.
11. Korobkin M. Computed tomography of the retroperitoneal vasculature and lymph nodes. *Semin Roentgenol* 1981;16:251–267.
12. Deutch SJ, Sandler MA, Alpern MB. Abdominal lymphadenopathy in benign diseases: CT detection. *Radiology* 1987;163:335–338.

13. Strijk SP. Lymphography and abdominal computed tomography in the staging of non-Hodgkin lymphoma. *Acta Radiol* 1987;28:263–269.
14. Nyman R, Rehn S, Glimelius B, et al. Magnetic resonance imaging, chest radiography, computed tomography and ultrasonography in malignant lymphoma. *Acta Radiol* 1987;28:253–262.
15. Breiman RS, Castellino RA, Harell GS, et al. CT-pathologic correlations in Hodgkin's disease and non-Hodgkin's lymphoma. *Radiology* 1978;126:159–166.
16. Brascho DL, Durant JR, Green LE. The accuracy of retroperitoneal ultrasonography in Hodgkin's disease and non-Hodgkin's lymphoma. *Radiology* 1977;125:485–487.
17. Nolan RL, Banerjee A, Adikio H. Castleman's disease with vascular encasement and renal sinus involvement. *Urol Radiol* 1988;10:173–175.
18. Lisbon E, Fields S, Strauss S, et al. Widespread Castleman's disease: CT and US findings. *Radiology* 1988;166:753–755.
19. Callen PW, Marks WM. Lymphomatous masses simulating cysts by ultrasonography. *J Can Assoc Radiol* 1979;30:244–246.
20. Koehler PR, Mancuso AA. Pitfalls in the diagnosis of retroperitoneal adenopathy. *J Can Assoc Radiol* 1982;33:197–201.
21. Callen PW, Filly RA, Sarti DA, Sample WF. Ultrasonography of the diaphragmatic crura. *Radiology* 1979;130:721–724.
22. Glazer HS, Lee JKT, Balfe DM, Mauro MA, Griffith R, Sagel SS. Non-Hodgkin lymphoma: computed tomographic demonstration of unusual extranodal involvement. *Radiology* 1983;149:211–217.
23. Stephens DH. Retroperitoneal masses. In: Taveras JM, Ferrucci JT, eds. *Radiology: diagnosis—imaging—intervention.* Philadelphia: JB Lippincott; 1990:Chapters 1–12.
24. Lane RH, Stephens DH, Reiman HM. Primary retroperitoneal neoplasms: CT findings in 90 cases with clinical and pathologic correlation. *AJR* 1989;152:83–89.
25. Morton DL, Eilber FR. Soft tissue sarcomas. In: Holland JF, Frei E, eds. *Cancer medicine,* 2nd ed. Philadelphia: Lea and Febiger; 1982:2141–2145.
26. Yiu-Chiu V, Chiu L. Ultrasonography and computed tomography of retroperitoneal liposarcoma. *CT* 1981;5:98–110.
27. Davidson AJ, Hartman DS, Goldman SM. Mature teratoma of the retroperitoneum: radiologic, pathologic, and clinical correlation. *Radiology* 1989;172:421–425.
28. Rowley VA, Cooperberg PL. The ultrasonographic appearance of abdominal leiomyosarcomas. *J Can Assoc Radiol* 1982;33:94–97.
29. Meyer HI. The reaction of the retroperitoneal tissues to infection. *Ann Surg* 1934;99:246–250.
30. Amis ES. Retroperitoneal fibrosis. *AJR* 1991;157:321–329.
31. van Sonnenberg E, Wittich GR, Casola G, et al. Lymphoceles: imaging characteristics and percutaneous management. *Radiology* 1986;161:593–596.

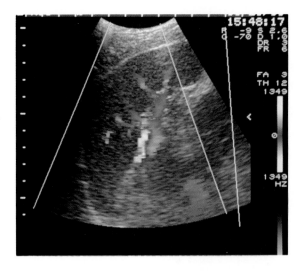

FIG. 6.6. *(See page 113 for the discussion of the figure.)* **Normal splenic vessels: CDU—coronal scan.**

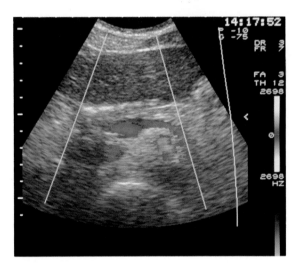

FIG. 6.7. *(See page 113 for the discussion of the figure.)* **Normal splenic vessels: CDU—transverse scan. Flow toward transducer is colored in blue. Red color indicates flow away from transducer. Intrasplenic vessels are well depicted in color Doppler scan, which allows accurate placement of cursor for PWD analysis.**

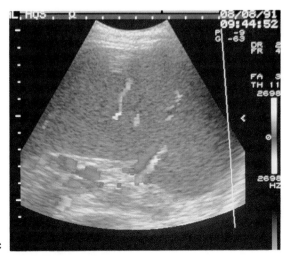

c

FIG. 6.11. Splenomegaly. *(See page 116 for parts **a** and **b**.)* **a:** parasagittal scan; **b:** transverse scan. This example illustrates moderate splenomegaly (SI = 1,274) in a patient with IM. **c: Massive splenomegaly: scan with CDU. SI measures >2,000 in this patient with cirrhosis. The varices at the splenic hilus are well demonstrated by CDU.**

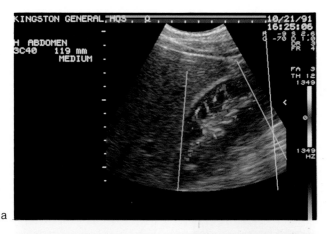

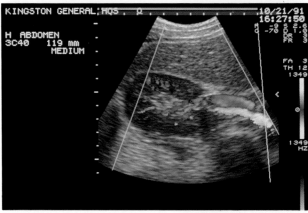

FIG. 8.3. Color Doppler of kidney in sagittal axis (**a**) and transverse axis (**b**). (*See page 148 for the discussion of the figure.*) **Color assignment is dependent on direction of flow and is indicated in color bar to right. Flow toward transducer is red, whereas flow away from transducer is blue. Note that arterial or venous structures may be red or blue on the same color Doppler picture depending on whether flow is toward or away from transducer. Arterial flow toward transducer will be depicted as red, whereas arterial flow away from transducer will be depicted as blue. The same is true of venous flow. One can discriminate between arterial and venous structures by PW spectral analysis and the pattern of pulsation. (Courtesy of Dr. Patrick Llewellyn.)**

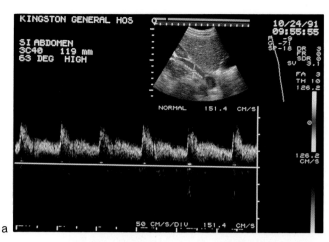
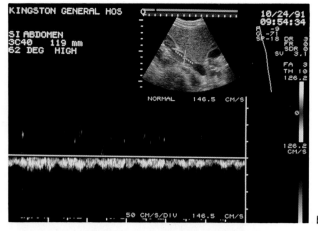

a

b

FIG. 8.7. Triplex (PW, color, real-time) scan of right renal hilum in transverse axis. (*See page 151 for the discussion of the figure.*) **a: PW sample is placed on renal artery. Renal artery flow is toward transducer and is red. b: PW sample is placed on renal vein. Renal vein flow is away from transducer and is blue. (Courtesy of Dr. Patrick Llewellyn.)**

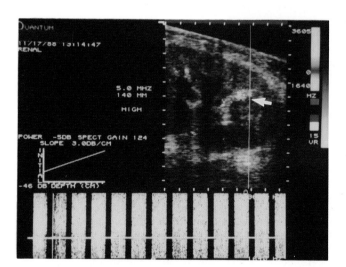

FIG. 8.111. Parenchymal AVM on color Doppler. (*See page 184 for the discussion of the figure.*) **This is same patient as in Fig. 8.110.** *Arrow* **indicates area of AVM with a small pseudoaneurysm. There is increased color saturation toward white caused by high velocity. There is also slight perivascular flow artifact in parenchyma caused by tissue vibration.**

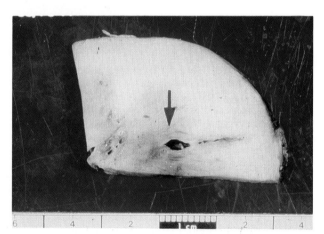

FIG. 8.112. Pseudoaneurysm at site of AVM. (*See page 184 for the discussion of the figure.*) **Same case as Figs. 8.110 and 8.111.**

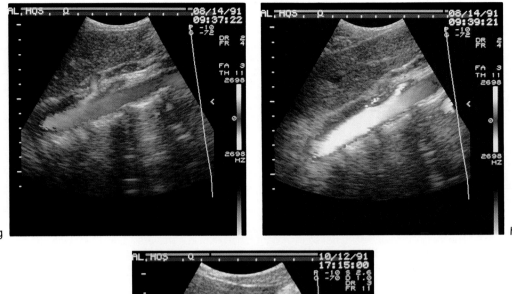

g   h

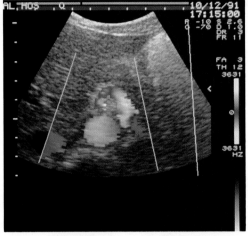

i

FIG. 10.2. Anterior branches of abdominal aorta. (*See page 209 for parts a–f.*) **a:** celiac artery and superior mesenteric artery. Sagittal scan demonstrates origin of SMA (*arrow*) and celiac artery (*ca*). *a*, aorta; *p*, pancreas; *s*, splenic artery. **b:** celiac axis. Transverse scan demonstrates tortuous celiac artery (*ca*) arising from aorta (*a*) and branching into common hepatic artery (*h*) and splenic artery (*s*). **c:** left gastric artery. Sagittal scan demonstrates proximal left gastric artery (*g*) arising from celiac artery (*ca*). **d:** aneurysm of common hepatic artery. Transverse scan of celiac axis demonstrates an aneurysm (*An*) of proximal common hepatic artery. Doppler cursor is in celiac artery. Doppler spectrum demonstrates forward flow in systole and diastole (*D*). *s*, splenic artery; *Ao*, aorta. **e:** celiac artery and sma with lymphadenopathy. Multiple enlarged lymph nodes (*n*) surround celiac artery (*ca*) and SMA (*sma*). Note small left gastric artery (*g*). *a*, aorta. (**f**) celiac axis with lymphadenopathy. Transverse scan of same patient as **e** demonstrates enlarged lymph nodes (*n*) stretching celiac artery (*ca*) and its branches. *a*, aorta; *i*, IVC. **g: color Doppler of celiac axis and SMA: diastole. Sagittal scan during ventricular diastole demonstrates forward blood flow (red) in aorta, celiac artery, and superior mesenteric artery. Note white in center of celiac artery, indicating higher velocity in center of lumen compared with edges of lumen. Note also blue color in left gastric artery, which arises from celiac axis. Blue indicates flow away from probe.**

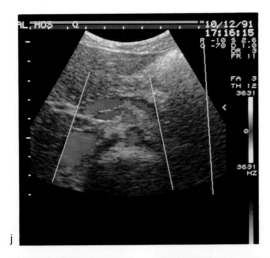

j

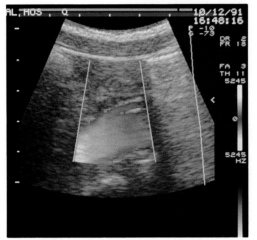

k

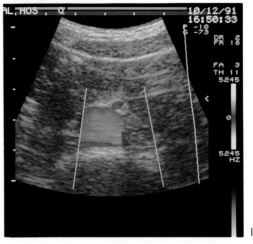

l

FIG. 10.2. *continued.* h: color Doppler of celiac axis and SMA: systole. Sagittal scan during ventricular systole demonstrates higher velocity flow (white versus red) in aorta and superior mesenteric artery. Celiac artery is less well visualized in this scan. i: celiac axis—missing hepatic artery (color). Transverse scan demonstrates forward flow in celiac artery (red) and splenic artery (blue because artery courses away from probe). Common hepatic artery is absent (see g). j: SMA—replaced common hepatic artery. Transverse scan through proximal SMA demonstrates common hepatic artery arising from right side of SMA and coursing toward porta hepatis (see i). k: inferior mesenteric artery: sagittal, color Doppler. Sagittal scan of distal aorta demonstrates origin of IMA at anterior aspect of aorta with forward flow (red) in both vessels. l: IMA: transverse, color Doppler. Transverse scan through distal aorta demonstrates IMA along anterior aspect of aorta. Blood flow is toward probe (red) because probe was angled toward head. (Scans c, i, j, k, and l are courtesy of Mr. Tyler Sauerbrei.)

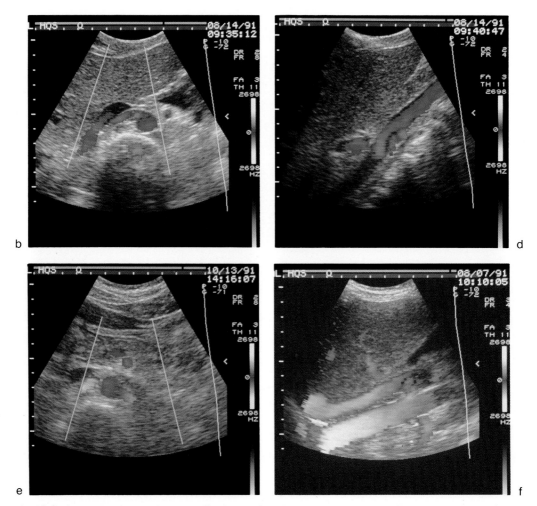

b

d

e

f

FIG. 10.3. Normal right renal artery. (*See page 211 for parts **a** and **c**.*) **a:** Transverse scan of upper abdominal aorta (*a*) demonstrates right renal artery (*r*) originating from aorta and coursing posterior to IVC (*i*). There was congenital absence of left kidney and left renal artery in this patient. *s*, splenic vein; *sma*, superior mesenteric artery. **b: Right renal artery: transverse, color Doppler same patient as a. Flow in proximal right renal artery is coded red because it is toward the probe. Flow in portion of artery behind IVC is blue because it is away from probe. Note red flow (i.e., toward probe, away from right kidney) in right renal vein into IVC. c:** IVC and right renal artery: sagittal. Sagittal scan of IVC (*i*) demonstrates right renal artery (*r*) posterior to IVC. Right portal vein (*p*) lies anterior to IVC in liver parenchyma. **d: IVC and right renal artery: sagittal, CDU. Flow in IVC is coded blue because it is away from probe, toward heart. Flow in right renal artery behind IVC is also coded blue because it is away from probe in this case. Red color adjacent to right renal artery represents swirling blood flow in IVC after stream passes over artery. Note also blue coded flow in portal vein anterior to IVC. e: Right and left renal arteries: transverse, color Doppler. Origins of right and left renal arteries are visualized and blood flow (blue) is away from probe. Note also flow in SMV (blue) and SMA (red). f: Right and left renal arteries: coronal, CDU. Scan through right hepatic lobe demonstrates blood flow in IVC (blue) and aorta (red). Flow in right renal artery (adjacent to IVC) is red (toward probe), whereas flow in origin of left renal artery is a small patch of blue (away from probe). Red flow adjacent to blue is left renal vein (flow toward probe and toward IVC).**

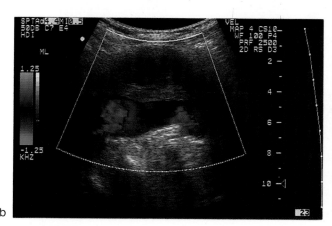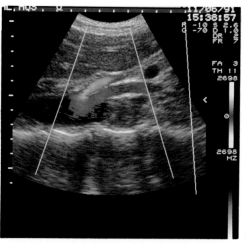

b   f

FIG. 10.7. Thrombosis in aortic aneurysms. (*See page 215 for parts **a, c–e.***) **a:** Transverse scan demonstrates thrombus (*t*) in anterior portion of aneurysm. Anterior and posterior walls of aorta are well defined, whereas lateral walls are poorly defined. Therefore width is more difficult to measure accurately than anteroposterior diameter. *l*, patent lumen. **b: CDU of aortic aneurysm. CDU demonstrates blood flow (red and blue) in residual lumen of aneurysm. Large amount of clot occupies anterior portion of aneurysm. Note lack of color in middle of scan of lumen because ultrasound beam is perpendicular to direction of blood flow. c and d:** Transverse and sagittal scans of an aortic aneurysm with complete thrombosis of lumen. This patient had poor left ventricular function, and slow blood flow predisposed to thrombosis of aortic lumen. *arrows*, margins of recent thrombus formation within "patent lumen"; *s*, splenic vein; *i*, inferior vena cava. **e:** Recanalization of intraluminal thrombus, mimicking a periaortic fluid collection. Cescent-shaped fluid collection (*f*) represents a blood-filled channel between intraluminal thrombus (*t*) and wall of the aorta. No periaortic fluid collection was found at surgery. *ivc*, inferior vena cava; *l*, patent lumen. **f: Total occlusion of aorta by thrombus. CDU demonstrates blood flow in proximal aortic lumen (red) and in two major anterior branches (celiac artery and SMA). Just interior to SMA origin, aortic lumen is filled with thrombus. There was no evidence of flow in distal aorta.**

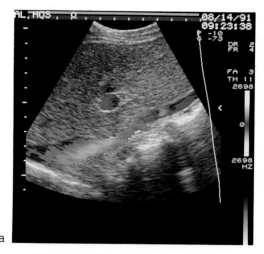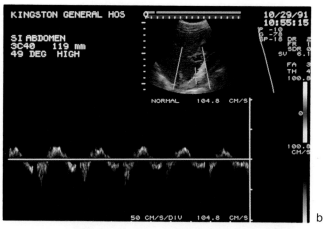

a   b

FIG. 10.14. Doppler of normal IVC and branches. (*See page 222 for the discussion of the figure.*) **a: CDU demonstrates net flow (blue) toward chest. Red color in distal IVC represents local turbulence with net flow toward ultrasound probe. Note blood flow in right portal vein and smaller adjacent right hepatic artery (red color). b: Normal Doppler spectrum from IVC. Doppler cursor lies in middle of IVC lumen (blue represents flow away from probe at the point in time). Doppler spectrum demonstrates two peaks directed below baseline and one above baseline in opposite direction. First negative peak represents right atrial diastole, and second negative peak represents right ventricular diastole. Positive peak (flow away from chest) represents right atrial contraction.**

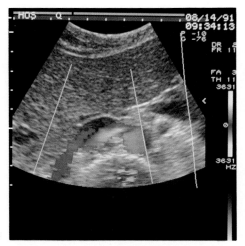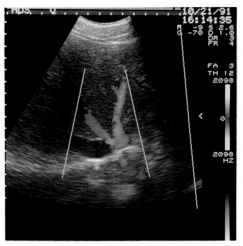

c   d

FIG. 10.14. *continued.* c: CDU of right renal vein. Blood flow in right renal vein is coded red (toward probe), as it flows into IVC. Right renal artery (blue) passes posterior to IVC. d: CDU of hepatic vein. Transverse scan demonstrates flow toward IVC (blue) in middle and left hepatic veins. (Scans b and d are courtesy of Dr. Patrick Llewellyn, Resident in Radiology, Queen's University, Kingston, Canada.)

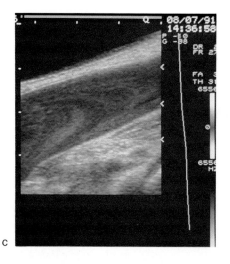

c

FIG. 10.16. IVC dilatation and echogenic blood. (*See page 224 for parts **a** and **b**.*) **a:** Sagittal scan demonstrates dilatation of IVC (anteroposterior diameter is 2.8 cm in supine position). There was very little variation in size with respiration. This patient had right heart failure. **b:** Sagittal scan of IVC demonstrates multiple low-level echoes within lumen of IVC. These are due to aggregates of red blood cells (Rouleaux formation). **c: Scan of a partially obstructed internal jugular vein demonstrates a similar phenomenon. Real-time scanning demonstrated very slow blood flow within jugular vein. Slow flow and enlarged vein both predispose to clumping of red blood cells and thus to visible echogenic blood.**

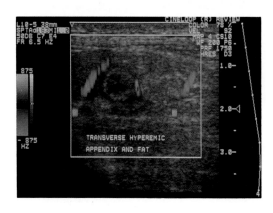

FIG. 12.20. Appendicitis: color Doppler ultrasound. (*See page 253 for the discussion of the figure.*) Note increased blood flow (*arrows*) in appendiceal wall and surrounding tissue. [Scan is courtesy of ATL (Advanced Technology Limited).]

CHAPTER 12

Bowel and Mesentery

INTRODUCTION

The tubular portion of the alimentary tract begins in the abdomen at the gastroesophageal junction and ends at the rectum in the pelvis. It consists of the stomach, duodenum, jejunum, and colon. The mesentery is a fan-shaped sheet of serous membranes. Its root, extending from the duodeno-jejunal flexure (ligament of Treitz) to the ileo-cecal valve, provides attachment of the bowel to the posterior abdominal wall. The small bowel is thus suspended in the peritoneal cavity by the mesentery, which is mainly composed of fat and connective tissues surrounding blood and lymph vessels and nerves. Arterial supply to the bowel is provided by the celiac axis and the superior and inferior mesenteric arteries, which are branches of the abdominal aorta. Venous drainage is by way of the mesenteric veins, which join the splenic vein to form the portal vein.

The bowel lumen and mucosa are usually investigated by means of endoscopy and barium studies that cannot assess the bowel wall and surrounding tissues. Sonography allows quite detailed imaging of the wall in many parts of the gut and may detect various pathologies that affect the bowel wall and the surrounding mesentery. In

selected conditions such as appendicitis, diverticulitis, and HPS, ultrasound is assuming a dominant role for imaging assessment.

This chapter will discuss the sonographic features of the normal bowel and the common pathologies that may be detected by ultrasound.

12.1 SCANNING TECHNIQUES

The stomach is best scanned after oral ingestion of about 400 cc of tap water and using a 5- or 7.5-MHz transducer. Intravenous glucagon may also be given to induce gastric relaxation. The patient should also be fasting before the examination. Scanning is performed with the patient assuming different positions (1).

Scanning for HPS requires first a cooperative infant or child. This can usually be achieved by a pacifier or a juice bottle. When feeding the patient with fluid, care must be taken to avoid overdistending the stomach, because this will make the infant more uncomfortable and will prevent optimal measurements of the pylorus. Pressure on the abdomen with the transducer should be applied gently (2).

The appendix is best evaluated using the graded compression technique with a 5- or 7.5-MHz linear array probe. By applying and gradually increasing the pressure with the transducer, gas-filled bowel loops can be dis-

---

Abbreviations: **CT,** computed tomography; **GI,** gastrointestinal; **HPS,** hypertrophic pyloric stenosis; **MHz,** megahertz; **NHL,** non-Hodgkin's lymphoma.

placed from the right lower quadrant or from the area of maximal tenderness. This maneuver helps also to reduce the distance from the transducer to the appendix (3).

Scanning the small bowel, colon and mesentery is often difficult because of the presence of bowel gas or mesenteric fat or both (4). Attempts should be made during scanning to observe bowel peristalsis and to estimate bowel wall thickness.

12.2 NORMAL ANATOMY

Stomach

The gastroesophageal junction can usually be visualized by scanning through the left hepatic lobe. In large patients or patients with a small left lobe, the gastroesophageal junction may be difficult to see. It is best detected on a longitudinal scan to the left of the midline. It typically appears as a "target" or "bull's-eye" structure, lying posterior to the left lobe of the liver, anterior to the proximal abdominal aorta, and caudal to the diaphragm (Fig. 12.1).

The fluid-filled gastric fundus appears as a round cystic structure in the left upper epigastrium in the supine position. In some patients, it is very posterior in location, simulating a cystic mass adjacent to the splenic hilus. By turning the patient to the right, fluid can be seen to flow from the fundus to the more dependent distal stomach. The collapsed prepyloric antrum is typically seen in a right parasagittal scan inferior to the edge of the liver (Fig. 12.2).

Using the fluid-filled stomach technique and high-resolution transducers, it is possible to identify five layers in the wall of the normal stomach (Fig. 12.3a,b). The innermost echogenic line corresponds to the interface between the lumen and mucosa, the second hypoechoic layer corresponds to the mucosa itself, the third echo-

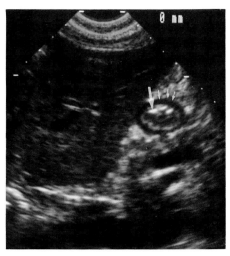

FIG. 12.2. Normal gastric antrum: parasagittal scan. Seen in cross section, collapsed normal antrum has a "target" or "bull's-eye" appearance. Thin sonolucent peripheral rim (*thin white arrows*) represents muscularis propria. Air bubbles (*thick white arrow*) appear as floating echoes within the lumen.

genic layer to the submucosa, the fourth hypoechoic layer to the muscularis propria, and the fifth echogenic line to the outer serosa and its interface with surrounding soft tissue (fat). The appearances are similar to those seen in endoscopic ultrasound as described by Strohm and Classen (5).

The gastric wall thickness is measured from the innermost echogenic layer to the outermost echogenic layer. Normal mean measurement is 2.5 mm (±1 mm). Maximum normal wall thickness should not exceed 5.0 mm in the fluid-distended stomach (6). Gastric rugae can be identified in the nondistended stomach.

Pylorus

The normal pylorus in infants and children can be identified using high-frequency transducers, by scanning below the xiphoid and to the right of the midline. It is medial to the gallbladder and lateral to the pancreatic neck. The pylorus should be scanned in its long and short axes. Figures 12.4a and b demonstrate the technique for measuring the pyloric length, cross-sectional diameter, and wall thickness. Ranges of normal measurements are given in Table 12.1 (2,7,8).

Duodenum and Small Bowel

When there is fluid in the lumen, small bowel appears as a tubular structure in long-axis view and as a target structure in cross section. Valvulae conniventes can be identified in a fluid-filled jejunal loop. The ileum typically appears featureless. Fleischer et al. (9) have found

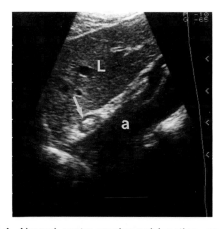

FIG. 12.1. Normal gastroesophageal junction: parasagittal scan. GEJ appears as a "target" structure (*arrow*) lying posterior to left lobe of liver (*L*) and anterior to proximal abdominal aorta (*a*).

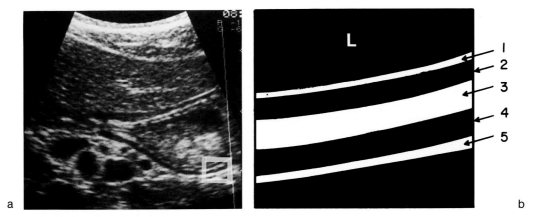

FIG. 12.3. Normal gastric wall. **a:** sonogram; **b:** diagram of area encased in box. (*1*), interface between lumen and mucosa; (*2*), mucosa; (*3*), submucosa; (*4*), muscularis propria; (*5*), interface between serosa and peritoneal fat. *L*, lumen.

that normal small bowel wall thickness should not exceed 3 mm.

Colon

This part of the GI tract is normally filled with gas and fecal material and thus makes ultrasound evaluation difficult. However, it is often possible to evaluate the anterior wall of the colon with ultrasound and assess for focal or diffuse wall thickening. This is especially useful when scanning for possible appendicitis in the right lower quadrant and acute diverticulitis in the left lower quadrant. Normal thickness of the colonic wall should not exceed 5 mm (6,10).

Appendix

This organ, lying in the right iliac fossa, is scanned along its long and short axes. It appears tubular in long-axis view and as a "target" structure in cross section (Fig. 12.5). It is compressible, with an hypoechoic wall surrounding a central echogenic line representing the mucosa. Maximal outer diameter of the appendix should not exceed 6 mm (3,11).

Fetal Bowel

The fetal stomach can be detected *in utero* during obstetric scanning. It appears in the left upper quadrant as a

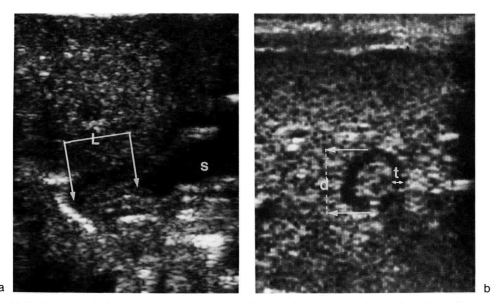

FIG. 12.4. Normal pyloric measurements. **a:** long-axis view; **b:** short-axis view. *L*, length; *d*, diameter; *t*, muscle thickness; *s*, stomach.

TABLE 12.1. *Range of normal measurements of pyloric muscle*

	Ranges (mm)	Maximum (mm)
Pyloric length	5–18	18
Pyloric diameter	6–13	13
Muscle thickness	1–4	4

fluid-filled structure that serves as a landmark to identify the fetal left side.

The fetal bowel is usually isoechoic or hypoechoic compared with the fetal liver (Fig. 12.6) (12). Small bowel loops are seen in only 30% of fetuses after 34 weeks gestation, and they should not exceed 6 mm in diameter. The colon is detectable in all fetuses after 28 weeks gestation. It appears as a tubular structure around the periphery of the abdomen, measuring from 4-6 mm at 22 weeks to 10-18 mm in diameter at term.

Meconium is routinely seen in the colon but not in the small bowel. It is usually hypoechoic, but sometimes echo-free, as compared with the bowel wall.

Mesentery

Normal mesenteric fat and blood vessels may be seen by ultrasound with careful scanning. Flow in smaller mesenteric vessels may be demonstrated by using Doppler techniques. When ascites is present, bowel loops can be seen arranged around the periphery of the fan-shaped echogenic mesentery.

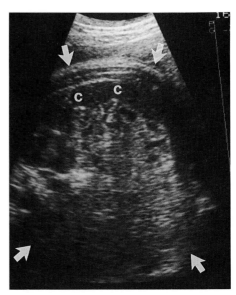

FIG. 12.6. Normal fetal bowel (30 weeks gestation). In this cross-sectional view, colon (*c*) appears as hypoechoic tubular structures around periphery of abdomen (*arrows*).

12.3 PATHOLOGY

Congenital Anomalies

Duodenal Atresia and Stenosis

According to current concepts, these conditions result from failure of recanalization during development. One third of the patients are seen in infants with Trisomy 21. Other associated anomalies of the GI tract and biliary tree are common (13). Clinically, abdominal distension and bilious vomiting are seen in the immediate postnatal period when complete atresia is present. In case of stenosis, symptoms usually appear later in life, depending on the degree of the obstruction. Traditionally, the diagnosis is made by radiographs of the abdomen, showing the "double-bubble" sign, which represents the dilated gas-filled stomach and duodenum. Sonography can detect duodenal obstruction *in utero* (14,15) by showing the dilated fluid-filled stomach and duodenum in the fetus (Fig. 12.7).

When duodenal atresia is associated with esophageal atresia without fistula, the stomach and duodenum are obstructed at both ends. The diagnosis cannot be made on the plain radiograph, which shows only a gasless abdomen. In this situation, sonography is the diagnostic tool of choice, by demonstrating the distended fluid-filled stomach and duodenum (16).

One should be aware that duodenal obstruction in the neonate may be due to other causes such as annular pancreas, Ladd's Bands, duodenal diaphragm, and duplication cysts (17).

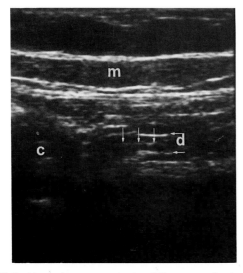

FIG. 12.5. Normal measurements of the appendix: long-axis view. *d,* diameter; *c,* cecum; *m,* abdominal wall. Echogenic white line (*long white arrows*) represents mucosal layer.

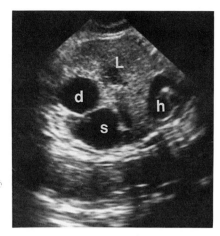

FIG. 12.7. Duodenal atresia seen *in utero*. Two round fluid collections (*double-bubble sign*) are seen in upper abdomen of this 28 weeks fetus. They represent dilated stomach (*s*) and duodenum (*d*). Note liver (*L*) and heart (*h*).

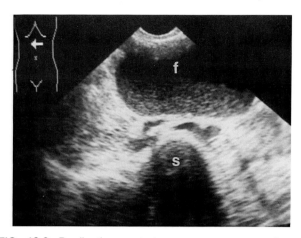

FIG. 12.8. Duplication cyst: transverse sonogram. Large fluid collection (*f*) containing layering debris was seen in upper abdomen of this 2-year-old child who presented with a palpable mass. At surgery, this proved to be a duplication cyst of jejunum. Most duplication cysts are usually smaller than this one. *s*, spine.

Duplication Cysts (Neurenteric Cysts)

Duplication cysts are thought to result either from failure of canalization or from faulty separation of the primitive neurenteric canal during development. They may occur anywhere along the tubular GI tract, but they are seen most commonly in the small bowel. Association with vertebral anomalies is relatively frequent. The cyst may also extend into the spinal canal, but it usually does not communicate with the lumen of the gut. It is often lined with gastric or intestinal mucosa. Patients usually present with abdominal pain and a mobile palpable mass (18).

Small bowel duplication may be multiple and may be mistaken for loculated ascites (19,20). Ultrasound readily identifies the cystic nature of the lesions, which often occurs on the mesenteric border of the bowel. Identification of the mucosal layer of the cyst by ultrasound and by Technetium⁹⁹ᵐ pertechnetate scanning help to establish the diagnosis. Omental and mesenteric cysts do not have mucosal lining in their wall (19,20). The duplication may contain septations and floating debris (Fig. 12.8) (21). It may be the leading point in intussusception.

Omental and Mesenteric Cysts

The exact etiology of omental and mesenteric cysts is still obscure. They may be due to congenital obstruction of the lymphatics or possibly hamartomas (22). The majority of patients present with a palpable abdominal mass that may be mistaken for ascites or solid neoplasms. Omental cysts usually follow the contour of the bowel; mesenteric cysts often occur in the root of the mesentery. They contain fluid that may be serous, chy-

lous, bloody, or mixed. Occasionally, a "cheesy-white" material is obtained from aspiration, and this is probably inspissated chyle (23).

Ultrasound readily demonstrates the cystic nature of the lesions (Fig. 12.9a,b), which are often unilocular but may be septated and may contain low-amplitude echoes representing chyle or blood particles from hemorrhage (24,25). An unusual appearance is the demonstration of a fat–fluid level within the cyst. This is thought to be due to the presence of chyle associated with an inflammatory exudate (26). Differentiation from a duplication cyst is difficult but is possible by identifying the echogenic mucosal layer in the wall of the duplication cysts (27).

Hypertrophic Pyloric Stenosis (HPS)

Traditionally, before real-time sonography and the original paper by Tunell and Wilson (28) in 1984, diagnosis of HPS was made by clinical findings and upper GI barium studies.

Hypertrophic pyloric stenosis is a disease with familial tendency and unknown pathogenesis. Recently, it is considered an acquired condition, which is suspected to be caused by prolonged pylorospasm (29,30). It affects most commonly infants after the first week of life and before 3 or 4 months of age. Eighty percent of patients are male. Most patients present with projectile vomiting and a mass the size of an olive palpable in the right upper quadrant. However, the clinical diagnosis is uncertain in 15% to 25% of cases. The barium study is inconclusive in 5% to 10% of cases (31).

Pathologically, HPS is due to thickening of the circular layer of the pyloric muscle, which also elongates and constricts the pyloric canal. The thickening is usually

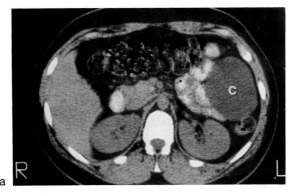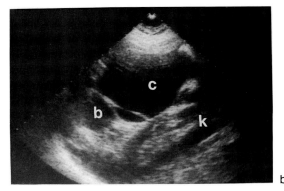

FIG. 12.9. Mesenteric cyst. **a:** CT scan; **b:** parasagittal sonogram. CT scan showed a low-density mass (c) displacing bowel around it. Sonogram demonstrated cystic nature of the lesion. Diagnosis was made at surgery. *b,* bowel; *k,* kidney.

concentric but may at times be asymmetrical, resulting in atypical findings on barium study (32).

The hypertrophied pyloric muscle is imaged and measured in the longitudinal and transaxial planes (Fig. 12.10a,b). Its sonographic appearances mimic a "doughnut" (target) or an "empty cervix" (33). Sonographically, the diagnosis of infantile HPS is established when the measurements shown in Table 12.2 are obtained.

The following points should be kept in mind:

1. The normal pylorus is detectable in almost all infants. If the pylorus cannot be seen by sonography and the patient's symptoms suggest HPS, a barium meal should be performed.
2. There is some overlap between normal and HPS in the measurement of pyloric diameter, muscle thick-

ness, and pyloric length (28,31,33). In cases in which measurements are equivocal, calculation of pyloric volume is useful. Westra et al. (34) found that this is the only value that has no overlap between normal and HPS.
3. When borderline measurements are obtained, follow-up studies should be performed.
4. During scanning, it is useful to observe the ancillary signs associated with HPS (Fig. 12.11): fluid distension of the stomach, hyperperistalsis, poor-to-absent gastric emptying, and thickened antropyloric muscle. They help to reinforce the diagnosis.
5. Sonography is also used to monitor the postoperative results. Sauerbrei and Paloschi (35) found that pyloric measurements usually become normal within 6 weeks after surgery.

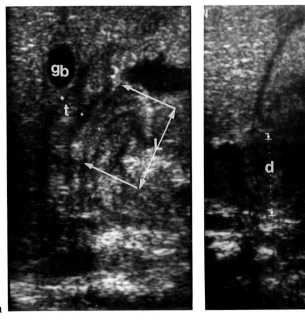

FIG. 12.10. HPS. **a:** long-axis view **b:** short-axis view. Pyloric length (*L*) measures 30 mm, muscle thickness (*t*) measures 10 mm, and pyloric diameter (*d*) measures 28 mm in this child with typical HPS. *gb,* gallbladder; *s,* stomach.

TABLE 12.2. *Measurement in HPS*

Pyloric diameter (*PD*)	> 13 mm
Muscle thickness	> 4 mm
Pyloric length (*PL*)	> 18 mm
Pyloric volume (*PV*)	> 1.40 ml

$$PV = \pi \left(\frac{PD}{2}\right)^2 \times PL$$

From Teele and Smith, ref. 2; Tunell and Wilson, ref. 28; Ball et al., ref. 33; Westra et al., ref. 34.

Bowel Obstruction

The most common causes of bowel obstruction are intussusception in children (36), hernias, and postsurgical adhesions in adults (37). Traditionally, diagnosis is made by clinical findings and abdominal radiographs.

Sonography is particularly useful in the investigation of the gasless abdomen. The absence of bowel gas optimizes the examination, which can easily determine whether the abdominal distension is due to ascites, dilated fluid-filled bowel, presence of a mass, or a combination of the above (36). The technique may also help to distinguish between adynamic ileus and mechanical obstruction. In adynamic ileus, very little if any peristalsis is seen, whereas in obstruction, significant contractile activity is usually identified with real-time ultrasound (37).

Obstructed bowel loops appear on ultrasound as dilated fluid-filled structures that appear tubular when scanned along their long axis and round when seen in cross section. Identification of the valvulae conniventes distinguishes jejunum from a loop of colon or ileum (Fig. 12.12).

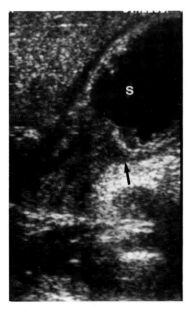

FIG. 12.11. HPS: secondary signs. Note distended fluid-filled stomach (*s*) and thickened antropyloric muscle (*arrow*).

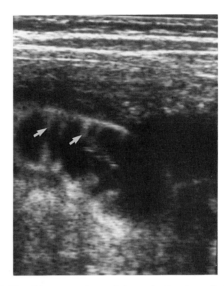

FIG. 12.12. Obstructed small bowel—keyboard sign. This loop is dilated and fluid-filled. Presence of valvulae conniventes (*arrows*) helps to identify this as a loop of small bowel.

When a single "U"- or "C"-shaped dilated bowel loop is seen, closed loop obstruction or volvulus should be suspected (38,39). Afferent loop obstruction in a Billroth type II anastomosis (39) can also be diagnosed by ultrasound, which typically shows a large cystic tubular structure containing layering debris in the upper abdomen (Fig. 12.13a,b).

Intussusception

This is defined as telescoping of one part of the intestine into the lumen of a contiguous adjoining segment. The intussusceptum is the central invaginated part, which is surrounded by the external layer of the distal segment called the *intussuscipiens*. Four major types are recognized: colocolic, ileoileal, ileoileocolic, and ileocolic. The last one is the most common, accounting for 75% to 95% of cases (40). Intussusception occurs most frequently in children between the ages of 6 months and 4 years. In children, there is a male preponderance with a 2:1 male–female ratio (40,41). It is occasionally seen in adults, where it is often associated with a lead point such as a Meckel's diverticulum or a neoplasm.

In most centers, contrast enema (e.g., barium, water-soluble contrast media, air) remains the diagnostic and therapeutic procedure of choice. However, in children with vague clinical findings, ultrasound may be performed as an initial test, and thus recognition of the possible ultrasound abnormalities is important.

Scanned in cross section, the apex of the intussusception appears as a target lesion, with the outer hypoechoic rim representing the edematous wall of the intussuscipiens and the echogenic center representing the compressed interfaces of the intussusceptum (Fig. 12.14a,b).

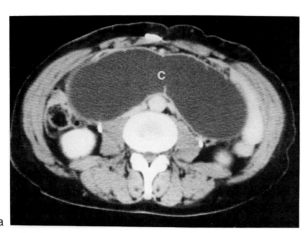
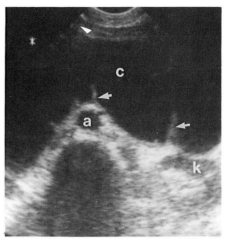

FIG. 12.13. Obstructed afferent loop. **a:** CT scan; **b:** transverse sonogram. CT scan shows a large sausage-shaped mass of low density (*c*) lying across abdomen. Sonogram identifies it as a dilated fluid-filled bowel loop by presence of valvulae conniventes (*arrows*). Patient had a previous remote Billroth type II operation. At surgery, afferent loop was obstructed by adhesions. *a*, aorta; *k*, kidney.

More proximal to the apex, three concentric rings may be seen. The outer and more inner hypoechoic ring represent the returning and the entering wall of the intussusceptum, respectively. The intervening echogenic ring represents the interface between the walls. Scans along the long axis of the intussusception show a characteristic appearance, with two echogenic stripes sandwiched among three hypoechoic ones (42). If a cyst or solid tumor forms the leading point to the intussusceptum, it may also be detected by sonography (43).

Inflammatory and Infectious Diseases

Gastritis and Ulcer Disease

Mucosal disease of the stomach and duodenum may be detected by ultrasound with careful scanning and par-

ticular attention to technical details. Thickened gastric rugae may be seen by scanning the stomach after it is partially filled with water (usually 300–400 cc). Further gastric distension may compress and efface the folds. The list of possible causes of thickened abnormal gastric folds is long. This ranges from gastritis of all sorts (e.g., infectious, eosinophilic, varioliform, Menetrier's disease) to infiltration by malignancies (e.g., carcinoma, lymphoma, breast metastases) (44,45). Diagnosis is established by clinical and endoscopic findings.

Peptic ulcer disease also can be evaluated with ultrasound when the stomach is carefully scanned after water ingestion using a 5- or 7.5-MHz transducer (46). Positive findings include thickening of the gastric wall (>5 mm), poor definition of the normal five sonographic layers, and presence of ulcer craters showing as depressions on the mucosal surface. Perforation should be suspected

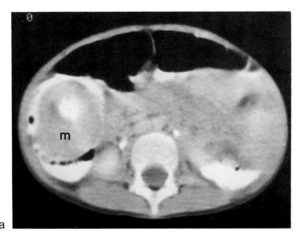
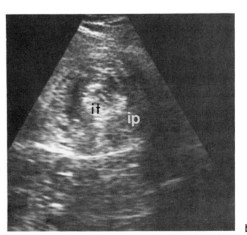

FIG. 12.14. Intussusception (ileocecal). **a:** CT scan; **b:** sonogram. CT scan was performed to look for enlarged nodes in this 4-year-old boy with known Burkitt's lymphoma. A mass (*m*) with target appearance was found in right iliac fossa. Sonogram showed characteristic appearance of intussusception, with outer hypoechoic rim (*ip*) representing intussuscipiens and echogenic center (*it*) representing intussusceptum.

when an ulcer crater is seen communicating with a fluid collection adjacent to the stomach (46). A "target" (or bull's-eye) appearance has been described in connection with duodenal ulcers (47). The hypoechoic rim represents the edematous duodenal wall surrounding the strongly reflective center, which is probably the ulcer crater. However, ulcer disease remains the domain of endoscopy and barium studies. Sonography offers a possible alternate way to detect and monitor gastric ulcers in patients in whom endoscopy and barium studies could not be performed for one reason or another.

Bowel Hematoma

This may be caused by a large number of conditions, including trauma, surgery, anticoagulant medication, blood dyscrasia, Henoch-Schonlein purpura, and inflammatory and neoplastic disease of the bowel. In children, child abuse should be suspected in the appropriate clinical setting (48).

The hematoma is usually intramural, producing eccentric thickening of the bowel wall (49,50). In blunt abdominal trauma, the duodenum, because of its fixed position, is the most commonly injured part of the GI tract. The sonographic appearance of a bowel hematoma depends on the stage of its evolution, as with hematoma occurring elsewhere. Fresh hematoma is often hyperechoic. It becomes hypoechoic as the hematoma resorbs. During lysis and fragmentation of the clot, it appears cystic and septated (49–51). Sonography is used to detect and monitor the hematoma. Conservative management is the rule, unless complications (e.g., infection, obstruction, marked increase in size) supervene.

Granulomatous Enterocolitis (Crohn's Disease)

This is an inflammatory disease of the GI tract of unknown etiology, characterized by granulomatous ulcers involving all layers of the bowel wall. The terminal ileum is most frequently affected, but any part of the GI tract may be involved in a segmental distribution. Complications include malabsorption, fibrosing strictures with or without bowel obstruction, internal and external fistulas, abdominal abscess, and increased incidence of gallstones and renal stones caused by abnormal reabsorption of bile salts. The disease affects patients of all ages, with a peak at 15 and 25 years. Clinical findings are usually nonspecific, consisting of crampy abdominal pain, bloody diarrhea, and weight loss. The diagnosis is made by endoscopy and biopsy. Extent of the disease is usually evaluated by means of barium studies (52).

Lutz (53) in 1972 was the first to describe the sonographic "target" or "bull's-eye" appearance of a bowel loop involved by Crohn's disease seen in cross section. Small bowel wall measuring more than 3 mm (Fig. 12.15) and colonic wall measuring more than 5 mm are

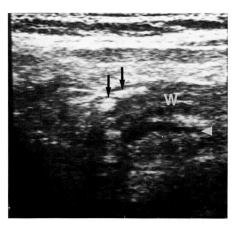

FIG. 12.15. Crohn's ileitis: long-axis view. Note thickened wall (*w*). Bright echoes (*black arrows*) represent probably areas of fibrosis. *Arrowhead,* fluid in lumen of ileum.

considered abnormal (6,7). The thickened wall, caused by edematous mucosa and submucosa, appears as a thick band of inhomogeneous texture. It is surrounded peripherally by a thin hypoechoic layer representing the muscularis propria. In the center is a reflecting layer representing air in the bowel lumen. This appearance is, however, seen in many other conditions including other inflammatory diseases and bowel neoplasms (54–56). Figure 12.16 illustrates the sonographic appearance of ischemic colitis.

In 1989, Limberg (57) claimed a high accuracy in differentiating Crohn's colitis from ulcerative colitis by sonographic criteria. However, it is apparent from the experimental work of Kimmey et al. (58) that, although sonography is accurate in distinguishing normal from inflamed bowel, it is not useful in determining the cause of the inflammation. There is also no significant correlation between bowel wall thickness and disease activity.

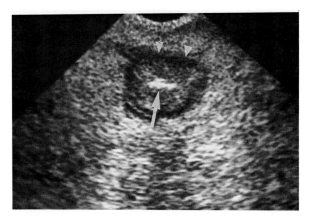

FIG. 12.16. Ischemic colitis: short-axis view. Note marked diffuse thickening of colonic wall (*arrowheads*). Innermost linear white echo (*thick arrow*) represents air in compressed lumen. Note also marked increase in echogenicity of tissue surrounding colon. This represents pericolonic edema and inflammation.

Ultrasound is useful in detecting complications in patients with documented Crohn's disease. The complications include gallstones with or without biliary obstruction, renal stone with or without hydronephrosis, abscess collections, bowel obstruction, and inflammation of adjacent organs such as the liver, ureters, or urinary bladder (Fig. 12.17) (59).

Typhlitis (Neutropenic Colitis, Ileocecal Syndrome)

This is a necrotizing inflammation of the cecum of unknown etiology, often complicated by secondary bacterial infection. It is most commonly seen in leukemic patients on chemotherapy, usually in the terminal stage of the disease. Neutropenia is often present. Diagnosis in the past was suggested by barium enema (60). The condition usually responds to antibiotics.

The sonographic findings of typhlitis have been described in two reports (61). They consist mainly of echogenic polypoid thickening of the mucosa and edema of the cecal wall. There may be necrosis of adjacent mesenteric fat showing as an hypoechoic mass.

Differential diagnosis with appendicitis and other inflammatory bowel diseases may be difficult but should be suspected in the appropriate clinical setting and by identifying the normal ascending colon, terminal ileum, and appendix on ultrasound.

Acute Appendicitis and Appendiceal Abscess

In children, this remains the most common cause of the acute surgical abdomen. History is often unobtainable, and symptomatology is often confusing because of many other conditions that mimic appendicitis. False-positive surgical rate is high, up to 32% in one study (62).

Since the first report by Puylaert (3) in 1986, graded compression technique using high-frequency linear

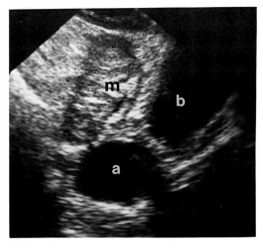

FIG. 12.17. Cystitis and abscess in Crohn's disease. Note inflamed bowel mass (m) adherent to dome of urinary bladder (b), which is thick-walled. Patient complained of dysuria and frequency. Round fluid collection (a) represents an interloop abscess posterior to the bowel.

array transducer has become an established noninvasive technique in the investigation of suspected appendicitis.

The acutely inflamed appendix can be diagnosed sonographically by using the following criteria (Fig. 12.18a,b): (a) maximal outer diameter greater than 6 mm; (b) muscular wall thickness exceeding 3 mm; (c) presence of appendicalith (Fig. 12.19); (d) appendix not compressible (62–64). Measurements are obtained in the cross-section scan of the appendix. Occasionally, increased blood flow is detected in the inflamed appendiceal wall and surrounding tissue by color Doppler ultrasound (Fig. 12.20).

The criteria are fairly specific for acute appendicitis and are valid for both children and adults (62,65). We concur with Worrell et al. (63) that sonography should not replace clinical screening. It should be used to confirm the diagnosis and to look for alternate pathology

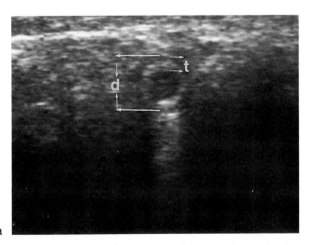

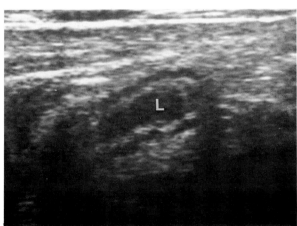

a

b

FIG. 12.18. Acute appendicitis. a: short-axis view; b: long-axis view. Note edematous irregular wall (t) and fluid-filled lumen (L). External diameter (d) measures 22 mm.

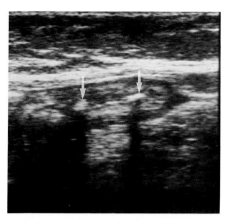

FIG. 12.19. Appendicitis with fecalith: long-axis view. Thick-walled appendix contains intraluminal echoes with posterior acoustic shadowing (*arrow*). Fecaliths were found at surgery. Air bubbles may have similar appearance.

that may simulate appendicitis such as ruptured ectopic pregnancies, ovarian torsion, hemorrhage in ovarian cysts, hydronephrosis, inflammatory bowel disease, or mesenteric lymphadenitis in children (66).

In patients with borderline measurements (maximal diameter 6 mm or less, wall thickness 3 mm or less) and with equivocal clinical findings and no other abnormalities detected by ultrasound, it is wise to perform follow-up scans. In this way, unnecessary surgery may be avoided. In experienced hands and with careful technique, diagnostic accuracy may attain 87% to 96%, with sensitivities of 75% to 90% and specificities of 86% to 100% (63–65,67).

Perforation of an inflamed appendix remains a common complication, occurring in more than 42% of cases, frequently in children and in patients older than 50 years of age. Most often the perforation results in a localized walled-off abscess, but occasionally free intraperitoneal spill may occur, causing severe acute peritonitis.

On ultrasound scan, appendiceal abscess usually appears as a complex mass in the right iliac fossa surrounding a swollen appendix. The mass may contain highly reflective echoes with or without acoustic shadowing, which may represent a fecalith or gas bubbles (Fig. 12.21). Free fluid around the cecum and loss of the echogenic mucosal layer in the fluid-filled appendix may also be seen (68). If percutaneous drainage is contemplated, it is wise to confirm the findings by CT scanning, which offers safer guidance for percutaneous access.

Diverticular Disease

The term encompasses diverticulosis and diverticulitis. Diverticula are formed by herniation of mucosa and muscularis mucosa through points of weakness in the muscular wall of the colon. Increased intracolonic pressure is the mechanical etiologic factor. Nearly 2% of the patients will require hospitalization. Half a percent will require surgery (69).

The condition affects most commonly people older than 50 years of age and the left-sided colon. Diverticula on the right-sided colon are more frequently seen in Orientals and are more prone to hemorrhage. Diverticula on the left-sided colon are more frequently seen in Caucasians and are more prone to inflammation and infection. Diverticulitis is often self-limited, responding usually to medical treatment.

Sonography demonstrates circumferential or asymmetric thickening of the colonic wall, usually at the site of maximum tenderness (Fig. 12.22). Gas-filled diverticula usually appear as focal echogenic sacs in or adjacent to the thickened wall. In most cases of diverticulitis, the surrounding fat is edematous (Fig. 12.23a,b). This gives a diffuse hyperechoic texture to the pericolic tissue, which has been likened to the appearance of thyroid parenchyma ("thyroid in the abdomen" appearance) (70).

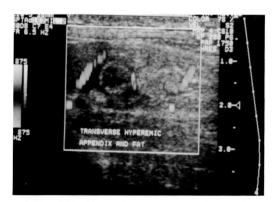

FIG. 12.20. Appendicitis: color Doppler ultrasound. (*See color image in color plate section B, which follows page 242.*) Note increased blood flow (*arrows*) in appendiceal wall and surrounding tissue. [Scan is courtesy of ATL (Advanced Technology Limited).]

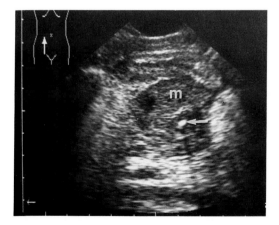

FIG. 12.21. Appendiceal abscess. Note fecalith (*arrow*) in inflammatory mass (*m*). Quite often, an appendiceal abscess appears as a complex mass containing fluid.

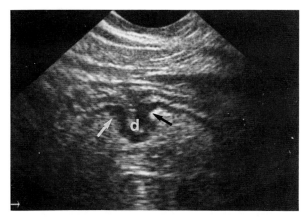

FIG. 12.22. Diverticulitis. Note thickening of bowel wall (*arrows*) adjacent to diverticulum (*d*) and increased echogenicity in tissue around diverticulum. This represents peridiverticular edema and inflammation.

On CT scan, the inflamed pericolic fat assumes increased density. If perforation occurs with abscess formation, a cystic or complex pericolic mass is seen (Figs. 12.24 and 12.25).

Ultrasound can be performed as the initial imaging test in patients suspected of having acute diverticulitis. If uncomplicated diverticulitis is demonstrated by sonography, nonsurgical therapy can be instituted and maintained. When a pericolic abscess is found, a drainage procedure is probably required. This can be performed under CT guidance.

Mesenteritis

Diffuse or focal mesenteric edema is seen in acute pancreatitis, appendicitis, diverticulitis, hypoalbuminemia, and superior mesenteric vein thrombosis (71). The mesenteric leaves appear thickened and strongly echogenic

(Fig. 12.26). The changes are better demonstrated by CT scanning (71).

Mesenteric fat necrosis and sclerosing (retractile) mesenteritis are rare conditions appearing as hypoechoic masses that may be mistaken for neoplastic lesions (72,73).

Neoplastic Diseases

Gastrointestinal Carcinoma

Carcinoma is the most common malignancy of the stomach, accounting for 90% to 95% of all gastric cancers. Next is lymphoma (3–5%) and lymphosarcoma (2%). During the past 50 years, two changes in the statistical profile of gastric carcinoma have been noted: its incidence has declined steadily in North America; and its anatomical distribution in the stomach has shifted with a decrease in incidence of antral lesions and a marked increase in lesions of the esophagogastric junction (Fig. 12.27a,b) (74). Symptomatology is frequently vague; patients usually present late with large palpable mass or disseminated disease. This accounts in large part for the dismal low 5-year survival rate of 10% to 20% (75).

Early gastric cancers (i.e., cancer confined to the mucosa or submucosa) can be detected by barium study and endoscopy. Endoscopic ultrasound offers significant prognostic contribution by determining accurately the depth of invasion (76). Careful transabdominal scanning of the fluid-filled stomach with a 7.5-MHz transducer may also reveal early cancer, which appears as a small hypoechoic mucosal elevation with preservation of wall layers (1). Carcinoma in more advanced stages appears as "target" lesion caused by wall thickening (Fig. 12.28a,b) or as a fungating extraluminal mass that may be confused with a leiomyosarcoma or lymphoma. It is

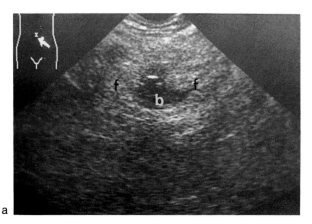

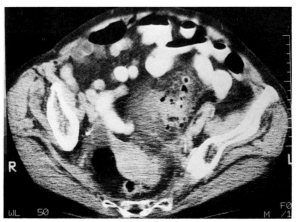

FIG. 12.23. Diverticulitis. **a:** sonogram; **b:** CT scan of pelvis. Note edema in fat (*f*) surrounding bowel (*b*). This has same echogenicity as that of a normal thyroid. This has been described as "thyroid in the abdomen" appearance. This is well seen in corresponding CT scan.

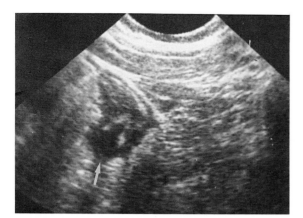

FIG. 12.24. Diverticular abscess. Small focal fluid collection (*arrow*) is seen surrounding ruptured diverticulum.

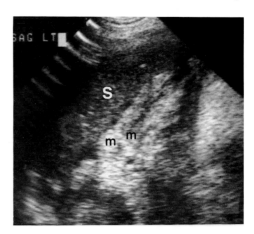

FIG. 12.26. Inflamed mesentery: sagittal scan. Leaves of mesentery filled with echogenic fat (*m*) are grossly thickened in this patient with acute pancreatitis. *S*, spleen.

possible to distinguish gastric carcinoma from lymphoma by the sonographic appearances, with gastric carcinoma being usually more echogenic than lymphoma (77). In practice, however, biopsies are required to make the diagnosis. Local spread to surrounding organs and distant metastases to the liver and ovaries (Krukenberg tumor) can be detected by sonography.

Adenocarcinomas of the small intestine are less common and more difficult to detect, affecting most frequently the duodenojejunal junction and the jejunum. This is in contrast to small bowel lymphoma, which occurs more frequently in the terminal ileum. Sonography usually reveals a target-like lesion or a fungating complex mass. Diagnosis should be established by barium studies and biopsies.

It is estimated that about one in 40 deaths will be due to carcinoma of the colon each year in the United States. It is now an established opinion that colonic cancers arise from preexisting adenomatous polyps, 60% of which are found in the rectum and sigmoid colon (78).

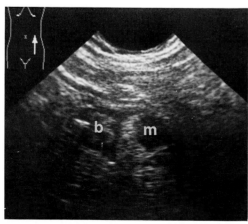

FIG. 12.25. Diverticular abscess: parasagittal scan. Inflammatory mass (*m*) is seen adjacent to thickened mesentery and sigmoid colon (*b*).

Mass screening is performed by stool testing for occult blood followed by barium enema and colonoscopy. There is an increased incidence of colon cancers in patients with long-standing ulcerative colitis, a family history of colon cancer, history of previous polyps or carcinoma, and the polyposes syndromes. These high-risk patients should have regular survey. In recent years, it appears that cancers of the right-sided colon have increased in incidence, whereas the rate of rectal cancers has decreased (78). Detection of early colon cancer is important, because there is a cure rate approaching 90% with Duke's A tumors (78). Patients with cancers in the right-sided colon often have iron deficiency anemia; those with cancers in the left-sided colon usually present with rectal bleeding.

Most colon cancers found by sonography are usually advanced and symptomatic. They show either a target-like appearance (bull's-eye) (pseudo-kidney sign) (Fig. 12.29a,b) or as a fungating complex mass filling the bowel lumen (Fig. 12.30a,b) (79). Barium enema and colonoscopy are usually indicated to look for another synchronous carcinoma, which is seen in about 5% of patients (80). Sonography is performed to detect metastatic disease in regional lymph nodes and the liver.

Gastrointestinal Lymphoma

The tubular GI tract may be the primary site of lymphoma or may be involved as part of disseminated systemic lymphoma. In either situation, about one half of all GI lymphomas occur in the stomach; one third involve the small bowel, most often the terminal ileum. Sixteen percent are found in the colon (81).

Both sexes are equally affected. There are two age-related peaks, one in children younger than 10 years, the other in adults in their 50s. Association with long-standing ulcerative colitis, Crohn's disease and celiac

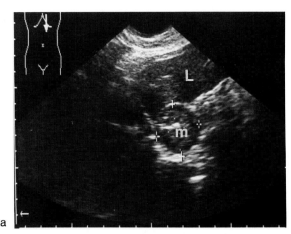
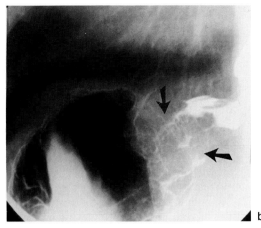

FIG. 12.27. Carcinoma of gastroesophageal junction. **a:** sagittal sonogram; **b:** barium meal (prone view). Gastroesophageal junction (*m*) appears too prominent in this patient with dysphagia. Barium meal confirmed presence of an annular mass at the cardia (*arrows*). *L,* liver.

disease have been described. Abdominal pain, anemia, weight loss, malabsorption, and a palpable abdominal mass are the usual clinical findings, but not all patients have all the findings and symptomatology is often vague (81).

Pathologically, the malignancy originates from the lymphoid tissue in the lamina propria and submucosa. Eighty percent of GI lymphoma are NHL, which includes the Burkitt's variety. Isolated Hodgkin's disease of the GI tract is exceptionally rare (81). The gross anatomy ranges from thickened mucosal folds, shallow ulcerative plaques to submucosal polypoid nodules, annular constricting lesions, and fungating extraluminal masses.

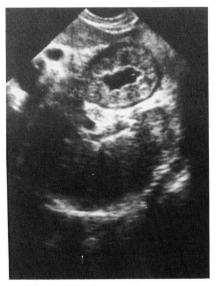

FIG. 12.28. Carcinoma of stomach: cross-sectional view of antrum. Striking circumferential thickening of gastric wall is typical of linitis plastica. A similar appearance may be seen in metastatic infiltration of the stomach.

Diagnosis is usually made by means of barium and endoscopic studies. The primary role of sonography is to determine the extent of the disease in patients with documented GI lymphoma. Occasionally, however, sonography detects lymphomatous GI masses during routine abdominal scanning for vague complaints. One should be able to recognize the abnormalities and recommend appropriate further investigation.

In the stomach, thickened mucosal folds, ulcerative lesions, and submucosal nodules can be detected transabdominally using the fluid-filled stomach technique. Depth of invasion can be determined by endoscopic sonography. When the gastric folds are grossly thickened, a characteristic sonographic appearance is seen. In cross section, their interface produces linear echogenic strands radiating from a central core within the round sonolucent gastric mass, like spokes of a wheel. This is the "spoke-wheel" pattern (Fig. 12.31) described by Derchi et al. (82). Infiltrating circumferential mural lesions produce the target-like appearance previously described. They are better detected by ultrasound and CT than by endoscopy. Unfortunately, the sonographic findings of gastric lymphoma are also seen in other conditions such as hypertrophic gastritis, Menetrier's disease, gastric carcinoma and metastases, and submucosal neoplasms such as leiomyosarcomas (83). In most instances, the diagnosis, which may be suggested in certain cases by the sonographic findings, should be confirmed by appropriate biopsies.

Small bowel lymphoma is more difficult to identify by ultrasound than gastric lymphoma. Six appearances based on barium study findings have been described: the aneurysmal, ulcerative, mesenteric, nodular, constrictive, and sprue-like forms. Ultrasound can detect the first three: target-like lesions caused by bowel wall thickening ("aneurysmal" form) (Fig. 12.32a,b), extraluminal excavated masses (ulcerative form) (Fig. 12.33a,b), and

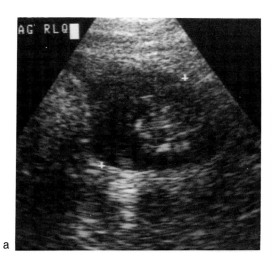
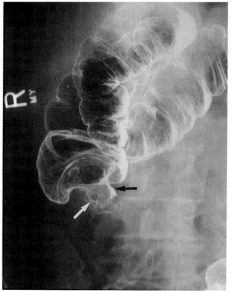

FIG. 12.29. Carcinoma of cecum—"pseudokidney" sign. **a:** sonogram; **b:** barium enema. Annular mass encircling cecum has sonographic appearance of a kidney (pseudo-kidney sign). Note typical "apple core" deformity of cecum (*arrows*) associated with this type of lesion.

the "sandwich" sign (Fig. 12.34), which refers to mesenteric lymphoma, in which entrapped mesenteric vessels are surrounded by hypoechoic masses (84). A similar appearance may be seen in primary lymphoma of the colon (85). Differentiation with carcinoma is usually not possible by ultrasound appearance alone.

Rare GI Neoplasms

Leiomyoma, leiomyosarcoma, and metastases are uncommon GI neoplasms (86,87). Gastric leiomyoma and leiomyosarcoma, when submucosal, may be detected by scanning the fluid-filled stomach transabdominally with

a 7.5-MHz transducer. A submucosal mass shows lifting of the mucosal, submucosal, and serosal layers around the lesion. This is called the mucosal and serosal "bridging layers" sign described by Miyamoto et al. (88). Large exophytic gastric leiomyosarcomas may cause diagnostic confusion. They often appear as lobulated masses with central excavation, which is due to necrosis, hemorrhage, and myxoid degeneration.

Metastases to the GI tract occur chiefly by intraperitoneal spread, hematogenous dissemination, or direct invasion by neoplasms in adjacent organs. Embolic metastases, most often from melanoma, breast and lung carcinoma, grow in the submucosa along the antimesenteric border of the bowel. They usually produce submu-

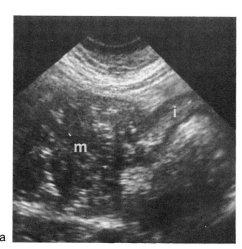
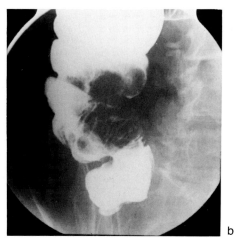

FIG. 12.30. Carcinoma of cecum—intraluminal mass. **a:** sonogram; **b:** barium enema. Lobulated mass (*m*) fills and distends cecum. There is no apparent wall thickening. Note normal terminal ileum (*i*) joining the mass.

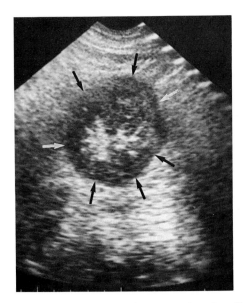

FIG. 12.31. Gastric lymphoma: cross-section view ("spoke-wheel" pattern). *Arrows* outline stomach seen in cross section. Markedly thickened folds are seen radiating from echogenic center, giving appearance of spokes in a wheel.

cosal nodules. The usual sonographic appearance is either a target-like lesion or a fungating mass (89,90). In the stomach, marked thickening of the gastric rugae or of the wall may be seen (Fig. 12.35). Diagnosis is usually made by clinical findings and appropriate biopsies.

Appendiceal Mucocele

This rare lesion is defined as an appendix abnormally distended with mucoid material. Four types are recog-

nized: retention cyst, mucosal hyperplasia, mucinous cystadenoma, and mucinous cystadenocarcinoma. The sonographic appearances reflect the internal characteristics of the lesion. A purely cystic mass corresponds to a mucocele containing thin and watery fluid. A mucocele containing thick and gelatinous material usually appears as a hypoechoic mass (Fig. 12.36a,b). Thin calcification and polypoid excrescence may be occasionally seen in the wall (91). Barium enema often shows nonfilling or partial filling of the appendix.

Preoperative diagnosis is rarely made. The lesion has been mistaken for ovarian cysts and cystic neoplasms, inflammatory and neoplastic bowel mass, and pelvic inflammatory masses (92). It is therefore important to include appendiceal mucocele in the differential diagnosis of a cystic or complex mass in the right iliac fossa. If the diagnosis is suspected, percutaneous aspiration biopsy should be avoided, for fear of causing peritoneal seeding (pseudomyxoma peritonei).

Mesenteric Neoplasms

Primary mesenteric neoplasms are uncommon. Whether benign or malignant, they tend to grow to massive proportion. The histologic types of the tumors include lipoma/liposarcoma (Fig. 12.37a,b), leiomyoma/leiomyosarcoma, hemangiopericytoma, neurofibroma, and mesenchymoma (93). Desmoid tumors, found most often in the abdominal wall, may also occur in the mesentery. They usually appear as well-circumscribed hypoechoic masses encasing the mesenteric vessels, thus simulating the "sandwich" sign seen in mesenteric lymphoma (94).

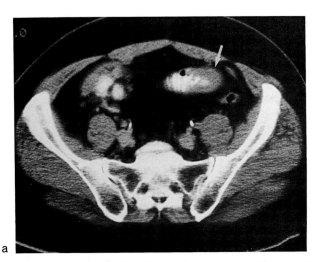

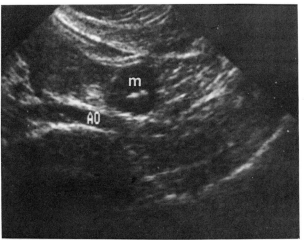

a   b

FIG. 12.32. Small bowel lymphoma. **a:** CT scan; **b:** sagittal sonogram. CT scan shows a loop of small bowel with asymmetrical wall thickening (*arrow*) in this patient with anemia and abdominal pain. This, however, may be artifactual, related to peristalsis or partial averaging volume effect. Corresponding sonogram confirms true thickening of bowel wall (*m*), giving bowel the typical "target" or "bull's-eye" appearance. *Ao,* aorta.

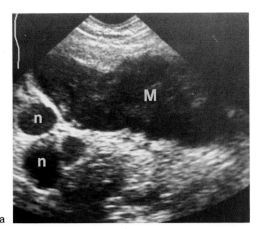
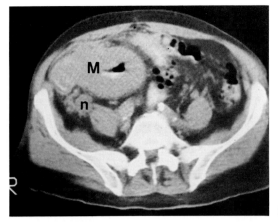

FIG. 12.33. Ileocecal lymphoma. **a:** sonogram; **b:** corresponding CT scan. Note enlarged nodes (*arrows*) adjacent to lymphomatous mass (*M*) in cecum. There is good correlation between the two scans. Lymphomatous masses and nodes are often hypoechoic.

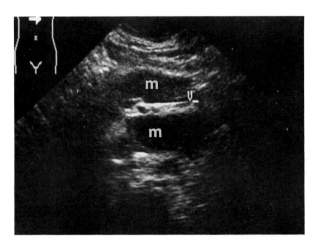
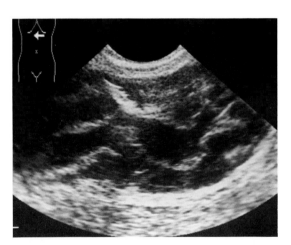

FIG. 12.34. Mesenteric lymphoma—"sandwich" sign. Mesenteric vessels (*V*) are encased by a hypoechoic mass (*m*). This appearance is typical of mesenteric lymphoma.

FIG. 12.35. Metastases to stomach: transverse sonogram. In this patient, gross thickening of gastric folds is due to infiltration by breast carcinoma secondaries. A similar appearance may be seen in Menetrier's disease, in gastritis, or in lymphoma.

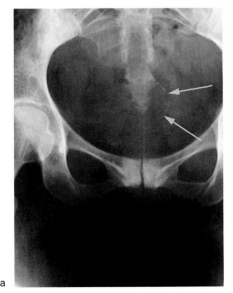
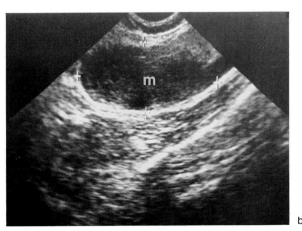

FIG. 12.36. Appendiceal mucocele. **a:** radiograph; **b:** sonogram. Faint curvilinear calcification (*arrows*) was seen in this radiograph of the pelvis. Patient presented with a palpable pelvic mass. Sagittal sonogram showed a fluid collection filled with irregular echoes in right iliac fossa extending into pelvis (*m*). At surgery, an appendiceal mucocele was found.

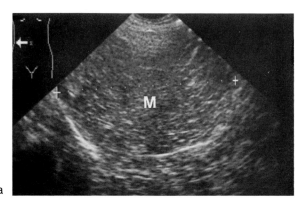 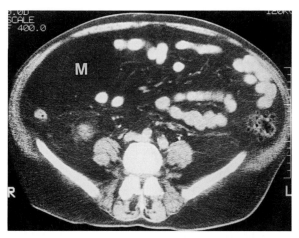

a   b

FIG. 12.37. Mesenteric lipoma. **a:** transverse sonogram; **b:** CT scan. Echogenic mesenteric mass (*M*) corresponds to fatty mass seen on CT. This was found incidentally during scanning for suspected gallbladder disease.

Mesenteric mesothelioma and metastases have been discussed in Chapter 2.

Enlarged Mesenteric Nodes—Lymphoma

Mesenteric lymphadenopathy is most frequently seen in lymphoma and metastatic disease, but it may also be due to reactive hyperplasia. It is seen in 50% of patients with NHL and in only 5% of patients with Hodgkin's disease (95).

In thin patients without a large amount of bowel gas, ultrasound performs as well as CT and often better in detecting isolated enlarged lymph nodes (>15 mm) in the porta hepatis and around the celiac axis (Fig. 12.38). Computed tomography, of course, obtains better results in large or obese patients. Conglomeration of enlarged mesenteric nodes shows the characteristic "sandwich"

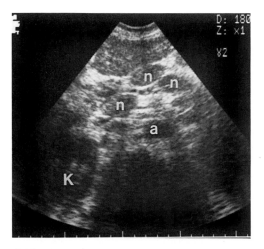

FIG. 12.38. Enlarged mesenteric nodes. A few enlarged nodes (*n*) are seen in this transverse sonogram around celiac axis. Patient had carcinoma of stomach. *K,* kidney; *a,* aorta.

sign already described: the mesenteric vessels are encased by hypoechoic lobulated masses. This sign is more commonly seen in lymphoma than in metastatic disease (84). Yoshinaka et al. (96) found that failure to visualize the celiac axis in esophageal or gastric cancer patients is associated with extensive metastases to the celiac lymph nodes in 73% of cases.

12.4 SPECIAL TECHNIQUE: ENDOSCOPIC ULTRASOUND

Endoscopic ultrasound is a relatively recent innovation that requires the expertise of an endoscopist and a sonologist. The earliest published work on the technique was by Di Magno et al. in 1982 (97). The endoscope is fitted with a 5-MHz, 7.5-MHz, or high-frequency transducer, which allows direct visualization of the esophageal, gastric, and duodenal wall. The procedure can detect mucosal and submucosal lesions, either benign or malignant. Its main advantage is to determine depth of invasion and local spread of a known malignancy. It is also useful in detecting adjacent enlarged lymph nodes and tumor recurrence.

12.5 PITFALLS, ARTIFACTS, AND PRACTICAL TIPS

1. The stomach may contain residual foods or foreign bodies (e.g., phytobezoars, trichobezoars) that may simulate neoplasms on sonography (98,99). Ideally, the patient should be fasting from midnight before the day of examination. The diagnosis of a bezoar is easily confirmed with a barium meal.

2. Apparent thickening of the gastric wall is seen when the stomach is collapsed. The gastric wall should be scanned with the stomach distended with fluid.

3. Fecal material or obstructed large bowel loops may mimic colonic carcinoma (100). It is important in doubtful situations to correlate the findings with plain radiographs of the abdomen or barium enema.

4. It is helpful to avoid overdistending the stomach with fluid when scanning for HPS. In addition to making the patient more uncomfortable, the distended stomach may prevent optimal measurement of pyloric length and thickness of the antro-pyloric muscle, particularly with a posteriorly directed antrum (101).

5. When the pyloric muscle or mucosa is scanned tangentially, it may appear thickened in the long-axis view (101). This artifactual thickening disappears in a true midline scan.

6. The colon may be interposed between the liver and the right hemidiaphragm. Most often, the interposition is anterior; occasionally, it may be posterior (102). When performing percutaneous procedures, one should recognize this normal variant, which is easily diagnosed by CT scanning, to avoid puncturing the colon.

7. Scanning for appendicitis may be time-consuming and requires perseverance and patience. As a general rule, if a normal appendix is seen, the diagnosis of acute appendicitis is unlikely.

8. A few lesions such as ovarian teratoma and periaortic hematoma may simulate the target appearance usually associated with bowel pathology (103).

9. Gas in the bowel, in the biliary tree, or in an abscess is the cause of ring-down artifacts, which appear as parallel strong echogenic bands radiating away from the gas collection (Fig. 12.39). Avruch and Cooperberg (104) postulated from their experiment that the source of the artifact is a horn- or bugle-shaped fluid collection that is entrapped between a cluster of four gas bubbles (bubble tetrahedron). When excited by an ultrasound pulse, this fluid collection vibrates and emits sound toward the transducer as a continuous sound wave that manifests as a series of echogenic bands seen in the ring-down artifact (104,105).

10. Comet-tail artifact is associated with abdominal foreign bodies, particularly metallic objects. This is due to reverberation of the sound beam within the foreign body and between it and the transducer. The artifact resembles the ring-down artifact, consisting of a series of strong echogenic parallel bands posterior to the foreign body, looking like a comet tail (106).

REFERENCES

Scanning Techniques

1. Worlicek H, Dunz D, Engelhard K. Ultrasonic examination of the wall of the fluid-filled stomach. *JCU* 1989;17:5–14.
2. Teele RI, Smith EH. Ultrasound in the diagnosis of ideopathic hypertrophic pyloric stenosis. *N Engl J Med* 1977;296:1149–1150.
3. Puylaert JBCM. Acute appendicitis: US evaluation using graded compression. *Radiology* 1986;158:355–360.
4. Bree RL, Shwab RE. Contribution of mesenteric fat to unsatisfactory abdominal and pelvic ultrasonography. *Radiology* 1981;140:773–776.

Normal Anatomy

5. Strohm WD, Classen M. Benign lesions of the upper GI tract by means of endoscopic ultrasonography. *Scand J Gastroenterol* 1986;21(suppl 123):41–45.
6. Needleman L. Ultrasound measurements of the bowel. In: Goldberg BB, Kurtz AB, eds. *Atlas of ultrasound measurements.* Chicago: Yearbook Medical Publisher; 1990:139–144.
7. Blumhagen JD, Nobel HGS. Muscle thickness in hypertrophic pyloric stenosis: sonographic determination. *AJR* 1983:140:221–223.
8. O'Keeffe FN, Stansberry SD, Swischuk LE, Hayden CK Jr. Antropyloric muscle thickness at US in infants: what is normal? *Radiology* 1991;178:827–830.
9. Fleischer AC, Muhletaler CA, James AE Jr. Sonographic assessment of the bowel wall. *AJR* 1981;136:887–891.
10. Fleischer AC, Dowling AD, Weinstein ML, James AE Jr. Sonographic patterns of distended, fluid-filled bowel. *Radiology* 1979;133:681–685.
11. Puylaert JBCM, Rutgers PH, Lalisang RI, et al. A prospective study of ultrasonography in the diagnosis of appendicitis. *New Engl J Med* 1987;317:666–669.
12. Nyberg DA, Mack LA, Patten RM, Cyr DR. Fetal bowel—normal sonographic findings. *J Ultrasound Med* 1987;6:3–6.

Pathology

13. Boychuk RB, Lyons EA, Goodhand TK. Duodenal atresia diagnosed by ultrasound. *Radiology* 1978;127:500.
14. Lees RR, Alford BA, Brenbridge A, Buschi AJ, Williamson BR. Sonographic appearance of duodenal atresia *in utero. AJR* 1978;131:701–702.
15. Zimmerman HB. Prenatal demonstration of gastric and duodenal obstruction by ultrasound. *J Can Assoc Radiol* 1978;29:138–141.
16. Hayden CK Jr, Schwartz MZ, Davis M, Swischuk LE. Combined esophageal and duodenal atresia: sonographic findings. *AJR* 1983;140:225–226.
17. Cremin BJ, Solomon DJ. Ultrasonic diagnosis of duodenal diaphragm. *Pediatr Radiol* 1987;17:489–490.

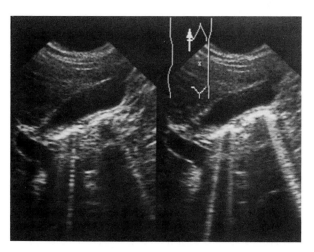

FIG. 12.39. Ring-down artifact (*arrows*). In this example, air in bowel adjacent to gallbladder causes the artifact.

18. Teele RL, Henschke CI, Tapper D. The radiographic and ultra-sonographic evaluation of enteric duplication cysts. *Pediatr Radiol* 1980;10:9–14.

19. Moccia WA, Astacio JE, Kandi JV. Ultrasonographic demonstration of gastric duplication in infancy. *Pediatr Radiol* 1981;11:52–54.

20. Kangarloo H, Sample WF, Hansen G, Robinson JS, Sarti D. Ultrasonic evaluation of abdominal gastro-intestinal duplication in children. *Radiology* 1979;131:191–194.

21. Warkit JM, Goldman MA, Fagelman D. Ultrasound and computed tomographic demonstration of a duplication cyst of the ileum. *J Ultrasound Med* 1984;3:565–566.

22. Fragoyamis SG, Anagnostopulos G. Hemangiolymphomatous hamartoma of the mesentery. *Am J Dis Child* 1974;128:233–234.

23. Walker AR, Putnam TC. Omental, mesenteric and retroperitoneal cysts: a clinical study of 33 new cases. *Ann Surg* 1973;178:13–19.

24. Geer LL, Mittelstaedt CA, Staab EV, Gaisier G. Mesenteric cyst: sonographic appearance with CT correlation. *Pediatr Radiol* 1984;14:102–104.

25. Mittelstaedt C. Ultrasonic diagnosis of omental cysts. *Radiology* 1975;114:673–676.

26. van Mil JBC, Laméris JS. Unusual appearance of a mesenteric cyst. *Diagn Imaging* 1983;52:28–32.

27. Bender TM, Ledesma-Medina J, Kook Sang Oh. Radiographic manifestations of anomalies of the gastrointestinal tract. *Radiol Clin North Am* 1991;20:335–349.

28. Tunell WP, Wilson DA. Pyloric stenosis: Diagnosis by real time sonography, the pyloric muscle length method. *J Pediatr Surg* 1984;19:795–799.

29. Friesen SR, Pearce AGE. Pathogenesis of congenital pyloric stenosis, histochemical analyses of pyloric ganglion cells. *Surgery* 1963;53:604–608.

30. Welin SL, Grand RJ, Drum DE. Congenital hypertrophic pyloric stenosis: the role of gastrin re-evaluated. *Pediatrics* 1978;61:881–885.

31. Shuman FI, Darling DB, Fisher JH. The radiographic diagnosis of hypertrophic pyloric stenosis. *J Pediatr* 1967;71:70–74.

32. Swischuk LE, Hayden CK Jr, Tyson KR. Atypical muscle hypertrophy in pyloric stenosis. *AJR* 1980;134:481–484.

33. Ball TI, Atkinson GO Jr, Gay BB Jr. Ultrasound diagnosis of hypertrophic pyloric stenosis: real time application and the demonstration of a new sonographic sign. *Radiology* 1983;147:499–502.

34. Westra SJ, de Groot CJ, Smits NF, Staalman CR. Hypertrophic pyloric stenosis: use of the pyloric volume measurement in early US diagnosis. *Radiology* 1989;172:615–619.

35. Sauerbrei EE, Paloschi GGB. The ultrasonic features of hypertrophic pyloric stenosis, with emphasis on the postoperative appearance. *Radiology* 1983;147:503–506.

36. Seibert JJ, Williamson SL, Galladay ES, Mmollitt DL, Seibert RW, Sutterfield SL. The distended gasless abdomen: a fertile field for ultrasound. *J Ultrasound Med* 1986;5:301–308.

37. Scheible W, Goldberger LE. Diagnosis of small bowel obstruction: the contribution of diagnostic ultrasound. *AJR* 1979;133:685–688.

38. Hayden CK Jr, Boulden TF, Swischuk LE, Lobe TE. Sonographic demonstration of duodenal obstruction with mid-gut volvulus. *AJR* 1984;143:9–10.

39. Hopens T, Coggs GC, Goldstein HM, Smith BD. Sonographic diagnosis of afferent loop obstruction. *AJR* 1982;138:967–969.

40. Bisset GS, Kirks DR. Intussusception in infants and children: diagnosis and therapy. *Radiology* 1988;168:141–145.

41. Agha FP. Intussusception in adults. *AJR* 1986;146:527–531.

42. Burke LF, Clarke E. Ileocolic intussusception: a case report. *JCU* 1977;5:346–347.

43. Pandher D, Sauerbrei EE. Neonatal ileocolic intussusception with enterogenous cyst: ultrasonic diagnosis. *J Can Assoc Radiol* 1983;34:328–330.

44. Stringer DA, Daneman A, Brunelle F, Ward K, Martin DJ. Sonography of the normal and abnormal stomach (excluding hypertrophic pyloric stenosis) in children. *J Ultrasound Med* 1986;5:183–188.

45. Morrison S, Dahms BB, Hoffenberg E, Czinn SJ. Enlarged gastric folds in association with *Campylobacter* pyloric gastritis. *Radiology* 1989;171:819–821.

46. Tomooka Y, Onitsuka H, Goya T, et al. Ultrasonography of benign gastric ulcers. Characteristic features and sequential follow-up. *J Ultrasound Med* 1989;8:513–517.

47. Tuncel E. Ultrasonic features of duodenal ulcer. *Gastrointest Radiol* 1990;15:207–210.

48. Filiatrault D, Longpré D, Patriquin H, et al. Investigation of childhood blunt abdominal trauma: a practical approach using ultrasound as the initial diagnostic modality. *Pediatr Radiol* 1987;17:373–379.

49. Hayashi K, Futagawa S, Kozaki S, Hirao K, Hombo Z. Ultrasound and CT diagnosis of intramural duodenal hematoma. *Pediatr Radiol* 1988;18:167–168.

50. Hernanz-Schulman H, Genieser NB, Ambrosino M. Sonographic diagnosis of intramural duodenal hematoma. *J Ultrasound Med* 1989;81:273–276.

51. Derchi LE, Iearace T, De Pra L, Solbiati L, Rizzatto G, Musante F. The sonographic appearance of duodenal lesions. *J Ultrasound Med* 1986;5:269–273.

52. Engleholm L, DeToeuf J, Herlinger H, Maglinte DDT. Crohn's disease of the small bowel. In: Herlinger H, Maglinte D, eds. *Clinical radiology of the small intestine.* Philadelphia: WB Saunders; 1989:295–334.

53. Lutz H, Rettenmaier G. Sonographic pattern of tumours of the stomach and the intestine. In: *Proceedings of the 2nd World Congress on Ultrasound in Medicine.* Rotterdam, 1972. Amsterdam: Excerpta Medica; 1973:67.

54. Albano O, Carrieri V, Vinciguerra V, et al. Ultrasonic findings in Whipple disease. *JCU* 1984;12:286–288.

55. Bolondi L, Ferrantino M, Trevisani F, Bernardi M, Gasbarrini G. Sonographic appearance of pseudo-membranous colitis. *J Ultrasound Med* 1985;4:489–492.

56. Downey DB, Wilson SR. Pseudomembranous colitis: sonographic features. *Radiology* 1991;180:61–64.

57. Limberg B. Diagnosis of acute ulcerative colitis and colonic Crohn disease by colonic sonography. *JCU* 1989;1:25–31.

58. Kimmey MB, Wang KY, Haggitt RC, Mack LA, Silverstein FE. Diagnosis of inflammatory bowel disease with ultrasound—an *in vitro* study. *Invest Radiol* 1990;25:1085–1090.

59. Boag GS, Nolan RL. Sonographic features of urinary bladder involvement in regional enteritis. *J Ultrasound Med* 1988;7:125–128.

60. McNamara MJ, Chalmers AG, Morgan M, Smith SEW. Typhlitis in acute leukemia: radiological features. *Clin Radiol* 1987;37:83–86.

61. Alexander JE, Williamson SL, Seibert JJ, Golladay ES, Jimenez JF. The ultrasonographic diagnosis of typhlitis (neutropenic colitis). *Pediatr Radiol* 1988;18:200–204.

62. Jeffrey RB Jr, Laing FC, Townsend RR. Acute appendicitis: sonographic criteria based on 250 cases. *Radiology* 1988;167:327–329.

63. Worrell JA, Drolshagen LF, Kelly TC, Hunton DW, Durmon GR, Fleischer AC. Graded compression US in the diagnosis of appendicitis: a comparison of diagnostic criteria. *J Ultrasound Med* 1990;9:145–150.

64. Brown JJ. Acute appendicitis: the radiologist's role. *Radiology* 1991;180:13–14.

65. Vignault F, Filiatrault D, Brandt ML, Garel L, Grignon A, Ouimet A. Acute appendicitis in children: evaluation with US. *Radiology* 1990;176:501–504.

66. Gaensler EHL, Jeffrey RB Jr, Laing FC, Townsend RR. Sonography in patients with suspected acute appendicitis: value in establishing alternative diagnoses. *AJR* 1989;152:49–51.

67. Abu-Yousef MM, Bleicher JJ, Maher JW, et al. High-resolution sonography of acute appendicitis. *AJR* 1987;149:53–58.

68. Borushuk KF, Jeffrey RB Jr, Laing FC, Townsend PR. Sonographic diagnosis of perforation in patients with acute appendicitis. *J Ultrasound Med* 1985;4:489–492.

69. Bartram CI. Diverticular disease. In: Laufer I, ed. *Double contrast gastro-intestinal radiology.* Philadelphia: WB Saunders; 1979:583–599.

70. Parulekar SG. Sonography of colonic diverticulitis. *J Ultrasound Med* 1985;4:659–666.
71. Silverman PM, Baker ME, Cooper C, Kelvin FM. CT appearance of diffuse mesenteric edema. *J Comput Assist Tomog* 1986; 10:67–70.
72. Kordan B, Payne SD. Fat necrosis simulating a primary tumor of the mesentery: sonographic diagnosis. *J Ultrasound Med* 1988;7:345–347.
73. Bendon JA, Poleynard GD, Bordin GM. Fibrosing mesenteritis simulating pelvic carcinomatosis. *Gastrointest Radiol* 1979;4: 195–197.
74. Meyers WC, Damiano RJ, Postlethwait RW, Rotolo FS. Adeno-carcinoma of the stomach: changing patterns in the last four decades. *Ann Surg* 1987;205:1–8.
75. Kurtz RC, Sherlock P. The diagnosis of gastric cancer. *Semin Oncol* 1985;12:11–18.
76. Botet JF, Lightdale C. Endoscopic sonography of the upper gastro-intestinal tract. *AJR* 1991;156:63–68.
77. Brady LW, Ashell SO. Malignant lymphoma of the gastrointesti-nal tract. *Radiology* 1980;137:291–298.
78. Laufer I. Tumors of the colon. In: Laufer I, ed. *Double contrast gastrointestinal radiology*. Philadelphia: WB Saunders; 1979: 517–559.
79. Gooding GAW. Ultrasonography of the cecum. *Gastrointest Ra-diol* 1981;6:243–246.
80. Kremer H, Lohmueller G, Zollner N. Primary ultrasonic detec-tion of a double carcinoma of the colon. *Radiology* 1977;124:481–482.
81. Dodd GD. Lymphoma of the hollow abdominal viscera. *Rad Clin North Am* 1990;28:771–783.
82. Derchi LE, Bonderali A, Bossi MC, et al. The sonographic appear-ance of gastric lymphoma. *J Ultrasound Med* 1984;3:251–256.
83. Goerg C, Schwerk WB, Goerg K. Gastrointestinal lymphoma: sonographic findings in 54 patients. *AJR* 1990;155:795–798.
84. Mueller PR, Ferucci JT, Harbin WP, Kirkpatrick RH, Simeone JF, Wittenberg J. Appearance of lymphomatous involvement of the mesentery by ultrasonography and body computed tomogra-phy; the "sandwich" sign. *Radiology* 1980;134:467–473.
85. Parker LA, Vincent LM, Ryan FP, Mittelstaedt CA. Primary lymphoma of the ascending colon: sonographic demonstration. *JCU* 1986;14:221–223.
86. Nanert TC, Zormoza J, Ordonez N. Gastric leiomyosarcomas. *AJR* 1982;139:291–297.
87. Rowley VA, Cooperberg PL. The ultrasonographic appearance of abdominal leiomyosarcomas. *J Can Assoc Radiol* 1982;33: 94–97.
88. Miyamoto Y, Tsujimoto F, Tada S. Ultrasonographic diagnosis of submucosal tumours of the stomach: the "bridging layers" sign. *JCU* 1988;16:251–258.
89. De Wilde V, Voel D, Dhont M, DeRoose J, Vallaeys J, Afschrift M. Ultrasound diagnosis of a solitary gastric metastasis. *JCU* 1989;17:678–681.
90. Morgan CL, Trought WS, Oddson TA, Clark WM, Rice RP. Ultrasound patterns of disorders affecting the gastrointestinal tract. *Radiology* 1980;135:129–135.
91. Athey PA, Hacken JB, Estrada R. Sonographic appearance of mucocele of the appendix. *JCU* 1984;12:333–337.
92. Batria JO, Wilson MH. Mucocele of the appendix presenting as an adnexal mass. *JCU* 1989;17:62–66.
93. Yannopoulos K, Stout AP. Primary solid tumors of the mesen-tery. *Cancer* 1963;16:914–927.
94. Baron RL, Lee JK. Mesenteric desmoid tumors: sonographic and computed tomographic approach. *Radiology* 1981;140:777–779.
95. Levitt RG, Koehler RE, Sagel SS, Lee JKT. Metastatic disease of the mesentery and omentum. *Radiol Clin North Am* 1982;20:501–510.
96. Yoshinaka H, Nishi M, Kajisa T, Kuroshima K, Morifugi H. Ultrasonic detection of lymph node metastases in the region around the celiac axis in esophageal and gastric cancer. *JCU* 1985;13:153–160.

Endoscopic Ultrasound

97. Di Magno EP, Regan PT, Clain JE, James EM, Buxton JL. Hu-man endoscopic ultrasonography. *Gastroenterology* 1982;83: 824–829.

Pitfalls, Artifacts, and Practical Tips

98. Bidula MM, Rifkin MD, McCoy RI. Ultrasonography of gastric phytobezoar. *J Clin Med* 1986;14:49–51.
99. Malpani A, Ramani SK, Wolverson MK. Role of sonography in trichobezoars. *J Ultrasound Med* 1988;7:661–663.
100. Flanagan M, Dubbin PA. An unusual bowel pseudotumour. *JCU* 1984;12:296–298.
101. Swischuk LE, Hayden CK Jr, Stansberry SD. Sonographic pitfalls in imaging of the antro-pyloric region in infants. *Radiographics* 1989;9:437–447.
102. Auh YH, Pardes JG, Chung KB, Rubenstein WA, Kazam E. Posterior hepatodiaphragmatic interposition of the colon: ultra-sonographic and computed tomographic appearance. *J Ultra-sound Med* 1985;4:113–117.
103. Chisholm HL, Raptopoulos V, Fabian TM. The sonographic tar-get pattern in non-gastrointestinal abnormalities. *JCU* 1985;13:42–44.
104. Avruch L, Cooperberg PL. The ring-down artifact. *J Ultrasound Med* 1985;4:21–28.
105. Scanlan KA. Sonographic artifacts and their origins. *AJR* 1991;156:1267–1272.
106. Thickman DI, Ziskin MC, Goldenberg NJ, et al. Clinical mani-festations of the comet-tail artifact. *J Ultrasound Med* 1983;2:225–230.

CHAPTER 13

Invasive Procedures

INTRODUCTION

Ultrasound technology is now advanced to the degree that it is a safe and efficacious guidance technique for many interventional procedures. Most biopsies and some catheter drainage procedures can be performed with US guidance only. It is the preferred technique for pregnant patients. In some cases, US must be combined with fluoroscopy. Ultrasound can be used for the initial localization and puncture for biliary and renal procedures, whereas subsequent guidewire and catheter insertion are preferably performed under fluoroscopic guidance to provide direct visualization so that compli-

cations can be minimized. Percutaneous nephrostomy can be performed via US guidance as the only imaging guidance if the collecting system is dilated. The latter is recommended only if absolutely necessary and should only be attempted by an experienced and skilled interventionalist. Occasionally, the area of interest is obscured by gas or bone or not adequately visualized because of extreme obesity. In these instances, CT is the preferred mode of guidance. Computed tomography is usually recommended in interloop abscesses when optimal visualization of needle tip and contiguous bowel is necessary before inserting a catheter (1). The interventionalist must use his or her judgment in choosing the best guidance technique.

Ultrasound has a number of advantages over other guidance systems. It is inexpensive and readily available. There is no ionizing radiation, which is of greatest im-

Abbreviations: **ASA,** acetylsalicylic acid; **CT,** computed tomography; **g,** gram(s); **PNB,** percutaneous needle biopsy; **PT,** prothrombin time; **PTT,** partial thromboplastin time; **US,** ultrasound; **WBC,** white blood cell.

portance to the operator and pregnant patients. It provides multiple instantaneous scan planes. Most importantly, it permits dynamic interaction between the operator, the needle (± guidewire ± catheter), and the area of interest in the patient. Ultrasound also tends to be more sensitive than CT for determining the internal characteristics (e.g., debris, septation) of a mass or fluid collection.

13.1 INFORMED CONSENT, PRELIMINARY INVESTIGATIONS, AND PATIENT CARE

Informed Consent

It is mandatory that informed consent be obtained for all interventional procedures. This includes a discussion of

1. procedure
2. anticipated benefits
3. potential risks and complications
4. alternate investigations or therapy

Hematology

Preliminary testing is recommended when

1. there is a clinical suspicion or history of a bleeding disorder (e.g., hemophilia, disseminated intravascular coagulopathy)
2. a drainage procedure is planned
3. a large-gauge biopsy is planned (>20-gauge)

Preliminary testing should include (2,3)

1. hemoglobin (should be >100 g/L)
2. PT (normal within 3 sec of control value)
3. PTT (normal within 6 sec of control value)
4. Platelets (should be >100,000/mm^3).

Specific medications and disease processes may affect blood coagulation. These include ASA, heparin, warfarin, nonsteroidal anti-inflammatory agents, uremia, liver disease, and vitamin K deficiency (caused by parenteral nutrition, biliary obstruction, malabsorption, and antibiotics). Appropriate questions regarding these specific disease processes and medications need to be asked at the time of history taking and consultation (2,3).

If the preliminary investigations are abnormal or if there is clinical history or suspicion of a bleeding disorder, then hematologic consultation is recommended before any elective procedure. If the procedure is performed on an emergency basis, a careful risk–benefit analysis should be completed before the procedure. Blood transfusion, platelet transfusion, and vitamin K administration may be necessary.

Urine

Preliminary investigations for any elective genitourinary procedure should include (3)

1. routine urinalysis
2. culture and sensitivity

If these are abnormal, the patient may require further investigation or antibiotic therapy to achieve urinary sterilization. This may be impossible to achieve if the patient has infection associated with calculi, particularly staghorn calculi.

Antibiotic Coverage

Infection is a potential risk of any radiologic interventional procedure. High-risk patients (e.g., immune-compromised) and high-risk procedures should be identified for antibiotic prophylaxis (4–6). Antibiotics will not prevent bacteremia or endotoxemia (3).

Procedures with a high risk of infection include

1. percutaneous biliary procedures: 22% to 46% are complicated by infection (e.g., cholangitis, septicemia)
2. percutaneous genitourinary procedures: approximately 7% risk of shock and 15% risk of fever
3. percutaneous abscess drainage: 5% incidence of sepsis

In some cases of aspiration of simple hepatic or renal cysts, one can safely predict a sterile collection, and antibiotic prophylaxis is not recommended. In cases of fluid collections of unknown etiology (including lymphocoele, urinoma, pancreatic pseudocyst, loculated ascites), it may be difficult to predict or exclude infection. Therefore, one should exercise clinical judgment and use prophylactic antibiotic coverage if there is a high clinical suspicion.

Prophylactic antibiotics should start before the procedure and continue for 48 hr. Therapeutic antibiotics for documented infection should be continued for at least 7 days or the recommended course of therapy for the particular organism and antibiotic based on the sensitivity studies.

Recommendations for Prophylactic Antibiotics (3–6)

1. Biopsy	No
2. Aspiration of cyst, peritoneal fluid, or retroperitoneal fluid	No if no evidence of clinical infection Yes if clinical infection
3. Abscess drainage	Yes
4. Biliary procedure	Yes
5. Genitourinary procedure	Yes

One should consult infectious disease specialists or current literature (4) for specific antibiotics, dosages, route of administration, and duration of antibiotic therapy.

Sedatives, Analgesics, and Antiemetics

Sedatives, analgesics, and antiemetics will depend on the anxiety level of the patient, age, and the complexity of the procedure. Many procedures can be performed with only local analgesics. Sedatives (e.g., diazepam), analgesics (e.g., fentanyl, morphine), and antiemetics (e.g., promethazine) may need to be added. The Compendium of Prescription Specialists or current literature is recommended for specific information on specific medications, dosages, route of administration, and adverse effects (3).

Patient Preparation

The following sequence may be used as a general guideline for US-guided invasive procedures but will vary depending on the procedure and potential complications:

1. informed consent
2. localization and planning access
3. sterile gloves
4. skin preparation with chlorhexidine gluconate (e.g., Hibitane) for biopsy or providone–iodine (Proviodine) for catheter procedures
5. patient draping—minimal for biopsy but needs to be more extensive for catheter procedures to avoid potential contamination of guidewires and needles
6. masks—worn for all catheter procedures and biopsies of immune-compromised patients
7. local analgesia (xylocaine 1% without epinephrine) for the skin puncture site and peritoneum

13.2 SCANNING TECHNIQUES

Localization and Planning Access

The area of abnormality is localized with the highest-frequency transducer possible for optimal visualization. Lesions that are deep or in very obese patients may require lower-frequency transducers (e.g., 3-MHz) (1).

One should select the most direct field of view for localization. This is not necessarily the most desirable path for needle access. The needle path must avoid vascular structures, gallbladder, and bowel. Therefore, one may have to plan a less direct access that avoids structures that should not be punctured. The ideal situation would permit

1. the shortest path to the abnormality
2. minimal angulation
3. avoidance of all other organs or structures if possible

Major vascular structures must be avoided in all circumstances. Bony structures may deflect the needle. Bowel or stomach should be avoided if possible. If they cannot be avoided, one should use only needles that are 20-gauge or smaller to minimize the risk of complications. Of necessity, the US transducer may need to be remote to the puncture site to permit visualization of the needle as it enters the area of interest. The optimal orientation is to have the US beam perpendicular to the needle as it enters the tissue.

The major advantage of US is that it permits instantaneous dynamic visualization of the needle as it passes through the tissues. This permits fine adjustments in angulation and depth to ensure optimal needle position. It also permits the operator to avoid undesirable structures (e.g., pleura, lung, vascular structures, spleen, bowel, and gallbladder) (1).

If possible, one should not transgress extraperitoneal and intraperitoneal spaces to do a biopsy or drainage procedure unless absolutely necessary. This will minimize the number of structures that may be inadvertently punctured and also reduce the risk of contaminating another space.

Percutaneous cholecystostomy is sometimes done for acute cholecystitis. This procedure should only be performed by skilled and experienced interventionalists. A transhepatic approach is used that will avoid porta hepatis vascular structures. The procedure may be performed by Seldinger or trochar technique. The initial localization and access route can be completed under US guidance. The subsequent guidewire and catheter insertion are best performed under direct fluoroscopic guidance. Many experienced interventionalists prefer to do the complete procedure under US guidance.

Guidance

Freehand Technique

This method avoids the need for sterile transducers, as the transducer contact point is remote from the needle entry point into the skin (Fig. 13.1). The needle path of entry should be perpendicular to the sound beam. This permits optimal visualization of the needle in the tissues. Subtle changes in direction can be made by dynamically scanning the needle as it enters the soft tissues (1).

Visualization of the needle tip is of the utmost importance (Fig. 13.2). It may be enhanced by gently moving the needle tip in the tissues ("bobbing" the needle), by moving the stylet within the shaft of the needle, and by using needles that have roughened surfaces with Teflon coating (1). The needle should be advanced with the patient breath-holding. If possible, the operator should scan in the long axis of the patient so that the needle path can be followed more easily during patient respiration (1).

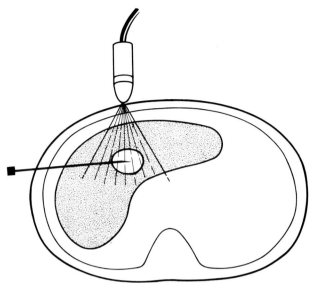

FIG. 13.1. Freehand technique of percutaneous biopsy. Transducer is held at a position remote from biopsy site. Needle tip is most easily visualized if axis of sound beam is perpendicular to axis of needle.

Needle Guides

Needle guides are attached to the transducer and are discussed below. The screen will display the anticipated needle path. Once the area of interest is localized within the field, the needle can be advanced through the needle guide to the desired depth. The needle tip should be visible within the area of interest (7).

13.3 INSTRUMENTATION

Transducers

Sector transducers may be mechanical or phased array. Their major advantage is their small size and con-

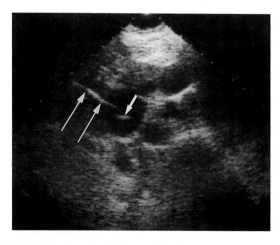

FIG. 13.2. Freehand technique. Tip of needle (*small arrow*) is seen in center of retroperitoneal mass. *Long arrows*, needle.

tact surface area. This permits scanning through small acoustic windows. Curved array transducers are larger than sector transducers but smaller than most linear array transducers. They produce a sector-like image. Linear array transducers have a relatively large contact surface area, which may limit the access with a small acoustic window (7).

Biopsy Guides

Some linear array transducers have a slot to serve as a needle guide. This results in a defect in the image at the site of the missing crystal. The needle is inserted through the slot to the desired depth. The localization of the needle tip in relation to the area of interest must be confirmed by moving the transducer to scan at a different angle. Some other linear transducers have attachable biopsy guides. Most sector and curved array transducers have attachable biopsy guides. These will electronically display the expected needle path on the screen as well as the needle tip as it enters the field of view (Figs. 13.3 and 13.4). Because the needle puncture site is entering the patient at a site adjacent to the transducer, one must ensure that there are no structures beneath the skin that one should avoid (e.g., bone, bowel) (7).

In general, whenever one uses an attachable biopsy guide, the transducer and needle guide must be sterilized before the procedure. This should be completed according to the manufacturer's specifications to avoid damage to the crystal from heat or liquid seepage. Some transducers require gas sterilization. Others can be soaked in a sterilization fluid such as Cidex. One major disadvantage is the loss of use of the transducer while it is being sterilized (7).

An alternate approach is to use a sterile sheath, sterile glove, or Opsite dressing with gel over the transducer. The sterile biopsy guide can then be attached to the transducer. This avoids problems associated with sterilizing the transducers.

Needles

There is a large variety of needles from which to choose (Fig. 13.5). They vary in length, caliber, and design. Needles of 20-gauge (0.9-mm outer diameter) or smaller are optimal for cytology, whereas 19-gauge or larger (1.0-mm outer diameter) cutting tip needles are optimal for histology. Some manufacturers now produce cutting tip needles for small core histology. The success of these needles will depend on the consistency of the tissue (7).

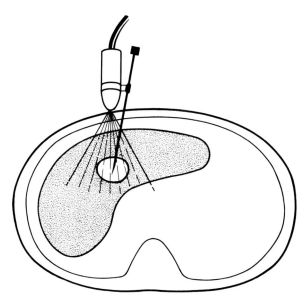

FIG. 13.3. Biopsy guide for percutaneous biopsy. Needle passes through a slot in biopsy guide that is attached to transducer. Tip of the needle is readily visualized as it enters into field of view.

In vitro testing (8) showed

1. The size and quality of tissue samples increase as the needle bore increases.
2. The needles with a more acute bevel angle produce a better specimen especially with small bore needles.
3. Some cutting tip designs obtain better specimens. The Lee (slotted cutting gap) and Franseen (trephine tip) were best in an *in vitro* situation (8).

We recommend that you select only a few needles for use so that one becomes familiar with the technique of use of these particular needles. Needles for fine needle biopsy for cytology usually have a varying degree of bevel (e.g., Chiba needle) rather than a cutting tip. This

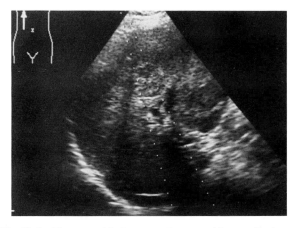

FIG. 13.4. Biopsy guide for percutaneous biopsy. Projected path of needle is electronically displayed on screen. Dots also represent distance in centimeters. A lesion that is displayed between lines of dots can be accurately localized for biopsy.

needle is introduced to the site of lesion. The stylet is removed, a syringe is attached, and negative pressure is created by the syringe. The needle and syringe are gently moved in and out of the tissue to aspirate clumps of cells into the needle shaft. The negative pressure is then released and the needle is removed. The aspirate is spread on slides for immediate fixation by the cytology technologist or cytologist.

Some needles are designed for small core histology. These have a cutting tip. They may be beveled, have a cutting slot, or have a trephinated tip (Fig. 13.5). Depending on the design, they may require an in–out motion while under negative pressure (via a syringe) or a rotational motion while being advanced under negative pressure.

A recent modification of an Otto design (two sharpened cutting teeth) allows creation of a negative pressure without a syringe. The Vacu Cut needle has a rubber vacuum seal for the stylet as it enters the shaft (Fig. 13.5). Once appropriately placed, one creates negative pressure by withdrawing the stylet part way out of the shaft. The needle is rotated while being slowly advanced within the tissue. The 18-gauge needle gave better specimens than the smaller 21-gauge needle size during *in vitro* testing (9).

Small-gauge needles are relatively flexible and may bend easily within the soft tissues. It is sometimes useful to use a standard 18-gauge needle in the superficial soft tissues to act as a "needle guide" and stabilizer for the more flexible biopsy needle. The fine needle is inserted through the lumen of the larger needle. Biopsies may be repeated with only one skin puncture.

Some physicians have saline within the syringe to prevent drying of the aspirated specimen. This is not necessary if the specimen can be immediately spread onto a slide for fixation. Needles for core biopsy of either the thin- (20-gauge or smaller) or large-bore needles (19-gauge or larger) are available. The specimens should be injected via syringe, pushed by stylet or dropped into fixation solution for later preparation into cell blocks. Most radiologists prefer fine needle aspiration biopsy over the large-core biopsy needles because of the lower risk of complications.

When a drainage procedure is anticipated or planned, the interventionalist may first aspirate with a thin needle to confirm location (e.g., kidney), to inject contrast for fluoroscopic guidance (e.g., hydronephrosis), or to collect a sample to confirm the nature of the contents (e.g., pus, urine). Some interventionalists prefer to use a Mittey-Pollick needle in this circumstance. The Mittey-Pollick needle is a coaxial 22-18-gauge needle that allows one to convert a small needle aspiration procedure into a drainage procedure by advancing the 18-gauge needle coaxially over the 22-gauge needle. A guidewire can then be inserted through the 18-gauge needle after the 22-gauge needle has been removed. This does not permit the

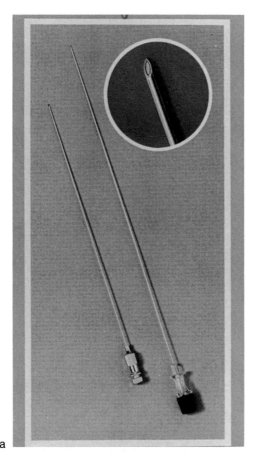

a

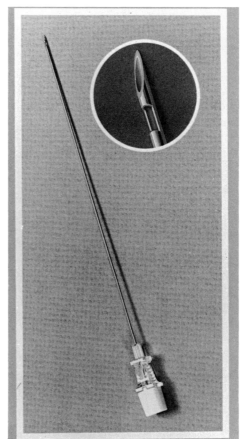

b

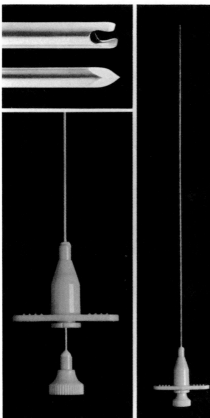

c

FIG. 13.5. Needles for biopsy. Many designs are available. **a:** Chiba needle with sharpened bevel tip. (Courtesy of Medi-tech.) **b:** notched aspiration needle with a slot. Tissue is drawn into slot by vacuum created with the syringe. (Courtesy of Medi-tech.) **c:** Percu Cut-A with sharpened cutting tip. This needle has a sealing diaphragm between needle and stylet that maintains a negative pressure effect when stylet is partially withdrawn. (Courtesy of E-Z-EM, Inc.)

operator to choose the optimal site of puncture, which may be of some importance with some procedures. An example of the latter is percutaneous nephrostomy for nephrolithiasis, in which the access must be optimal to reach the calculus. Therefore, we prefer to decompress the collecting system, inject contrast media for direct fluoroscopic guidance, and then do a selective puncture with an 18-gauge needle.

Biopsy Gun

Several hand-triggered biopsy devices are now available. Some are disposable, whereas others are dedicated units for use with disposable needles (9) (Fig. 13.6). These are designed to obtain core biopsies with minimal crush artifact. The design permits very rapid puncture and cutting action of the tissue. The puncture is so rapid that the organ tends not to push away from the needle tip. The needle must be advanced to the lesion. When triggered, the needle is advanced a fixed distance, tissue becomes entrapped into the biopsy slot, and the cutting sleeve is advanced rapidly to produce a specimen with minimal crush artifact.

Guidewires and Dilators

There is a large variety of guidewires available. We prefer a stiff Teflon-coated guidewire for easier catheter insertion. The interventionalist must make sure that the guidewire will be of the correct size for the needle used.

Dilators are tapered plastic devices that are inserted over a guidewire to facilitate subsequent catheter insertion. The interventionalist usually dilates up to the size of the catheter that will be used.

Catheters

There are many drainage catheters available, which are made of various materials (Fig. 13.7). Sizes vary from 6 to 14 French. A 6 French catheter has an internal diameter of 2 mm, while a 14 French catheter has an internal diameter of 4.7 mm. Larger-bore 10 to 14 French double lumen catheters (i.e., van Sonnenberg Sump, Ring-McLean catheters) are preferred for drainage of thick material and debris. All the side holes must be within the space being drained. These permit simultaneous irrigation and air circulation, as well as suction without catheter collapse. Medium-bore 8 to 9 French single lumen catheters are suitable for most purposes but may need frequent irrigation if the aspirated material is thick. Small-bore 6 to 7 French catheters are suitable for nonviscous fluid drainage or small superficial collections.

13.4 PERCUTANEOUS NEEDLE BIOPSY

Techniques of PNB

This may be for cytology or histology depending on the choice of needle and tissue consistency. The operator may choose to use a manually triggered biopsy gun, needle biopsy guide, or freehand technique (10). The following steps are a suggested approach:

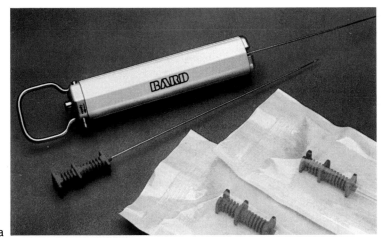

a

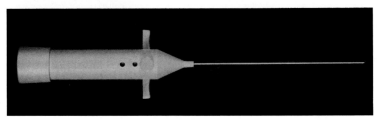

b

FIG. 13.6. Automated biopsy devices include reusable type (**a**) biopsy gun (courtesy of BARD) and disposable-type (**b**) Autovac (courtesy of Angiomed).

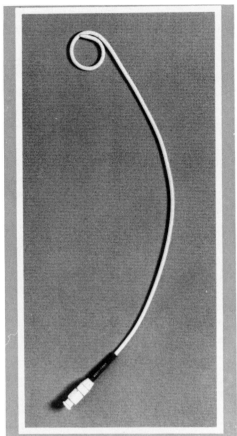

a

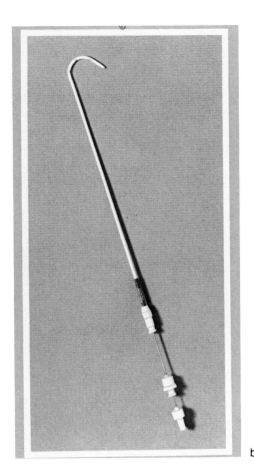

b

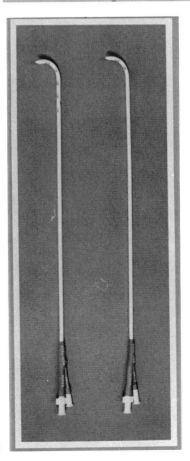

c

FIG. 13.7. Multiple types of catheters of various diameter, length, design, and materials. **a:** pigtail drainage catheter, which is usually inserted via Seldinger technique. (Courtesy of Medi-tech.) **b:** all purpose drainage catheter, which can be inserted by Seldinger or trochar technique. (Courtesy of Medi-tech.) **c:** van Sonnenberg sump drainage catheters, which can be inserted by Seldinger or trochar technique. These allow better drainage of thick material through larger lumen and allow air or fluid to circulate through sump lumen. This prevents catheter from collapsing when on suction. (Courtesy of Medi-tech.)

1. If a sterile biopsy attachment guide is used, the transducer must be sterilized or covered by a sterile glove, sheath, or Opsite dressing. If the freehand technique is employed, the transducer will be remote from the sterile needle. The needle path is followed under direct US guidance to the lesion. The needle should be advanced under suspended respiration. The needle tip will be best visualized if the sound beam is perpendicular to the shaft of the needle. Bobbing the needle, moving the stylet within the shaft, or using a needle with a roughened surface may aid in visualization of the needle tip.

2. Once the needle tip is within the lesion, perform the biopsy as recommended for the design of the needle. The needle in the biopsy gun needs to be advanced to the near edge of the lesion before firing. The distance of throw (2 cm or 0.9 cm) must be calculated for the specific biopsy gun. Other needles require the removal of the stylet and attachment of a syringe to create negative pressure within the needle. The needle is then moved in and out through the lesion or rotated during advancement, depending on the needle design. One must make the correct motion for the design of the needle. We usually obtain specimens from the edge and center of the lesion. The vacuum is released, and the needle is removed from the patient.

3. The aspirate should be immediately spread on slides for fixation by the cytotechnologist. This prevents drying and distortion of the cells. If the aspirate is inadvertently drawn into the syringe, fixative can be drawn into the syringe. The specimen can be spun down and later spread on a slide or made into a tissue block. If a core biopsy is obtained, it should be injected into fixative or fixative can be aspirated through the needle for later tissue block preparation. In ideal situations, the cytopathologist is available to determine the adequacy of the specimen. However, this is the exception rather than the rule.

Complications of PNB

Mortality rate 0.008–0.03%
Needle tract seeding 0.009–0.003%

The spectrum of complications include bile peritonitis, hematoma, peritonitis, and pancreatitis. Tumor tracking is extremely rare. Approximately 50% of all reported cases involved pancreatic cancer. Approximately 75% of all reported deaths were due to hemorrhage, with the remainder caused by pancreatitis, sepsis, and one case involving carcinoid crisis. Of the deaths, almost all involved biopsy of the liver or pancreas (11).

Needles of 20 gauge or smaller are recommended if bowel puncture is a significant risk. Aspiration biopsy of localized cystic gynecologic tumors is not recommended because of the risk of fluid spill into the peritoneal cavity.

Superficial subcapsular lesions of the liver may represent a hemangioma or other vascular lesion. Therefore, biopsy should ideally be performed with a PNB needle through normal parenchyma to reach the lesion. If blood is obtained, larger core biopsy should be avoided. If tissue is obtained, a larger-core biopsy can be performed with minimal risk. Biopsies of the liver or traversing the liver have a small risk of bile peritonitis. Puncture of the gallbladder has a similar risk if a thin needle is used and if there is no evidence of gallbladder obstruction. Biopsies traversing the pleura or lung have a risk of pleural effusion and pneumothorax.

Contraindications of PNB

There is no absolute contraindication. A relative contraindication is the presence of major clotting disorder. Anaphylactic reaction is a theoretical risk with *Echinococcus* infection. Hypertensive crisis is a theoretical risk with pheochromocytoma (11).

13.5 CYST OR FLUID ASPIRATION

Technique

1. Insert 22-18-gauge needle. The larger needle may be necessary for viscous fluid or debris. Aspirate with a syringe. Small collections can be completely aspirated.
2. Send specimen for desired tests:

If tumor is suspected	→ cytology
If pseudocyst is suspected	→ amylase
If infection is suspected	→ Gram's stain, culture and sensitivity (aerobic and anaerobic)
If *Echinococcus* is suspected	→ serology
If urinoma is suspected	→ BUN and creatinine
If bile leak is suspected	→ bilirubin
If lymphocoele is suspected	→ protein

Pitfalls of Cyst–Fluid Aspiration

1. Clear fluid may grow organisms.
2. Uninfected collections may appear cloudy if they contain blood, lymph, or necrotic debris.
3. Sterile abscesses may contain WBCs but no organisms on Gram's stain.
4. Abscesses should show WBCs and organisms on Gram's stain. Inadvertent puncture and aspiration of bowel may show organisms but not WBCs.

5. If an apparent fluid collection does not give free flow of fluid, the fluid may be viscous (blood or pus) or it may be a homogeneous solid structure that is hypo-echoic. In the former, insert a larger needle. In the latter, use an aspiration biopsy technique for cytology.

13.6 CATHETER DRAINAGE

Seldinger Technique

This often follows a diagnostic aspiration to confirm the presence of an abnormal fluid collection (e.g., abscess). It may also follow an US-guided limited antegrade pyelogram in an obstructed renal collecting system. Some experienced interventionalists will perform drainage procedures using only US guidance. However, in many instances it is safer to combine US guidance with fluoroscopic guidance. This usually necessitates injection of contrast medium for direct fluoroscopic guidance. An 18-gauge needle can then be inserted for subsequent guidewire, dilators, and catheter insertion (12).

Decompression of obstructed systems (e.g., renal, biliary) or abscesses is an essential component of the drainage procedure. This is done to minimize the risk of bacteremia and septic shock (Fig. 13.8) (4–6). At the initial procedure, "diagnostic" antegrade studies and excessive manipulation are to be avoided to minimize further the risk of bacteremia and endotoxic shock. These can be performed a few days later when a tract develops around the catheter (4–6).

Whenever a drainage procedure is planned, one should avoid transgressing the pleura, other organs, and bowel to get to the drainage site. It is contraindicated to traverse bowel to gain access to a collection. Perienteric (around small and large bowel) collections require an element of risk to contiguous bowel during drainage procedures. Some of these may be better performed under CT guidance if a safe access cannot be found by US.

The following steps are recommended for catheter drainage by Seldinger technique:

1. Superficial collections may be punctured directly with an 18-gauge special procedures needle or trochar-catheter set (Fig. 13.7). The trochar technique will be described in greater detail later.
2. Aspiration of the contents is performed to confirm the nature of the contents (e.g., urine, pus). Infected collections or systems should be partly decompressed. Contrast medium is injected into the collection or system to permit direct fluoroscopic visualization. Overdistention should be avoided.
3. Guidewires, dilators, and catheter are inserted in sequence. The guidewire is removed and the system is decompressed as much as possible. If the aspirate is rela-

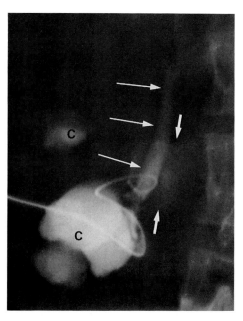

FIG. 13.8. Decompression of inflammatory collections: why it is important. Inflammation of wall of an infected collection can result in release of endotoxins and bacteria into circulation. This example of pyonephrosis secondary to a renal calculus demonstrates intravasation of contrast media during drainage procedure. There was no evidence of perforation of collecting system: *short arrows,* calculus in renal pelvis; *CM,* contrast media in dilated calyces; *long arrows,* intravasation of contrast media in inferior vena cava. Patient experienced an episode of septic shock after percutaneous nephrostomy procedure.

tively thick, small volumes of sterile saline (5–10 cc) may be necessary as irrigation fluid. The catheter should be attached to a sump drain or gravity-dependent drain, depending on the type of catheter used.

4. Secure the catheter by sutures, Molnar disc, and adhesive bandages. An adhesive bandage "mesentery" is useful to avoid direct traction on skin sutures.

This technique can be used for abscesses, hydronephrosis, and obstructed biliary tract. It is necessary to puncture through normal renal or liver parenchyma to support the catheter and to avoid leakage of urine or bile. With percutaneous nephrostomy, the skin puncture should be posterolateral to enter the renal parenchyma into a peripheral calyx. One must avoid posterior or lateral positional bowel (best seen under fluoroscopy). One must avoid large central and interlobar arteries by puncturing a peripheral calyx. Do not puncture the renal pelvis directly, as this will have an increased risk of urinoma formation. If the collecting system is not very distended, this may be difficult under US guidance alone. In these circumstances get assistance from a more skilled and experienced interventionalist or do the procedure under fluoroscopic guidance after an antegrade pyelogram has been performed.

Trochar Technique

The trochar set is a combination of catheter, stiffener, and trochar stylet (Fig. 13.7). It is usually used for superficial collections or situations in which there is direct access without intervening structures (12). The following steps are recommended:

1. Assemble stylet, stiffener, and catheter unit. Advance the assembled unit directly into the collection with a single stick maneuver.

2. Remove the central trochar stylet. Aspiration of fluid/pus confirms the entry of the tip of the catheter into the collection. One must avoid perforating the far wall of the collection. A guidewire is inserted through the catheter while the stiffener is in place.

3. The catheter and stiffener can be disassembled to permit the catheter to slide over the guidewire into the collection. Remove the guidewire and stiffener. The catheter will coil within the cavity. Secure the catheter by sutures, Molnar disc, and adhesive bandages. An adhesive bandage "mesentery" is useful to avoid direct traction on skin sutures. Irrigation may be necessary if the aspirate is thick.

Contraindications to Catheter Drainage

The only absolute contraindication is the absence of a safe access. Relative contraindications include contiguous bowel, intervening organs, contiguous vascular structures, and clotting disorder.

Complications of Catheter Drainage

This will vary depending on the skill and experience of the interventionalist. It also depends on the site of collection and the collecting system being drained.

Percutaneous nephrostomies have approximately a 2% failure rate, 4% significant complication rate, and 0.2% mortality rate (13). Abscess drainage has approximately 23% failure rate, 1.4% mortality rate, and 10% complication rate (14). Causes of limited success or failure include multiloculated collection, thick fluid (e.g., blood, pus, debris), fistula, phlegmon without liquifaction, and inadvertent catheterization of a solid mass that has been mistaken for an abscess. The latter is the reason for initial diagnostic aspiration that can be modified to do cytologic diagnosis if the observed mass is solid. Complications include bleeding, infection, shock (hemorrhagic or septic), and bowel perforation. Pleural effusion, pneumothorax, and empyema are risks if the pleura is transgressed.

13.7 PRACTICAL TIPS

Know Yourself

- Know your limitations based on skill, experience, and training.
- Know when you are in trouble. Stop. Get help.
- If you have limited experience, seek the advice and supervision of a more skilled and experienced colleague to assist you until you have sufficient experience and confidence to perform interventional procedures independently.

Know the Problem

- Know what you want to achieve: diagnosis versus drainage.
- Know how to do it before you start. Learn the essential information and seek expert advice before attempting new procedures.
- Know the indications, contraindications, and complications.
- Know the alternate approaches for diagnosis and therapy.
- Know how to deal with the complications.
- Be prepared to deal with the complications or ensure that someone else is prepared to do so.

Know the Technology

- Transducers
- Needle guides
- Guidewires
- Dilators
- Catheters
- Before you start the procedure, have available everything that you plan to use or might need.
- It helps to have someone assist you.

Know What to Avoid

- Bowel
- Bone
- Intervening organs
- Intervening bowel
- Pleura
- Lung
- Do not overdistend collections or collecting systems.

Respect Tissue Planes and Compartments

- Avoid transgressing tissue planes and compartments. This will minimize the risk of spreading infection.

Keep It Simple

- Do only what you feel competent to do.
- Simple procedures will minimize the risks to the patient.
- Become knowledgeable and comfortable with a few needles and catheters before trying other variations.
- The simpler the procedure, the easier it will be to perform while minimizing the risks for the patient.

REFERENCES

1. Matalon TAS, Silver B. US guidance of interventional procedures. *Radiology* 1990;174:43–47.
2. Silverman SG, Mueller PR, Pfister RC. Hemostatic evaluation before abdominal interventions: an overview and proposal. *AJR* 1990;154:233–238.
3. Barth KH, Matsumoto AH. Patient care in interventional radiology: a perspective. *Radiology* 1991;178:11–17.
4. Spies JB, Rosen RJ, Lebowitz AS. Antibiotic prophylaxis in vascular and interventional radiology: a rational approach. *Radiology* 1988;166:381–387.
5. vanWaes PFGM, Simoons-Smit IM. Use of antibiotics in interventional radiologic procedures: an important lesson still to be learned. *Radiology* 1988;166:570–571.
6. Hunter DW, Simmons RL, Hulbert JC. Antibiotics for radiologic interventional procedures. *Radiology* 1988;166:572–573.
7. Holm HH, Torp-Pederson S, Juul N, Larsen T. Instrumentation for sonographic interventional procedures. In: van Sonnenberg E, ed. *Interventional ultrasound*. New York: Churchill Livingstone; 1987:9–40.
8. Andriole JG, Haaga JR, Adams RB, Nunez C. Biopsy needle characteristics assessed in the laboratory. *Radiology* 1983; 148:659–662.
9. Hopper KD, Baird DE, Reddy VV, et al. Efficacy of automated biopsy guns versus conventional biopsy needles in the pygmy pig. *Radiology* 1990;176:671–676.
10. Rowley VA, Cooperberg PL. Ultrasound guided biopsy. In: van Sonnenberg E, ed. *Interventional ultrasound*. New York: Churchill Livingstone; 1987:59–76.
11. Smith EH. Complications of percutaneous abdominal fine-needle biopsy. *Radiology* 1991;178:253–258.
12. Casola G, van Sonnenberg E. Sonographic guidance for percutaneous drainage of abscesses and fluid collections. In: van Sonnenberg E, ed. *Interventional ultrasound*. New York: Churchill Livingstone; 1987:151–172.
13. Staples DP. Percutaneous nephrostomy: techniques, indications, and results. *Urol Clin North Am* 1982;9:15–29.
14. Lang EK, Springer RM, Glorioso LW, Cammarata CA. Abdominal abscess drainage under radiologic guidance: causes of failure. *Radiology* 1986;159:329–336.

Subject Index

Subject Index